Documentation *for* Rehabilitation

Documentation *for* Rehabilitation

A GUIDE TO CLINICAL DECISION MAKING IN PHYSICAL THERAPY

Fourth Edition

LORI QUINN, PT, EdD, FAPTA

Professor
Department of Biobehavioral Sciences
Teachers College, Columbia University
New York, New York

JAMES GORDON, PT, EdD, FAPTA

Professor and Associate Dean
Division of Biokinesiology and Physical Therapy
Herman Ostrow School of Dentistry
University of Southern California
Los Angeles, California

ELSEVIER

ELSEVIER
3251 Riverport Lane
St. Louis, Missouri 63043

DOCUMENTATION FOR REHABILITATION: A GUIDE TO CLINICAL
DECISION MAKING IN PHYSICAL THERAPY, FOURTH EDITION

ISBN: 978-0-323-69430-8

Notice

Practitioners and researchers must always rely on their own experience and knowledge in evaluating and using any information, methods, compounds or experiments described herein. Because of rapid advances in the medical sciences, in particular, independent verification of diagnoses and drug dosages should be made. To the fullest extent of the law, no responsibility is assumed by Elsevier, authors, editors or contributors for any injury and/or damage to persons or property as a matter of products liability, negligence or otherwise, or from any use or operation of any methods, products, instructions, or ideas contained in the material herein.

Previous edition copyrighted 2016

Content Strategist: Lauren Willis
Content Development Specialist: Shilpa Kumar
Content Development Manager: Somodatta Roy Choudhury
Publishing Services Manager: Deepthi Unni
Senior Project Manager: Kamatchi Madhavan
Design Direction: Brian Salisbury

Printed in India

Last digit is the print number: 9 8 7 6 5 4 3 2 1

Working together
to grow libraries in
developing countries

www.elsevier.com • www.bookaid.org

CONTRIBUTORS

Julie Fineman, PT, EdD
Clinical Assistant Professor and Director of Clinical Education
Doctor of Physical Therapy Program
Marist College,
Poughkeepsie, NY
Associated Faculty
Department of Biobehavioral Sciences, Motor Learning Program
Teachers College, Columbia University
New York, New York

Agnes McConlogue Ferro, PT, DPT, PhD
Clinical Associate Professor
School of Health Professions, Physical Therapy
Stony Brook University
Stony Brook, New York

John G. Wallace, PT, MS
SVP, Member Value
Compliance Officer
WebPT
Decatur, Georgia

Stephanie Woelfel, PT, DPT, CWS
Associate Professor of Clinical Physical Therapy & Surgery
Division of Biokinesiology and Physical Therapy
Department of Surgery
University of Southern California
Los Angeles, California

FOREWORD

Concepts, documents, ways of thinking and analyzing, and performance quality are closely interrelated. Furthermore, they evolve mutually; a new concept may alter documents, better documents may improve analysis, and they may suggest new concepts. The evolutionary process occurs in individuals and groups: I may alter my documents and improve my practice, and an organization may alter its documents and thus alter the performance of many people.

Evolution has an overriding selective force, survival, that tends to lead to improved species' survival in their environment. Unfortunately, in health care, no single selective force ensures clinical improvement. An organization may prioritize control over clinicians, financial performance, or convenience over improving clinical practice when developing or selecting documents.

This book is a substantial force for improving clinical practice. It draws on well-established concepts, but its principal value arises from its adaptation of concepts and documents to the daily practice of clinical staff. In effect, it allows clinicians to benefit from the hard-won experience of others and short-circuiting their need to evolve from a standing start.

This combination of scientific and practical excellence will enable individual clinicians to improve their practice; they can use the book to educate, persuade, and even compel their nonclinical managers to use better documents. The electronic patient record has many disadvantages, and an important one is the suppression of variation and the ability of individuals and teams to evolve better ways of working.

This book should guide the documents included in electronic patient records. Ideally, rehabilitation teams should also be encouraged to try different documents so that progress continues, and in another 8 years, a better edition of this book can be produced.

The scientific basis of the book is sound. It is based on many of the main concepts underlying effective rehabilitation.[1] For example, the biopsychosocial model of illness, manifested by the WHO *International Classification of Functioning*, is the central organization for rehabilitation and this book. Goal setting that prioritizes longer-term social participation is the second vital idea needed to ensure effective rehabilitation.

Multiprofessional teamwork is another critical idea and, though not a focus of the book, promoting good documentation and goal setting implies teamwork and, more importantly, significantly increases the team's coherence. Evaluation of individually tailored interventions is greatly improved by good documentation of outcomes.

Last, the book is unusually good at educating. The chapters are short and succinct, highlighting the essential information needed. The closely associated test material enhances the educational aspect. The reader is encouraged to test their understanding in each chapter. The questions must be based on years of actual teaching because they explore areas that are not always easily understood. Do not worry about failing the tests; failure is a potent way of learning, primarily when closely related to the material to be learned.

Derick Wade
Professor of Neurological Rehabilitation,
Oxford Brookes University

---

[1]Wade DT. What is rehabilitation? An empirical investigation leading to an evidence-based description. *Clin Rehabil.* 2020;34(5):571–583. https://doi.org/10.1177/0269215520905112

The main philosophical idea underlying this textbook is simple: not only is the logic of clinical reasoning reflected in documentation, but documentation itself shapes the process of clinical reasoning. Thus, we would argue that one of the best ways to teach clinical reasoning skills is by teaching a careful and systematic approach to documentation. This book is, therefore, not just a "how-to" book on documentation of physical therapy practice. Rather, it presents a framework for clinical decision making in physical therapist practice.

In this fourth edition, the International Classification for Functioning, Disability and Health (ICF) model is woven into the fabric of the text. We believe this framework provides a unique structure for understanding the complex relationships between a person's health condition and their ability to participate in life skills. The terms *participation*, *activities*, *impairments*, and *health condition* are incorporated into the vocabularies of contemporary physical therapists and certainly of entry-level physical therapy students. Nevertheless, for physical therapists to "walk the walk" rather than just "talk the talk," the framework exemplified by the ICF model must be incorporated into how they design and implement evaluations and interventions. This process is reflected in the documentation written by physical therapists. The outside world views physical therapy primarily through words that are written—as communicated in a medical record, progress notes given to a patient or physician, or forms completed for an insurance company. We believe that documentation shapes and reflects the advances in the science of physical therapy and therefore requires a contemporary framework that incorporates current knowledge regarding the disablement and rehabilitation process.

The purpose of this book is to provide a general approach to documentation—not a rigid format. It is, first and foremost, a textbook for entry-level physical therapist and physical therapist assistant students. It is intended to promote a style and philosophy of documentation that can be used throughout an entire physical therapy curriculum. However, it is also a book that we hope will appeal to practicing physical therapists and physical therapist assistants who are searching for a better structure for the note-writing process. We have provided examples and exercises related to wide-ranging areas of physical therapy practice, including pediatrics, rehabilitation, women's health, health and wellness, orthopedics, and acute care. This book was designed to help students and therapists organize their clinical reasoning and establish a framework for documentation that is easily adaptable to different practice settings and patient populations.

Although this book has many examples and exercises, it certainly does not include all possible types of documentation or all the details of how to document in different settings. Rather, this book provides a method for learning good documentation skills that can be adapted to different settings.

Although physical therapist assistants and physical therapist assistant students will find this book relevant, their practice is inherently limited to writing treatment notes. A large portion of this book focuses on the documentation of the initial evaluation. However, the components listed in each of these chapters, particularly the documentation of activities, are important components of the daily note documentation.

We believe one of the greatest strengths of this book is in the case presentations. We have made great efforts to address most areas of clinical practice, including different settings and patient populations. In this fourth edition, we have added cases related to COVID-19, telehealth, and post gender-affirming surgery, and updated all cases to be in line with the best available evidence for outcomes and interventions.

As much as possible, we have attempted to incorporate the terminology and main ideas of the newly revised *Guide to Physical Therapist Practice 4.0*. Readers should find this book "*Guide*-friendly," and we have reprinted figures and adapted components of the *Guide* into our documentation framework.

This book should be used in conjunction with other resources and references related to functional outcomes and documentation. Many of these resources are listed in the appendices of this book and at the end of each chapter. In particular, there are important legal aspects of documentation. We have provided a foundation for key elements related to the legal aspects of documentation; however, readers should consult state and federal laws to ensure that their documentation follows current guidelines.

Finally, we do not intend that this book should be the last word on documentation in physical therapy. On the contrary, we see it as a beginning. We hope that physical therapists will continue to explore new forms of documentation that will better reflect the changing patterns of practice and that will facilitate improvements in patient care. We invite readers to send comments, suggestions, and criticisms to us and to publish alternative approaches in journals and textbooks. Discussion and debate about the best ways to document will help us to find the true path to best practice.

Lori Quinn
James Gordon

ACKNOWLEDGMENTS

The authors would like to acknowledge the contributions of many people who provided examples, ideas, insights, and most importantly, critiques of this book at various stages of its inception. First, we owe a debt of gratitude to past students of the Physical Therapy Program at New York Medical College, Valhalla, New York. We have benefited so much from the thoughtful insights of the students for whom this material was first designed.

Next, we would like to thank the students, staff, and faculty of Teachers College, Columbia University; the Department of Biokinesiology and Physical Therapy at the University of Southern California; the Physiotherapy Program at Cardiff University, Wales; and the Program in Physical Therapy at Columbia University. Many of the students and faculty provided important comments for this book, wrote or reviewed case examples, or helped with editorial components. We specifically would like to thank Dr. Mahlon Stewart, Assistant Professor of Rehabilitation and Regenerative Medicine (Physical Therapy) at Columbia University Irving Medical Center, and students from the Doctor of Physical Therapy Program who offered insightful comments about the book for use in physical therapy education. Thank you:

Hilary Busick, PT, DPT
Sean Elliott, PT, DPT
Caitlin Gopie, PT, DPT
Joseph Graham, PT, DPT
Rachel Greenwell, PT, DPT
Audrey Hidacavage, PT, DPT
Jennifer King, PT, DPT
Deanna Madagan, PT, DPT
Breigh Sonnier, PT, DPT

We gratefully acknowledge the following individuals who provided insightful feedback and wrote or reviewed cases for this fourth edition:

Theresa Aversano, MSPT
Kathy Gill-Body, PT, DPT, MS, NCS, FAPTA
Chelsea MacPherson, PT, DPT, NCS
Kristin Mende, PT, DPT
James F. Ross, PT, DPT, CSCS
Stephanie Woelfel, PT, DPT, CWS

And from previous editions:

Janet Albanese, PT
Monica Busse, PhD, MSc (Med), BSc (Med), Hons BSc (Physio)
Kate Button, PhD, MSc, BSc Physiotherapy, MCSP
Stephanie Enright, PhD, MPhil, MSc, MCSP, PG Cert HE

Helene M. Fearon, PT, FAPTA
Jody Feld, DPT, MPT, NCS, C/NDT
Julie Fritz, PT, PhD, ATC
Tammy Goedken, DPT, ATP
Brenda Koepp, PT, MS
Janet Herbold, PT, PhD
Jacqueline Lamando, PT
Stephen M. Levine, PT, DPT, MSHA, FAPTA
Lori Michener, PT, PhD, ATC, SCS, FAPTA
Dan Millrood, PT, EdM
Barbara Norton, PT, PhD, FAPTA
Patricia Scheets, PT, DPT, NCS
Lori Schneider, PT, DPT, MS
Martha Sliwinski, PT, PhD
Karen Stutman, PT
Thank you for bringing to life the conceptual framework in this textbook.

We would also like to thank our contributors for their tireless work in writing and editing their respective chapters and cases.

Julie Fineman, PT, EdD, for acting as Case Coordinator and coauthor of the Outcomes Measure chapter, for providing some excellent case examples, and for masterfully coordinating the cases. We could not have done this without you. Thank you.

Agnes McConlogue Ferro, PT, MA, PCS, for revising the pediatrics chapter as only you could do. Your dedication to pediatric physical therapy and getting it right for students is unsurpassed.

Stephanie Woelfel, PT, DPT, CWS, for so carefully reviewing chapters and cases and being a great collaborator.

John Wallace, PT, OCS, for your extraordinary patience in getting this fourth edition out and for providing expert updates to the legal, payment, and Electronic medical record chapters.

We thank the many reviewers who carefully read and provided insightful comments about the book. We have made every effort to incorporate their suggestions into this fourth edition.

We also gratefully acknowledge the work of our editors, who provided great support and encouragement during this process. We would like to thank Shilpa Kumar, Lauren Willis, and Laura Klein, as well as the entire editorial and production staff for their expert assistance in completing this project.

Last, we thank our families for their never-ending support. With love and gratitude:

to Eric, Annabel, and Samantha
to Provi, Jason, Anita, and Maddie

Lori Quinn
James Gordon

CONTENTS

1

Disablement Models and the ICF Framework

LEARNING OBJECTIVES

After reading this chapter and completing the exercises, the reader will be able to:

1. Define a functional outcome, and discuss its importance in physical therapy documentation.
2. Explain the concept of disablement and its relevance to physical therapist practice.
3. Define the components of the International Classification of Functioning, Disability and Health (ICF) model.
4. Classify clinical observations and measurements according to the ICF.

This book outlines a method for physical therapy documentation and clinical decision-making based on the general principle that documentation should focus on functional outcomes. An *outcome* is a result or consequence of a physical therapy intervention. A *functional outcome* is one in which the effect of treatment is a change in an individual's ability to accomplish a goal that is meaningful for that individual. In this text we advocate that physical therapists (PTs) use a type of documentation format that is referred to as a *functional outcomes report* (Stamer, 1995; Stewart & Abeln, 1993). Functional outcomes should be the focus of physical therapy documentation for the following reasons:

1. Examination procedures should determine relevant limitations in functional activities and the impairments that cause those limitations.
2. Goals should be explicitly defined in terms of the functional activities that the patient will be able to perform.
3. Specific interventions should be justified in terms of their effects on functional outcomes.
4. Most importantly, the success of interventions should be measured by the degree to which desired functional outcomes are maintained or achieved.

This book has two main purposes: (1) to provide a framework for clinical decision-making that is based on a functional outcomes approach and (2) to provide guided practice in writing functional outcomes documentation.

There is no single correct way to write physical therapy documentation. Documentation must be adapted to the context in which it is written. The purpose of this book is not to present a rigid format for writing documentation but rather to provide a set of guidelines that are flexible and adaptable to different practice settings.

The framework for documentation presented in this text is based on the widely accepted International Classification of Functioning, Disability and Health (ICF)[1] model of how pathological conditions lead to disability. In 2008 the American Physical Therapy Association joined the WHO, the World Confederation for Physical Therapy, the American Therapeutic Recreation Association, and other international organizations in endorsing the ICF model. In addition, our framework is informed by and consistent with the terminology outlined in the *American Physical Therapy Association's Guide to Physical Therapist Practice.*[2]

In this chapter we discuss the importance of disablement models and the rationale for our focus on the ICF model. We also consider how this model can be used to understand the role of PTs in diagnosis and treatment planning. Finally, the importance of the ICF framework for documentation is discussed. The exercises at the end of this chapter provide practice in classifying conditions according to the ICF model.

---

[1]APTA Guide to Physical Therapist Practice 4.0. American Physical Therapy Association, 2023.

[2]https://guide.apta.org/

THE CONCEPT OF DISABLEMENT AND THE ICF MODEL

Clinical decision-making by PTs begins with an analysis of how a patient's3 health condition (disease or medical disorder) may lead to functional limitations and disability, a process that has been referred to as *disablement*. Disablement describes the consequences of disease in terms of its effects on an individual's body functions, the ability to perform meaningful tasks, and the ability to fulfill one's roles in life. Saad Nagi (1965) developed one of the most influential models of disablement. As shown in Fig. 1.1, this model provides a causal framework for analyzing the various effects of acute and chronic conditions on the functioning of specific body systems, basic human performance, and people's functioning in necessary, expected, and personally desired roles in the society (Jette, 1994).

The arrows in Fig. 1.1 imply a causal chain leading from active pathology to disability. The causal links between elements in the models are useful; they help to conceptualize the relationships between findings at different levels. Nevertheless, the arrows were often interpreted as indicating a temporal series of events, which many health professionals found problematic. Furthermore, many believed that these models did not capture the complexity of the relationships between different levels, which were often multidirectional.

In 2001, the WHO revised its disablement model to address these criticisms (Fig. 1.2). The ICF used the positive terms *activity* and *participation* to redefine what Nagi refers to as *functional limitation* and *disability*. Thus, although the general structure is similar to the original Nagi model, the focus of this new model is on what the patient can do, rather than what they cannot do.

In the ICF model (see Fig. 1.2) the process of disablement is a combination of (1) losses or abnormalities of *body function* and *structure*, (2) limitations of *activities*, and (3) restrictions in *participation* (Box 1.1). Of note, the terms *activity* and *participation* focus on a person's abilities. The ICF model relinquishes the notion of simple, unidirectional causal links between levels. The individual's pathological state (health condition) becomes a broader category that influences all other levels. Furthermore, contextual factors—both extrinsic (environmental) and intrinsic (personal)—are specifically identified as affecting the relationship between body structures and functions, and between activities and participation. Intrinsic personal factors can consist of such things as level of education, coping style, and family support, whereas extrinsic environmental factors might include social attitudes, architectural barriers, and social/legal structures. These important additions highlight the multiple factors that can be related to any one person's "disability."

The ICF is endorsed by the WHO as the international standard used to measure health and disability. In addition to the overall model presented in Fig. 1.2, the ICF provides

---

3The Guide to Physical Therapist Practice uses the term patient or client when referring to individuals who receive services from a PT. We have chosen to primarily use the term patient throughout this text to simplify writing and improve readability.

Nagi Model

Active pathology ⟹ Impairment ⟹ Functional limitation ⟹ Disability

FIG. 1.1 The Nagi model utilizes a causal framework of disablement. This model and its terminology have been largely replaced by the International Classification of Functioning, Disability and Health (ICF) model.

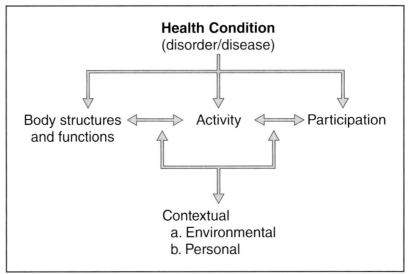

FIG. 1.2 The International Classification of Functioning, Disability and Health model of disablement.

BOX 1.1 Definitions of the Components of International Classification of Functioning, Disability and Health

- *Body functions* are physiological functions of body systems (including psychological functions).
- *Body structures* are anatomic parts of the body, such as organs, limbs, and their components.
- *Impairments* are problems in body function or structure such as a significant abnormality or loss.
- *Activity* is the performance of a task or action by an individual.
- *Participation* is involvement in a life situation.
- *Activity limitations* are difficulties an individual may have in performing activities.
- *Participation restrictions* are problems an individual may experience in involvement in life situations.
- *Environmental factors* make up the physical, social, and attitudinal environment in which people live and conduct their lives.

From World Health Organization. *Towards a common language for functioning, disability and health.* <https://cdn.who.int/media/docs/default-source/classification/icf/icfbeginnersguide.pdf>; 2002. Accessed 01.09.2024

definitions (see Box 1.1) and detailed descriptions of what each "level" encompasses. Within each of the ICF domains there is a hierarchy of descriptions. This ultimately leads to a code that can be used to refer to a specific domain. These definitions and codes provide common terminology that can be used by all health professionals, whether describing individual patient characteristics or conducting large-scale population-based research.

ICF is part of the WHO family of international classifications, which includes the *International Statistical Classification of Diseases and Related Health Problems* (ICD). ICD-11 (https://icd.who.int/en) is currently the version used by health professionals in the United States to classify diseases, disorders, or other health conditions. Each disease or health condition has its own ICD-11 code. These codes are used most frequently by PTs in the United States for patient classification for reimbursement purposes (see Chapter 5); however, they are designed to provide a common international language for communication and research.

REHABILITATION IS ENABLEMENT: THE REVERSE OF DISABLEMENT

Disablement models can be counterproductive if they lead to an overly reductionist approach to rehabilitation, that is, if improvements in impairments are assumed to lead to improvements in activity limitations. This is a subtle example of the so-called medical model, in which it is assumed that curing a disease will automatically improve the patient's quality of life. PTs fall victim to the same fallacy when they focus intervention exclusively on impairments.

This pitfall can be avoided if rehabilitation is conceptualized as enablement: the reverse and mirror image of disablement (Fig. 1.3). Whereas disablement begins with a disease/

disorder, rehabilitation begins with participation—specifying the desired result in terms of personal and social roles the patient is attempting to achieve, resume, or retain. These roles require the performance of skills or activities—from self-care to household to community to occupation. The therapist must determine how these skills are limited in such ways as to prevent the fulfillment of the individual's roles. Then the therapist must ascertain why the specified activities are limited by determining the critical neuromotor and musculoskeletal mechanisms that are impaired. These mechanisms can be considered resources that can be used in the performance of the skills.

Finally, the opposite of a disease/disorder is *health*. Health is not simply the absence of disease but an active process of recovery. In many instances, especially in the acute stages, the primary goal of therapy is to promote recovery by creating an optimal environment for tissue healing and system reorganization.

For example, in a patient with an acute injury to the rotator cuff musculature, the overall goal of therapy might be to prevent disability, such as the loss of a valued recreational activity. If the patient were a recreational tennis player, the ability to perform strong and accurate overhead service swings would be an activity-level goal. The immediate impairments would likely include pain, loss of passive range of motion, and weakness. Interventions initially would be planned to promote tissue healing by avoiding strong overhead swings and encouraging pain-free motion at the shoulder. In the postacute stage of the rehabilitation process, interventions would be designed to increase strength and range of motion. As soon as they are deemed practical and safe, the specific activities that are limited would be practiced. Isolated flexibility and strengthening exercises might be taught to the patient, but they would be validated by frequent retesting of the functional task at the activity level of the ICF model. Finally, the patient would be taught proper techniques to avoid reinjury. In both acute and chronic stages, the clinical decision-making process is initiated by determining, in consultation with the patient, the personal and social roles that the patient wishes to fulfill.

A primary goal of physical therapy is to minimize participation restrictions and activity limitations. Nevertheless, the emphasis on functional outcomes in documentation should not be assumed to imply that PTs should focus exclusively on measuring performance at the activity level and training in functional skills. PTs are trained to determine the causes of movement dysfunction, usually in terms of impairments of body structure/function. Ignoring or neglecting this aspect of physical therapy is as much a fallacy as neglecting functional outcomes. Furthermore, Fig. 1.3 emphasizes that the ultimate goal of physical therapy is to promote health and recovery from injury and disease.

FUNCTIONAL OUTCOMES: MORE THAN SIMPLY A DOCUMENTATION STRATEGY

The organizing principles chosen by a therapist for documentation exemplify the organizing principles chosen for diagnosis

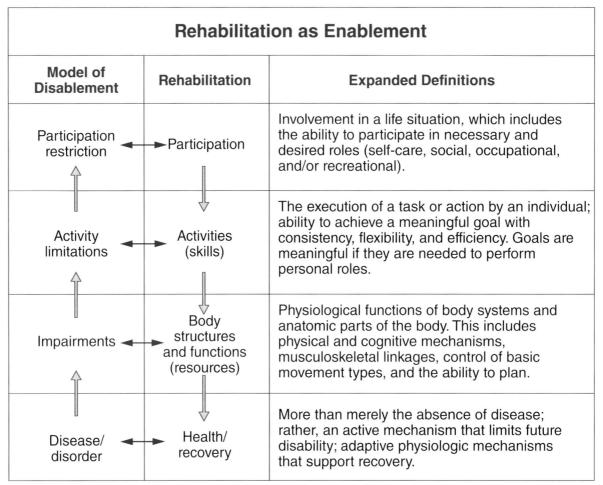

FIG. 1.3 Rehabilitation is a process of enablement.

and treatment. *A haphazard approach to documentation is likely to reflect a disorganized approach to physical therapy evaluation and intervention.* Therefore the organizational framework for documentation presented in this book represents more than simply a way to organize notes. The method of documentation is based on two assumptions: (1) the primary purpose of physical therapy evaluation is to define the specific functional outcomes that need to be achieved, and (2) the criterion for judging the effectiveness of treatment should be whether those outcomes are achieved.

In other words, if it is accepted that physical therapy documentation should be focused on functional outcomes at the activity level, then, logically, physical therapy evaluation and intervention should be focused on functional outcomes. Neither the format presented here nor any functional outcomes format should be viewed as simply an after-the-fact method for justifying payment for physical therapy services in the managed care environment. The purpose of functional outcomes documentation is to provide an explicit and prospective framework by which PTs can (1) analyze the reasons for disablement in their patients, (2) formulate enablement strategies for preventing or reversing that disablement, and (3) explain and justify the resulting clinical decisions they make.

TABLE 1.1	Classification of Measurement Using the ICF Framework	
ICF Framework	**Organizational Level**	**Level of Measurement**
Participation restrictions	Whole person in relation to society	Participation/level of assistance/quality of life
Activity limitations	Whole person	Performance/skill (goal attainment)
Impairments	Body functions or structures	Functions of specific body systems
Health condition	Tissue or cellular	Medical diagnosis

ICF, International Classification of Functioning, Disability and Health.

CLASSIFICATION ACCORDING TO THE ICF FRAMEWORK

Documentation requires the PT to develop skills in classifying the various aspects of the patient's condition using the ICF as a framework. The classification has two bases: the organizational level at which function is observed and the level of measurement (Table 1.1).

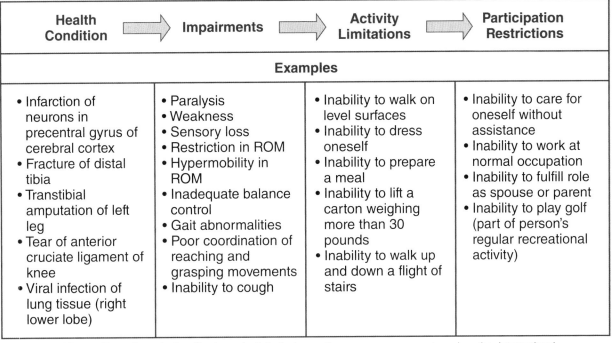

Health Condition →	Impairments →	Activity Limitations →	Participation Restrictions
Examples			
• Infarction of neurons in precentral gyrus of cerebral cortex • Fracture of distal tibia • Transtibial amputation of left leg • Tear of anterior cruciate ligament of knee • Viral infection of lung tissue (right lower lobe)	• Paralysis • Weakness • Sensory loss • Restriction in ROM • Hypermobility in ROM • Inadequate balance control • Gait abnormalities • Poor coordination of reaching and grasping movements • Inability to cough	• Inability to walk on level surfaces • Inability to dress oneself • Inability to prepare a meal • Inability to lift a carton weighing more than 30 pounds • Inability to walk up and down a flight of stairs	• Inability to care for oneself without assistance • Inability to work at normal occupation • Inability to fulfill role as spouse or parent • Inability to play golf (part of person's regular recreational activity)

FIG. 1.4 Examples of classification of clinical observations or measurements using the International Classification of Functioning, Disability and Health (ICF) framework. *ROM*, Range of motion.

For example, the observation that a patient has an infection of the femur (osteomyelitis) is an example of pathological information (at the tissue level, a health condition). The *health condition* usually includes the nature of the pathology (e.g., infection, tumor), its location, and the timing relative to onset (i.e., acute vs. chronic).

Weakness of the quadriceps muscle represents a reduction in body function (muscular); thus it is an *impairment of body structure/function*. It is measured in the frame of reference defined by the body system's function. The muscular system is defined by its ability to produce force over time. Weakness is measured in terms of the force output possible in a defined set of conditions.

An inability to walk is defined as an *activity limitation* because it is a deficit in the ability of the whole person to successfully perform an activity. Activity limitations are measured in terms of performance or skill. Considering whether—and to what degree—the goal of the activity has been attained is an essential component of measuring performance at the activity level.

A patient's inability to care for their child would be a *participation restriction*. It is measured at the level of the individual's social interaction, which can be quantified along three dimensions: (1) participation in desired or expected social roles, (2) the level of assistance required to achieve that participation, and (3) quality of life.

The ability to identify and classify patients' problems into each of the four main levels of the ICF model (health condition, body structures and function, activity, and participation) is a critical first step for therapists to "speak the same language" in both oral and written communication. Fig. 1.4 provides clinical examples of observations or measurements and classifies them according to the ICF framework. Exercise 1.1 provides an opportunity to practice classifying various statements within the ICF framework. Chapters 7-13 provide more extensive explanations and practices in classification and measurement within the framework.

■ SUMMARY

- This chapter has presented a conceptual framework for a specific documentation strategy organized around functional outcomes.
- Functional outcomes should be the focus of physical therapy documentation; this involves documenting limitations in activities, setting functional goals, justifying interventions, and measuring their success based on the effects of functional outcomes.
- Disablement describes the consequences of disease in terms of its effects on body structures and functions (i.e., impairments), the ability of the individual to perform meaningful tasks (i.e., activity limitations), and the ability to fulfill one's roles in life (i.e., participation restrictions).
- Rehabilitation is enablement, which is the reverse of disablement. Whereas disablement begins with disease/disorder, rehabilitation begins with participation—specifying the desired end result in terms of the personal and social roles that the patient is attempting to achieve, resume, or retain.
- Chapters 7-13 offer a set of guidelines for writing documentation in a functional outcomes format that should be adaptable to many different practice settings.

EXERCISE 1.1

Classify each statement according to the International Classification of Functioning, Disability and Health model it reflects: health condition/disease (HC), impairment in body structure/function (I), activity limitation (A), or participation restriction (P). Statements may reflect positive attributes.

Statement	Classification
1. Patient has 0°-120° of active abduction of the left shoulder.	_____
2. Patient can walk up to 50 feet on level surfaces indoors.	_____
3. Partial tear of right anterior cruciate ligament.	_____
4. Patient is unable to work at previous occupation as a salesperson.	_____
5. Strength right knee flexion 3/5 on manual muscle test.	_____
6. Patient needs minimal assistance to dress lower body.	_____
7. Transfemoral amputation of right lower extremity.	_____
8. Heart rate increases from 80 to 140 beats per minute after climbing one flight of stairs.	_____
9. Patient was diagnosed with multiple sclerosis in October 2020.	_____
10. Patient is able to eat soup from a bowl independently.	_____
11. Left lateral pinch strength is 15 lb.	_____
12. Patient transfers from bed to wheelchair independently with the use of a sliding board.	_____
13. Patient has a full passive range of motion in the left knee.	_____
14. Child is able to crawl a distance of 6 feet on living room floor to obtain a desired toy.	_____
15. Patient is able to reach for and grasp a cup located at shoulder height.	_____
16. Patient can stand at kitchen sink for 2 minutes.	_____
17. Patient is unable to perform a straight leg raise.	_____
18. Patient has pain in the right shoulder, rated 5/10, whenever he raises the arm above shoulder height.	_____

Statement	Classification
19. Patient has a personal aide for 4 hours a day to assist with daily care and household chores.	_____
20. Patient is unable to cook using the stove and needs moderate assistance to prepare all meals.	_____
21. Patient is able to transfer from floor to wheelchair within 1 minute.	_____
22. Patient was diagnosed with T8 spinal cord injury after a motor vehicle accident in 2019.	_____
23. Patient is able to enter most buildings in wheelchair, provided an appropriate ramp is present.	_____
24. Partial rotator cuff tear of right shoulder.	_____
25. Patient works as a bus driver with modified work duty with limitations of 4-hour shifts.	_____

Essentials of Documentation

After reading this chapter and completing the exercises, the reader will be able to:

1. Discuss the history of the medical record and documentation.
2. Identify the four basic types of physical therapy notes.
3. List the different purposes that documentation serves.
4. Discuss the pros and cons of different documentation formats.
5. Describe the strategies for concise documentation.
6. Appropriately use and interpret common rehabilitation and medical abbreviations.
7. Use people-first language in written and oral communication.

DOCUMENTATION: AN OVERVIEW

Physical therapists (PTs) and physical therapist assistants (PTAs) often view documentation as an onerous chore. Despite this view, the modern medical record is one of the most important achievements in the development of 20th-century medicine. At the beginning of the 20th century, the notion of a patient-centered chart that stayed with the patient was almost unheard of. Instead, records were kept by individual practitioners, and often the records were haphazard. The development of a comprehensive patient-centered chart, professionally written and clearly organized, enabled direct improvements in patient care by promoting accurate and timely communication among professionals. It also allowed improvements in patient care indirectly by facilitating a better review of the process. The medical chart is the collector and organizer of the primary data for clinical research. It is also an essential teaching device. Students and novice clinicians learn how to provide patient care by reading the documentation written by expert clinicians. It is doubtful that health care would have reached the present level of accomplishment without the changes in documentation over the past century. Moreover, future improvements in patient care will be associated with, and enabled by, changes in the way the process is documented. Documentation is, therefore, a dynamic, ever-changing phenomenon. The dominant formats can be expected to adapt to the changes in health care.

Despite its importance, documentation is often viewed negatively by therapists for at least two reasons. First, and most obvious, too little time is dedicated to documentation in the clinic.

Second, therapists are given relatively little training in documentation. When proper guidelines and adequate training are provided, appropriate outcomes-based documentation does not have to be extremely labor intensive. However, documentation is a skill that should be valued by therapists, educators, and supervisors, similar to any other physical therapy skill. Thus students and therapists must spend dedicated, focused time to learn the "skill" of documentation. Skill develops with practice, practice, and more practice.

Skill in documentation is the hallmark of a professional approach to therapy and is one of the characteristics that distinguishes a professional from a technician. Therapists should take pride in their professional writing; it is the window through which they are judged by other professionals. In fact, it could be argued that documentation of services rendered is just as important as the actual rendering of the services. Supervisors must recognize that good documentation takes time, and therapists must be provided with that time.

In this chapter, we address some of the essential aspects of documentation. Different classifications and formats for physical therapy documentation are presented, as well as critical aspects of information that should be included and the manner in which they should be reported.

TYPES OF NOTES

Four basic types of medical record documentation exist: the initial evaluation, session notes, reexamination or progress notes, and the discharge summary. The following list is adapted from

Guidelines: Physical Therapy Documentation of Patient/Client Management (American Physical Therapy Association [APTA]).[1]

The main aspects of this book focus on documentation of the initial evaluation components (see Chapters 7-13). Special considerations for writing session notes and progress notes are specifically covered in Chapter 14. Documentation of discharge summary and other types of documentation are discussed in Chapter 15.

Initial Examination/Evaluation (Written by Physical Therapist)

Documentation of the initial examination/evaluation is required at the onset of an episode of PT care. For the purposes of this book, we will use the term *initial evaluation* throughout. The initial evaluation should be a comprehensive report incorporating examination findings, a review of history and medical conditions, an assessment or evaluation of the findings and goals, and a plan of care. The format for the initial evaluation should follow this general guideline, which will be used throughout this text:
- Reason for referral
  - Health condition
  - Participation and social history
- Activities
- Impairments (including systems review)
- Assessment (including evaluation, diagnosis, and prognosis)
- Goals
- Plan of care

Session Notes (Written by Physical Therapist or Physical Therapist Assistant) for Each Treatment Session

Each visit or encounter with a patient requires documentation by the PT or PTA. These notes are sometimes referred to as daily notes, visit notes, session notes, or treatment notes. For the purposes of this book, we will use the term *session notes* throughout. The key components to be included in session notes are as follows:
- Patient self-report
- Specific interventions provided, including frequency, intensity, and duration as appropriate
- Changes in patient impairment, activity, and participation as they relate to the plan of care
- Response to interventions, including adverse reactions, if any
- Factors that modify the frequency or intensity of intervention and progression of goals, including adherence to patient-related instructions
- Communication/consultation with providers/patient/client/family/significant other

APTA Guide to Physical Therapist Practice 4.0. American Physical Therapy Association, 2023
[1]**GUIDELINES: PHYSICAL THERAPY DOCUMENTATION OF PATIENT/CLIENT MANAGEMENT BOD G03-05-16-41** (Amended BOD 02-02-16-20; BOD 11-01-06-10; BOD 03-01-16-51; BOD 03-00-22-54; BOD 03-99-14-41; BOD 11-98-19-69; BOD 03-97-27-69; BOD 03-95-23-61; BOD 11-94-33-107; BOD 06-93-09-13; Initial BOD 03-93-21-55) (Guideline), https://www.apta.org/siteassets/pdfs/policies/guidelines-documentation-patient-client-management.pdf

- Plan for ongoing provision of services for the next visit(s), which should include the interventions with objectives, progression parameters, and precautions, if indicated

Progress Notes (Written by Physical Therapist)

A progress note is often written based on a reexamination of a patient and provides an update on a patient's functional status and response to intervention. The key aspects of a progress note are as follows:
- Provide an update on the patient's status over a number of visits or a certain period
- Include selected components of examination to update patient's impairment, activities, and/or participation status
- Provide an interpretation of findings and, when indicated, revision of goals
- When indicated, include a revision of plan of care, as directly correlated with goals as documented

Discharge Summary (Written by Physical Therapist)

Discharge or discontinuation summaries are written at the completion of services by a PT. The discharge summary provides a final report covering the following information:
- Current physical/functional status
- The degree to which goals were achieved and reasons for any goals not being achieved or partially achieved
- Discharge/discontinuation plan related to the patient's continuing care and recommendations including home program, referral for additional services, family/caregiver training, and any equipment provided

PURPOSES OF NOTE WRITING

Documentation of physical therapy services serves many purposes. These include communication with health care professionals, health care administration, or a third-party payer; a guide to clinical decision-making; and provision of a legal record of PT management of a patient.

Communication With Other Health Care Professionals
- Ensures coordination and continuity of patient care
- Organizes the planning of intervention strategies

Communication With Health Care Administration
- Decides discharge and future placement
- Used as a quality assurance tool
- Used as data for research on outcomes

Communication With Third-Party Payers
- Can be used to determine how much should be billed for a visit
- Used as a record of services provided

Guide for Clinical Decision-Making
- Identify specific problems that may be amenable to physical therapy intervention so that an appropriate plan of care can be established

- Provide a structure to allow for evaluation of examination findings to determine a patient's prognosis, diagnosis, and appropriate goals

A Legal Record

- Specifies that the patient has been seen and that evaluation or intervention has occurred
- Serves as a business record
- Can be used as a legal record of services provided in case of legal dispute or malpractice

DOCUMENTATION FORMATS

Many possible formats can be used for writing notes. Sometimes a facility or institution mandates a particular format. Other times, the use of a particular format is not officially required but is instead established by tradition and the desire for consistency. In these cases, PTs, PTAs, and students should use the format in general use within the institution. A particular format does not guarantee well-written documentation; it just makes the process easier. The principles of well-written documentation can be applied in any format. This includes electronic medical records, which are used in most health care centers and many private physical therapy practices today (for further information on electronic medical records, see Chapter 6).

Narrative Format

The simplest form of documentation recounts what happened in a therapist-patient encounter. In this format, therapists can, and should, develop their own outline of information to cover. These outlines can be more or less detailed. The specific information listed in each heading is left to the writer's discretion, although some facilities provide guidelines for what should be covered under each heading. Because of the unstructured nature of narrative formats, the writer is prone to omissions, and there can be a high degree of variability (both within and among different writers). Furthermore, if information is not included, it is assumed it was not tested, whereas the writer may have inadvertently omitted the testing information. Thus, therapists must take particular care to be comprehensive in their documentation to minimize inconsistencies and maximize accuracy.

SOAP Format

The SOAP note is a highly structured documentation format. It was developed in the 1960s at the University of Vermont by Dr. Lawrence Weed as part of the problem-oriented medical record (POMR) (Weed, 1971). In this type of medical record, each patient chart is headed by a numbered list of patient problems (usually developed by the primary physician). When entering documentation, each professional would refer to the number of the problem he or she was writing about and then write a note using SOAP format. The SOAP format requires the practitioner to enter information in the order of the acronym's initials: *Subjective Objective Assessment Plan* (see Chapter 14 for more detailed information on writing SOAP notes).

The POMR was not widely adopted, perhaps because it was ahead of its time. Interestingly, however, the SOAP format did catch on and is now widely used by different professionals, despite the fact that it is no longer connected to its parent concept, the POMR. A major advantage of the SOAP format is its widespread acceptance and the resulting familiarity with the format. On the plus side, it emphasizes clear, complete, and well-organized reporting of findings with a natural progression from data collection to assessment to plan. On the other hand, it has generally been associated with an overly brief and concise style, including extensive use of abbreviations and acronyms, a style that is often difficult for nonprofessionals to interpret. On a more substantive note, Delitto and Snyder-Mackler (1995) have commented that the SOAP format encourages a sequential rather than integrative approach to clinical decision-making by promoting a tendency to simply collect all possible data before assessing it. Thus although the SOAP note does not provide the ideal format for an initial evaluation, it can be adapted to reflect functional outcomes and thus provides a useful framework for documenting session notes and progress notes (see Chapter 14).

Functional Outcome Report Format

The functional outcome report (FOR) format is a relatively new documentation format. It was developed in the 1990s as changes in the economics of health care led to increased emphasis on functional outcomes. The FOR format focuses on documenting the ability to perform meaningful functional activities rather than isolated musculoskeletal, neuromuscular, cardiopulmonary, or integumentary impairments. When the format is implemented properly, FOR documentation establishes the rationale for therapy by indicating the links between such impairments and the participation restrictions to which they are related. FOR documentation also emphasizes readability by health care personnel not familiar with PT jargon (at the expense of increased time to write the documentation). More importantly, it promotes a style of clinical decision-making that begins with the functional problems and assesses the specific impairments that cause the activity limitations or participation restrictions.

Several authors have presented frameworks for FOR documentation. The most well-developed and structured format is that of Stewart and Abeln (1993). Their book, now written more than 30 years ago, played a major role in promoting the idea that documentation should be focused on functional outcomes, and many of their ideas have been adapted in developing the format presented in this book.

WHAT CONSTITUTES "DOCUMENTATION"?

Documentation is any form of written communication related to a patient encounter, such as an initial evaluation, progress note, session note, or discharge summary. It encompasses the preparation and assembly of records to authenticate and communicate the care given by a health care provider and the reasons for giving that care.

Documentation can take many forms, including written reports, standardized assessments, graphs and tables, and photographs and drawings.

Written Reports

Most commonly, PTs use a written report to document their findings from an evaluation or convey what has occurred in a patient visit. The format of this report can take many forms; the two most common are a narrative format and a SOAP format. In this text, we use a narrative format for documenting an initial evaluation (see Chapter 7). For progress notes and session notes, we recommend using a SOAP format (see Chapter 14). Chapter 7 provides full-length examples of initial evaluation reports, and Chapter 14 provides examples of session notes and progress notes.

Graphs and Tables

Graphs can be used as a form of documentation to provide a visualization of a patient's progress in therapy. They can improve readability and readily focus a reader on the critical issues. Fig. 2.1 provides an example of a graph used to chart a patient's progress. In this figure, a patient's gait speed is charted over a period of about 3 weeks. This provides an easy visualization of progress for third-party payers, other health care professionals, and most important, the patient.

Tables are another format of documentation that can be used in the initial evaluation, both to document multiple findings of a similar impairment or functional skill and in progress reports to demonstrate changes over multiple sessions. Tables 2.1 and 2.2 show two examples of tables used in an initial evaluation report. Table 2.3 shows an example of a table used for a progress report, showing performance on the 6-minute walk test over multiple sessions.

Photographs, Drawings, and Graphics

Some aspects of patient care are difficult to describe narratively but may be best explained visually. Photographs (obtained with the patient's written consent) can be used very effectively for documenting impairments such as posture or wound size or for documenting functional abilities. Alternatively, drawings are typically used to document impairments such as extent of burn or pain. Fig. 2.2 shows the FACES scale, which can be used to document pain, particularly in younger patients.

TABLE 2.1	Example of Table Documenting Functional Skills	
Functional Skills	**Level of A**	**Comments**
Rolling in bed	Ind.	
Positioning in bed	Min A	Needs verbal cues to use L UE and LE to assist in movement
Supine sitting in bed	Mod A to R Sup. to L	Can bring legs over side of bed to R, unable to use L arm and trunk to push up to sit
Sitting supine in bed	Ind.	—
Transfer bed to wheelchair	Min A c̄ sliding board	Needs A for proper setup and to initiate movement

A, Assistance; *c̄,* with; *Ind.,* independent; *L,* left; *LE,* lower extremity; *Min,* minimal; *Mod,* moderate; *R,* right; *Sup.,* supine; *UE,* upper extremity.

TABLE 2.2	Example of Table Documenting Muscle Strength	
Muscle Group	**Strength (MMT)**	
	Right	**Left**
Knee extension	3 + /5	5/5
Knee flexion	3 + /5	4/5
Ankle dorsiflexion	4/5	4/5
Ankle plantarflexion	4/5	5/5

MMT, Manual muscle testing.

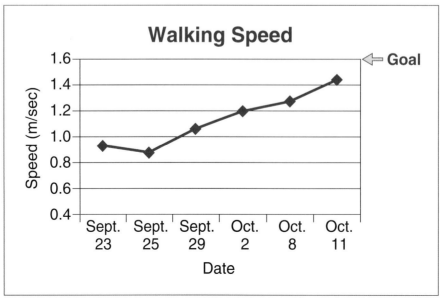

Fig. 2.1 Graphs can be very useful in providing a visualization of patient progress.

TABLE 2.3   A Table Used in a Progress Report Demonstrating the Results of the 6-Minute Walk Test Over a Period of 6 Weeks

	Results of a 6-Minute Walk Test			
	Feb. 5	Feb. 19	Mar. 5	Mar. 19
Distance walked (m)	205	262	301	355
Dyspnea (modified Borg)	4	4	2	2
O_2 sat pre/post	98/94	99/97	100/95	100/98

m, Meters; *sat*, saturation.

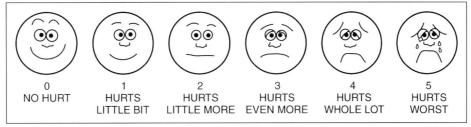

0	1	2	3	4	5
NO HURT	HURTS LITTLE BIT	HURTS LITTLE MORE	HURTS EVEN MORE	HURTS WHOLE LOT	HURTS WORST

Fig. 2.2 The Wong-Baker FACES rating scale. (From Arnold EC, Boggs KU. *Interpersonal Relationships: Professional Communication Skills for Nurses.* 6th ed. Saunders; 2011.)

EVIDENCE-BASED PRACTICE

The American Physical Therapy Association's (APTA) position on evidence-based practice HOD P06-19-10-05 (Amended: HOD P06-06-12-08; Initial: HOD P06-99-17-21, Position) states: "The American Physical Therapy Association supports the development and utilization of evidence-based practice that includes the integration of best available research, clinical expertise, and patient values and circumstances related to patient/client management, practice management, and health policy decision making." It is therefore critical that evidence-based practice be fully integrated into clinical documentation. This is most important in documentation of the initial evaluation and plan of care as well as during documentation of session notes, when specific intervention strategies are reported. The APTA recommends the following as key components of evidence-based practice in physical therapy (https://www.apta.org/patient-care/evidence-based-practice-resources/components-of-evidence-based-practice).

1. Using best available evidence, including clinical practice guidelines when available, to guide decision-making.
2. Using the physical therapist's knowledge and skills that are within scope of practice.
3. Incorporating patient's cultural considerations, needs, and values.

In certain situations, it may be useful for therapists to document specific evidence or provide references. This is particularly useful when a specific treatment is not standard or when providing justification for a certain plan of care to a third-party payer (see Chapter 15 for examples of letters to third-party payers).

TABLE 2.4   Examples of Using Concise Wording and Abbreviations

Too Wordy	Better
The patient can walk in the corridor for 50 ft with minimal assistance.	Pt. walks in corridor 50 c̄ min A
Manual muscle testing was performed for right knee extension, and the strength was 5 out of 5.	MMT R Knee/ 5/5

A, Assistance; *c̄*, with; *MMT*, manual muscle testing; *Pt.*, Patient; *R*, right; */*, extension; out of.

STRATEGIES FOR CONCISENESS IN DOCUMENTATION

Concise Wording

A written medical record has some specific characteristics that differentiate it from traditional narrative writing. For example, medical documentation should be appropriately concise. Time is often limited in health care settings; thus wordiness and undue lengthiness should be minimized (Table 2.4). One way to save time in medical documentation is by not using full sentence structures and using abbreviations. Also, eliminating the words *his, her, a, the, for,* and *an* can improve readability of a medical note.

Abbreviations and Medical Terminology

The first question that must be addressed regarding use of abbreviations is, "Who will be the reader of this note?" If the answer is "another physical therapist or physical therapist assistant (and no other person)," therapists can more freely use abbreviations and appropriate PT terminology. However, if only a slight possibility exists that the note might be read by another professional (e.g., physician or nurse) or by a nonprofessional (e.g., administrative staff, claims auditor, member of a jury), uncommon abbreviations and jargon almost certainly will impede understanding. Furthermore, if the writer is in doubt about the use of an abbreviation, it is best to spell out the word. The time saved writing an abbreviation may not be worth it if it cannot be interpreted by anyone else.

Clearly, common medical abbreviations can be useful time-saving devices (see Table 2.4). Appendix B provides a list of commonly accepted medical abbreviations that can be used for PT documentation in a medical chart. Although this list is not all encompassing, it represents abbreviations that are most likely to be understood by a range of medical professionals. Several books provide a more comprehensive listing of all types of medical abbreviations (Davis, 2019; Dorland 2023). Furthermore, hospitals and health care facilities often develop their own list of abbreviations that are considered acceptable in that institution, and those lists are likely to be more encompassing than those listed here. PTs and PTAs should follow guidelines set by individual institutions when considering the appropriateness of specific abbreviations. Importantly, the Joint Commission has provided a list of "Do not use" abbreviations,[2] which are also provided in Appendix B.

Certain types of documentation are intended for the primary readership of the patient. For example, a home exercise program should be written in lay terminology, avoiding abbreviations and medical jargon. Similarly, any documentation that is sent to third-party payers, and particularly to patients or their families, should make more limited use of abbreviations. If uncommon medical terminology is used, it should be defined in layperson's terms. Another example is note writing in pediatric practice, in which developmental evaluations are read primarily by parents, educators, service providers, and coordinators (Fig. 2.3). Professional notes should not be written in purely lay terminology, but they can be written in such a way as to be readable by those outside the profession.

---

[2]https://www.jointcommission.org/resources/news-and-multimedia/fact-sheets/facts-about-do-not-use-list/

The overuse of abbreviations and jargon is a symptom of a more serious problem: the use of a private language in which much of the rationale for treatment is left implicit. If it is assumed that the reader of a note is among the *cognoscenti*, in which he or she must be able to decipher the abbreviations and strange terms, then why bother explaining what was done and why? The critical elements of the clinical reasoning process cannot be omitted with the assumption that the reader will "fill in the blanks." The therapist has a professional responsibility to explain what has been done and what will be done, and why, in clear, unambiguous terms that will be understandable to all those authorized to read a therapist's notes.

Omit Unnecessary and Irrelevant Facts

The best way to write clear, concise notes quickly is to avoid unnecessary and irrelevant facts and conclusions. Merely because the therapist has observed something does not make it appropriate to include in the note. The note should include only those observations and interpretations that are essential for documenting the patient's reason for referral. Omitting nonessential items makes the note more readable and more efficient to write.

Therapists should generally avoid, or be very careful, when including the following information in a medical note:

- Detailed social history
- Detailed living situation
- Family history not directly related to current medical condition
- Detailed history of other medical conditions that have been resolved and do not affect the current condition

Therapists should use their knowledge of individual diseases to help guide what is considered pertinent for a medical note. In general, documentation should be kept focused to the information that directly affects that patient's current health condition.

Use of Templates

PTs often spend a good part of their working time doing documentation. Although "paperwork" can be extremely

MD/PT/PTA

Min A to transition from prone to sitting due to abdominal weakness and hypertonicity (2/5 on MAS) in hamstrings.

Parent

When lying on his belly, Jimmy needs help when trying to come to a sitting position. This may be due to abdominal weakness and increased muscle tone in his hamstring muscles.

Fig. 2.3 Note writing is audience specific. This figure shows two different wordings for documenting mobility skills in a young child with cerebral palsy. When a note will be read primarily by a parent or professional who is not familiar with common medical terminology, terms should be defined in an understandable and meaningful way. *MAS*, Modified Ashworth Scale; *MD*, medical doctor; *PT*, physical therapist; *PTA*, physical therapist assistant.

daunting—to the experienced and inexperienced clinician alike—the work can be streamlined without sacrificing quality. Although writing a long initial evaluation is not appealing to most PTs, it is equally unappealing for other medical professionals to read one. Therefore the more concise a PT's writing can be while covering all necessary and pertinent information, the better for everyone.

Templates are standard forms that therapists can use to essentially fill in the blanks, and they are standard practice in most electronic medical records. Templates ensure that pertinent items are covered and provide a consistent format for assessing different patients. Once the template is familiar to various professionals, pertinent information can be located readily within the report. Electronic medical records have facilitated the use of such templates in which therapists typically use a combination of narrative writing, check boxes, and pull-down menus from a prefabricated template to develop an individualized evaluation report. Chapter 6 provides an overview and sample templates used in computerized documentation.

If such forms are used, no line should be left blank. In this way, the evaluation cannot be altered by another party without the therapist's knowledge. Also, if a line is left blank, the reason it was left blank is unknown to the reader. The therapist must write one of the following on the line:

1. The results of the test, examination findings, or clinical opinion.
2. N/T (not tested) to indicate that this item was not tested. This entry in the note should be followed by a reason the item was not tested or a plan for testing in the future (e.g., "N/T 2° to time constraints—to be evaluated 11/1").
3. N/A (not applicable) to indicate that this test was not applicable for this particular patient given his or her diagnosis or condition. The therapist should state why the test or measure is not applicable (e.g., "N/A—Pt. is currently on ventilator and unable to get out of bed.").

PERSON-FIRST LANGUAGE

People-first language is language that is used in oral or written communication that describes the disease or medical condition a person *has* without it defining who the person *is* (Box 2.1). Terms such as *autistic*, *mentally retarded*, and *paraplegic* all focus on defining a person by his or her disability. The APTA supports the use of people-first language, as described in *Terminology for Communication about People with Disabilities* (HOD P06-91-25-34, Position).

Physical therapy practitioners have an obligation to provide nonjudgmental care to all people who need it. They should be guided in their written and spoken communication by the *Guidelines for Writing about People with Disabilities*.[3] PTs are encouraged to use appropriate terminology for specific disabilities as outlined in the *Guidelines*, which are available online. Patients should be thought of as people first, not their disability. Labeling patients according to their disability (e.g., stroke victim,

---
[3]https://adata.org/factsheet/ADANN-writing

BOX 2.1 Key Points in Writing People-First Language

Put People First Not Their Disability
Say a *woman with arthritis*, not *an arthritic woman*. This puts the focus on the individual and not on their disability or medical condition.

Emphasize Abilities, Not Limitations
Using the phrase: *Walks with leg braces*, or *uses a wheelchair for long-distance mobility*, is more accurate and positively focused than *confined to a wheelchair* or *wheelchair bound*.

Avoid Negative Labeling
Saying *afflicted with, crippled with, victim of* or *suffers from* devalues individuals with disabilities and portrays them as more helpless and defined by their disability.

Avoid Derogatory Statements
Avoid derogatory statements about patients, such as *Patient complains of...* Rather state *Patient reports...*

Adapted from *Research and Training Center on Independent Living.* Guidelines how to write about people with disabilities. <https://www.aucd.org/docs/phe/9%20ed%20guidelines%20pamphlet%207.24.pdf>; 2020.

TABLE 2.5 People-First Terminology

Write This...	Instead of This...	Example
Nondisabled	Able-bodied, normal, healthy	*Several nondisabled volunteers assisted in the dance program.*
Intellectual disability	Retarded, slow learner, handicapped	*Tom is a 12-year-old boy with an intellectual disability who attends Hawk Hill School.*
Survivor; person with ____ (e.g., autism, Down syndrome)	Victim	*Pt. is a 6-month stroke survivor. OR Pt. had a stroke on 6/1/23.*
Person with paraplegia	T12 para	*Lucy is a 53-year-old female with T12 level incomplete paraplegia.*
Person with amputation/person with limb loss	Amputee	*Pt. is a 76-year-old male with a right transtibial amputation.*

Adapted from *Research and Training Center on Independent Living.* Guidelines how to write about people with disabilities. <https://www.aucd.org/docs/phe/9%20ed%20guidelines%20pamphlet%207.24.pdf>; 2020.

---

amputee) suggests that their disability defines them. In contrast, therapists should strive to use person-first terminology in verbal and written communication (Table 2.5). Furthermore, when referring to individuals who do not have a disability, use of the term *able-bodied* (as well as *healthy* or *normal*) to contrast people without disabilities with people who have disabilities is considered inappropriate. Rather, use the term *nondisabled*.

Expressions such as *afflicted with, suffers from,* or *victim* focus unnecessarily on the negative aspects of a person's health condition. Rather, use a *man with post-polio syndrome* or a *stroke survivor*. Similarly, labeling patients with terms such as *confused*, *agitated*, or *noncompliant*, for example, focuses the reader on the label rather than the person, and the two become invariably linked. Rather, specific behaviors of a patient should be described. Simply because a patient may not be performing a home exercise program, he or she should not be identified as a "noncompliant patient." Instead, the patient might be described as *a patient*, *man*, or *woman*, and at some later point in the documentation, it could be noted that he or she *has not consistently complied with the home program*.

Therapists also should be careful to avoid derogatory statements about patients. Such statements as "*Patient complains…*" or "*Client suffers from…*" have negative connotations and should be avoided. Rather, "*Patient reports…*" or "*Client has a diagnosis of…*" reflect more objective statements.

SUMMARY

- Documentation in physical therapy takes many forms, mainly initial evaluations, progress notes, session notes, and discharge summaries.
- Documentation formats include narrative, SOAP notes, and FORs.
- Within these formats, therapists can use standardized forms, tables, graphs, photographs, and drawings to improve the readability of the documentation and highlight key aspects.

- Therapists can use several strategies to write medical notes in a concise manner: concise wording, use of abbreviations, avoidance of irrelevant facts, and use of documentation templates.
- All written and oral communication should avoid labeling patients and incorporate person-first language. Patients and clients are defined *as people*, not by their disability or disease.

EXERCISE 2.1 INTERPRETING ABBREVIATIONS

For the each of the following statements, write out the entire statement, interpreting the abbreviations. Use Appendix B for assistance with abbreviations. See Appendix C for Answer Key.

Statement

EXAMPLE: Pt. is I in all ADLs.

1. MMT 3/5 R quads

2. Pt. can stand $\bar{s}$ A for 30 sec $\bar{s}$ LOB

3. Pt. can transfer bed → w/c $\bar{c}$ mod A using SB

4. Pt. instructed in performing R SAQ, 3 sets × 10 reps

5. PROM R ankle DF 5°

6. Received Rx from MD for WBAT on L LE

7. Pt. instructed to perform HEP b.i.d., 10 reps each ex

Rewrite Statement

ANSWER: Patient is independent in all activities of daily living.

Statement   **Rewrite Statement**

8. Pt. admitted to ER 10/12/23 with GCS of 4 _____

_____

9. Medical dx: R hip fracture c̄ ORIF _____

_____

10. AROM B LEs WNL _____

_____

11. Pt. instructed in use of TENS unit, on prn basis _____

_____

12. CPT × 20 min; P&V RLL _____

_____

13. Pt. was d/c'd from NICU on 3/3/23 _____

_____

14. PMH: IDDM × 5 yr, HBP × 10 yr _____

_____

15. MRI revealed mod L MCA CVA _____

_____

EXERCISE 2.2 CONCISE DOCUMENTATION AND USE OF ABBREVIATIONS

Rewrite these notes as if you were writing them in a medical record. Consider condensing sentence structure, such as eliminating unnecessary words. Use abbreviations whenever possible. Use Appendix B for assistance with abbreviations. See Appendix C for Answer Key.

Statement   **Rewrite Statement**

EXAMPLE: Patient can walk a distance of 50 feet in the hospital corridors.   **ANSWER:** Pt. walks 50 ft in hospital corridors

1. Patient underwent a procedure called a coronary artery bypass graft on 3/17/21. _____

_____

2. Therapist will coordinate practice of activities of daily living training with occupational therapist and with nursing staff. _____

_____

Statement   **Rewrite Statement**

3. The patient's heart rate changed from 90 to 120 beats per
   minute after 3 minutes of walking at a comfortable speed.

4. The patient's obstetric/gynecologic doctor reported that this
   patient has been experiencing low back pain throughout her
   pregnancy.

5. Patient's daughter reports that patient has had a recent
   decrease in her functional abilities and has a history of falls.

6. The patient's breath sounds were decreased bilaterally.
   The patient was instructed in performing deep breathing
   exercises twice per day.

7. Patient's wife reports that the patient has had a history of
   chronic low back pain for the past 15 years.

8. The patient's long-term goal is to be able to walk using only
   a straight cane.

9. Deep tendon reflex of right biceps was recorded as a 2+.

10. Patient can ascend and descend one flight of stairs
    independently, using one hand on railing.

11. Prescription received for physical therapy to include
    therapeutic exercise and gait training.

12. Resident is 82 years old and has a primary medical
    diagnosis of congestive heart failure.

13. Electrocardiogram revealed ventricular tachycardia.

14. Patient suffered a cerebrovascular accident, with resultant
    hemiplegia of the right upper and lower extremity.

15. The home health aide was instructed in assisting patient to
    perform active-assistive range-of-motion exercises, which
    were straight leg raises and hip abduction in supine.

EXERCISE 2.3 PEOPLE-FIRST LANGUAGE

Therapists should avoid "labeling" patients and should always use people-first language in both oral and written communication. For each of the phrases here, decide first whether the phrase is appropriate. If it is, write "OK" in the space provided. If it is not, rewrite the phrase so that it reflects person-first language or restructure the sentence to provide a more objective or positive description of the patient. (Much of this exercise and the answers are adapted or reprinted with permission from Martin, 1999.)

Statement

1. A quadriplegic will require help with transfers.

2. The patient was afflicted with multiple sclerosis when she was in her 20s.

3. Many PTs are involved in foot clinics for diabetics.

4. Have you finished the documentation for that shoulder in room 316?

5. The patient complained of pain in the right upper extremity.

6. A care plan for patients with total knee replacements involves a strong element of patient education.

7. Although this computer program was designed for the disabled, able-bodied users will also find it helpful.

8. Because of a spinal cord injury, the patient was confined to a wheelchair.

9. Nine of 10 patients receiving physical therapy expressed interest in a group exercise session.

10. The patient is behaving like a child.

11. Which therapist is treating the brain-injured patient in room 216?

Rewrite Statement

Statement	Rewrite Statement
12. The stroke victim can often return to work.	_____ _____
13. The patient refused to modify her footwear choice even after the therapist told her not to wear 2-inch heels.	_____ _____
14. I'll put my 10:00 on the machine while my 10:15 gets a hot pack.	_____ _____
15. The patient suffers from Parkinson disease.	_____ _____

REFERENCES

Davis N.M. 2019. Medical Abbreviations: 55,000 Conveniences at the Expense of Communication and Safety 16th ed. Edition. Neil M. Davis Associates.

Dorland. 2023. Dorland's Dictionary of Medical Acronyms and Abbreviations. 8th Edition. Elsevier Publishers.

Legal Aspects of Documentation

John G. Wallace

LEARNING OBJECTIVES

After reading this chapter, the reader will be able to:
1. List and describe the key aspects of physical therapy documentation as a legal record.
2. Use the correct method for signing notes and correcting errors in documentation.
3. Describe the Health Insurance Portability and Accountability Act and the Privacy Rule and discuss the implication for physical therapy documentation.
4. Discuss the importance of appropriately documenting informed consent as part of a physical therapy evaluation.
5. Discuss the three legal reasons why a physical therapist's documentation may be scrutinized.

DOCUMENTATION AS A LEGAL RECORD

Documentation in a medical record is a legal document. A physical therapist (PT) should take their documentation very seriously and understand that documented notes may be scrutinized not only for payment of services but also for legal reasons.

State practice acts define the scope of practice for PTs in each state (see Recommended Resources at the end of this chapter). PTs should be familiar with their individual state practice acts and regulations to ensure they are in compliance and that their documentation reflects a practice that is within the legal and regulatory descriptions provided by their state. For example, if a state practice act has a requirement for an individual to obtain a referral from a physician for access to a PT, that information must be included in the medical record (regardless of whether it is required by a third-party payer). Box 3.1 contains definitions of important terms related to legal aspects of documentation.

Key Legal Aspects of Physical Therapy Documentation

Several key legal aspects pertinent to physical therapy documentation are outlined in the following sections.

Legibility of Handwritten Entries

Handwritten entries should be legible and written in ink. Many third-party payers, including Medicare, include legibility in their payment policy describing reasons for nonpayment. For this reason, electronic documentation is often recommended to eliminate this potential concern.

Intelligibility

In a medical record, whether handwritten or an electronic medical record (EMR), entries must be able to be understood by readers other than the author. Abbreviations (see Chapter 2 for information on abbreviations) must be clear and obvious. Identification of techniques and interventions should be clear and descriptive of the treatments performed. Avoid idiomatic names and colloquialisms that do not clearly describe the interventions used.

Dated in Month/Day and Year Format

All notes must be dated with the date the note was written. Backdating is illegal and should never be done. It is recommended that all notes be written or dictated on the date that an evaluation or intervention is performed. For notes in an interdisciplinary medical record, the time of day that the treatment was provided should also be recorded. An EMR typically time-stamps the date the documentation is signed and saved in the EMR; thus any late entries are automatically recorded. When documentation is missed or not written in a timely manner, the author should identify the new entry as a "late entry." An *addendum* is another type of late entry that is used to provide additional information in conjunction with a previous entry. In an EMR, an addendum is identified as such and the PT should include the reason for its creation. If the addendum refers to a previous day or date of service, that date should be noted.

Authentication

All physical therapy documentation must be authenticated by a PT or, when appropriate, a physical therapy assistant (PTA). All notes must be signed, followed by the provider's professional designation, and dated. The American Physical Therapy Association (APTA) House of Delegates (APTA, HOD, 2014, P06-03-17-14) has recommended the use of standard professional designations: PT for physical therapists and PTA for PTAs (Fig. 3.1A).

BOX 3.1   Important Definitions

Audit: a detailed review and evaluation of selected clinical records by qualified professional personnel for evaluating quality of medical care.

Authentication: identification of the author of a medical record entry by that author and confirmation that the contents are what the author intended.

HIPAA (Health Insurance Portability and Accountability Act) Privacy Rule: a component of a law passed in 1996 that is designed to protect the privacy of health care data and to promote more standardization and efficiency in the health care industry.

Informed consent: a voluntary, legally documented agreement by a health care consumer to allow performance of a specific diagnostic, therapeutic, or research procedure.

Malpractice: negligence or misconduct by a professional person, such as a doctor or physical therapist. The failure to meet a standard of care or standard of conduct that is recognized by a profession reaches the level of malpractice when a client or patient is injured or damaged because of error.

Medical necessity: services or items reasonable and necessary for the diagnosis or treatment of illness or injury or to improve the functioning of a malformed body member.

Notice of privacy practices (NPP): a notice or written document given to a health care consumer that explains the privacy policies related to his or her medical records. All patients must sign a statement acknowledging receipt of the NPP.

Third-party payer: an organization other than the patient (first party) or health care provider (second party) involved in the financing of personal health services.

Data from Reference.md (http://www.reference.md); Joint Committee on Administrative Rule (http://www.ilga.gov/commission/jcar); Centers for Medicare and Medicaid Services (http://www.cms.gov); Segan JC. *Concise Dictionary of Modern Medicine*. McGraw-Hill; 2006; The Free Dictionary (http://legal-dictionary.thefreedictionary.com/Malpractice); Physician's News Digest (http://www.physiciansnews.com/law); and *Mosby's Dental Dictionary*. 2nd ed. Mosby Elsevier; 2008.

Degrees and Certifications

The APTA supports the following preferred order when a therapist or assistant has additional degrees or designations (Fig. 3.1B). These are not relevant legally, but there are provisions in each state's practice act that are important for promoting consistent communication throughout the profession. The preferred order is as follows:

1. PT/PTA
2. Highest earned physical therapy-related degree
3. Other regulatory designation(s) issued by government entities
4. Other earned academic degree(s)
5. Optional fifth designation—FAPTA (Fellow of the American Physical Therapy Association)

In 2016 APTA's House of Delegates amended the position HOD P06-14-08-18 to limit the use of abbreviated designations after a PT's or PTA's name. Namely, the previously used abbreviations for American Board of Physical Therapy Specialties (ABPTS) are no longer recognized or used. Specialty certification through ABPTS should be spelled out whenever there is room to accommodate them.

Professional designation for PTs is described in detail in all state practice acts, and these should be consulted for any questions about the use of proper professional designators.

PTA Authentication

PTAs should sign any record where they participated in any aspect of the delivery of the service the documentation describes. Although all evaluations must be documented and signed by a PT, if a PTA, for example, takes and documents measurements as part of the PT's evaluation, the PTA should sign the record indicating this was done. If a PTA is involved in part of a treatment where the PT is also providing care, then both the PT and the PTA should sign that note. Depending on a state's practice act, PTs may be required to cosign each note written by a PTA, when the PTA is the only treating provider. Third-party payers

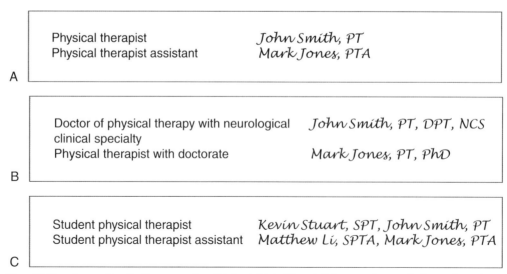

Fig. 3.1 Signature authentication examples. (A) The initials PT and PTA are to be used after a therapist or therapist assistant's name, separated by a comma. (B) Any advanced degrees or certifications should be listed after the designation PT or PTA. (C) Notes by a student physical therapist or physical therapist assistant must be cosigned by a licensed physical therapist or physical therapist assistant.

also may have requirements related to cosignatures that are stricter than a state's practice act requirements.

Student PT and PTA Authentication

Student PTs or student PTAs—individuals who are enrolled in a PT or PTA educational program—are allowed to write notes in the medical record. These notes must be signed and dated by the student and also must be authenticated by a supervising licensed PT or PTA (see also APTA Guidelines, Appendix A) (Fig. 3.1C).

If technicians or aides are performing tasks in a facility or practice, typically their tasks are not documented in the medical record but instead are guided through facility or practice policy and procedure manuals. If a technician is assisting the therapist in the delivery of care and he or she documents this in the medical record, that documentation should always be cosigned by the PT. Each state's practice act or third-party payer policy may have other signature requirements that should be reviewed, as these requirements may be stricter than those in APTA guidelines.

Errors

If an error is made in a handwritten note or a printed copy of an electronic note, the therapist should place a single line through the erroneous word and write his or her initials near the crossed-out word. The date and time of correction should also be included (Fig. 3.2).

Blank Lines or Spaces

Blank lines or large empty spaces should be avoided in the record. In a handwritten note, a single straight line should be drawn through any open spaces in a report.

Abbreviations

The writer should use only those abbreviations authorized by his or her facility. (Appendix B provides a list of commonly used abbreviations in rehabilitation settings.) Abbreviations should be kept to a minimum; if in doubt, write it out. (See Chapter 2 for information on using abbreviations.)

Information Included in a Session Note

From a legal perspective, the medical note should provide a record of everything that was done and how the patient responded to treatment during the therapy session. This includes specifics regarding the treatment techniques performed by the PT and/or PTA (e.g., therapeutic exercise technique, gait training, electric stimulation), how the patient responded (e.g., able to return demonstrate, noted change in condition), and the therapist–patient interaction while in direct contact. This comprehensive documentation approach, while helpful for purposes

of payment, is also very important for legal purposes. A therapist must ask whether his or her note, if referred to at a later date, would clearly establish what was done and why. If a therapist is involved in a professional liability action, for example, the medical record will be scrutinized to determine what interventions were performed, what the patient was able to do, and how the patient reacted to the interventions.

Only information that is directly relevant to the patient's medical condition, prognosis, or intervention plan should be documented in a medical record. Sometimes conflicts or personal issues arise between therapists and patients and between patients and their physicians or other medical professionals. Generally, information of this nature should not be included in clinical documentation but could be important to document in an administrative note that is separate from the medical record.

PRIVACY OF THE MEDICAL RECORD: HIPAA AND THE PRIVACY RULE

HIPAA stands for the Health Insurance Portability and Accountability Act. Congress passed this legislation in 1996. There are two parts to the law. The first part is involved with the portability of an individual's health care insurance in the event of a job loss. The second part, which is pertinent to medical documentation, was designed to protect the privacy of health care data and to promote more standardization and efficiency in the health care industry.

The US Department of Health and Human Services (HHS) implemented the Privacy Rule to comply with HIPAA. The Privacy Rule "address[es] the use and disclosure of individuals' health information—called *protected health information* (PHI) by organizations subject to the Privacy Rule—called *covered entities* as well as standards for individuals' privacy rights to understand and control how their health information is used" (HHS, 2003).

HIPAA rules govern only "covered entities." This includes any provider of medical or other health services, or supplies, who transmits any health information in electronic form (CMS, 2003). Therefore HIPAA applies to only those practices that submit or receive electronic documentation. In the near future, this most likely will apply to almost all physical therapy practice settings.

The Privacy Rule protects all individually identifiable PHI. This is information that is held or transmitted by a covered entity in any form (electronic, paper, or oral). Such information includes a patient's demographic data (e.g., name, address, birth date, Social Security number) and information related to the following:

- Individual's past, present, or future physical or mental health or condition
- Provision of health care to the individual
- Past, present, or future payment for the provision of health care to the individual

An important intention of the Privacy Rule is to limit the disclosure of any patient's PHI. A covered entity can use PHI only as the Privacy Rule permits or as the patient (or his or her representative) authorizes in writing.

Pt. reported pain in R hip (5/10) that is worse in the ~~evening~~ morning *LQ, 12/3/15; 3:25 pm*

Fig. 3.2 Error correction on a progress note.

BOX 3.2   Strategies for Maintaining Patient Confidentiality

The APTA (American Physical Therapy Association) Documentation Guidelines (https://www.apta.org/your-practice/documentation) recommends several general strategies for maintaining patient confidentiality, including the following:

- For paper charting, keep patient documentation in a secure area and never leave patient charts unattended.
- Do not discuss patient cases in open or public areas.
- Follow internal protocol and external regulations (including HIPAA [Health Insurance Portability and Accountability Act] privacy and security regulations) and policies relative to patient confidentiality, including when handling incoming calls related to an individual's condition and/or using electronic documentation. These regulations and policies may come from federal, state, and local governments, reimbursement sources, and other entities.
- When using electronic documentation, take steps to protect the confidentiality of the patient's record, and alert authorized users to their responsibility to maintain the confidentiality of the record at all times.
- Release records only upon consultation with your risk manager and in accordance with organizational/practice policies and laws.

Some basic guidelines for covered entities for maintaining patient privacy of medical records are as follows:

- Patients must be given a notice of privacy practice (NPP) document, which explains the privacy policies related to their medical records. All patients must sign a statement acknowledging receipt of the NPP.
- Therapists must obtain a patient's consent to access, use, or disclose any personally identifiable health information for purposes of treatment, payment, and health care operations. A patient's medical record should never be disclosed to a third party (including employers and family members) without specific permission from the patient.
- Parents or guardians must grant approval for access to a minor's medical record.

For more information on HIPAA rules and compliance, refer to https://www.hhs.gov/hipaa/for-professionals/privacy/laws-regulations/index.html, which provides detailed information on HIPAA and the Privacy Rule and is updated regularly.

In addition to the HIPAA ruling, therapists should take general precautions to ensure that any documentation remains private and is not shared with unauthorized persons (Box 3.2).

DOCUMENTATION OF INFORMED CONSENT

Components of Informed Consent

Informed consent is the process by which a health care consumer is given clear information about the risks and benefits of a proposed procedure or intervention and any alternatives, and the individual agrees to the proposed plan of care. To give informed consent, a person must have appropriate reasoning abilities and must have been provided with all relevant facts. As Purtilo (1984) states in her important publication on this topic, informed consent should help foster further trust between the health professional and the patient. The following information should be a part of spoken or written interactions, which are designed to enable the patient to make an informed decision:

1. A description of the patients' current status as it relates to the perceived need for physical therapy services
2. A description of the assessment procedure(s) or intervention(s) of choice indicated for clarifying the condition or treating it, as well as alternative procedures or interventions
3. A list of the risks and benefits of the procedures and interventions as far as the PT can judge them
4. Additional information that the PT believes will assist a particular patient to arrive at an informed choice
5. An offer to answer questions later as they arise
6. Any additional information recommended by policies or legal counsel of the institution

APTA Guidelines

The APTA's *Guide for Professional Conduct*, originally published in 1981 and last amended in November 2010 by the Ethics and Judicial Committee, states under Principle 2C, Patient Autonomy, that PTs shall provide the information necessary to allow patients or their surrogates to make informed decisions about physical therapy care or participation in clinical research. The underlying purpose of Principle 2C is to require a PT to respect patient autonomy. To do so, a PT shall communicate to the patient/client the findings of his or her examination, evaluation, diagnosis, and prognosis. A PT shall use sound professional judgment in informing the patient/client of any substantial risks of the recommended examination and intervention and shall collaborate with the patient/client to establish the goals of treatment and the plan of care. Ultimately, a PT shall respect the patient's/client's right to make decisions regarding the recommended plan of care, including consent, modification, or refusal.

Components of Documenting Informed Consent

In addition, documentation of informed consent should include the following information:

1. A statement that the PT gave the patient the necessary information to provide informed consent
2. A statement that the patient understood the information and consented to the plan of care

A statement such as the following is an example of documentation of informed consent in an initial evaluation:

The findings of this evaluation were discussed with the patient, and they consented to the above intervention plan.

The patient/client should therefore be asked to acknowledge understanding and consent before intervention is initiated. Many facilities have a separate form for this purpose. If a separate form is not used, a statement should be included in all physical therapy evaluations typically at the end of the documentation of the plan of care (see case examples in Chapter 7).

POTENTIAL LEGAL ISSUES

Although one could argue that the fear of litigation may be exaggerated, PTs and other health care professionals are under continued scrutiny and potential risk for liability and malpractice. Furthermore, billing of third-party payers, such as Medicare,

Medicaid, commercial insurance companies, and workers' compensation carriers, opens up therapists to claims of billing improprieties or fraudulent charging.

The following sections summarize the potential legal reasons why a PT's documentation could be scrutinized.

Malpractice

Malpractice suits against therapists, although rare, typically occur when an accident happens in the course of a therapy session. A patient who is recovering from an ankle injury could over exercise in therapy and reinjure the affected area, for example. Alternatively, a patient who had a stroke could fall and sustain a fracture during gait training or transfer training.

Keeping comprehensive and up-to-date medical records is critical to minimizing liability risk. For example, if a patient reported an increase in pain during the course of a treatment, the therapist should document the current and previous level of pain, whether the plan of care was altered, and if contact with a physician or other health care professional was made. If this information is not documented, then from a legal perspective it *did not happen*. If a patient experiences any mishap when attending therapy (e.g., tripping over a piece of equipment and falling), this should be written up as an incident report with clear documentation of the incident, the reaction to the incident (patient and therapy staff), and steps taken after the incident to attend to the patient's needs. All follow-up regarding the incident should be documented and that record maintained until the matter is resolved.

Documentation When Lawsuits Are Involved

A patient may be involved in a lawsuit related to an accident that he or she had, such as a workplace accident or a motor vehicle accident. In such cases, the PT's records will serve as a legal record and will be scrutinized to determine the necessity of the intervention and the degree of impairments and activity limitations for a patient that are direct results of the incident that is the subject of the lawsuit. The determination of cause and the related care being provided will be, in part, supported by the therapist's documentation of the evaluation (examination and plan of care) and follow-up. All documentation performed by a health care provider is considered a legal document, but in the case of lawsuits there is additional scrutiny placed on the information due to the process involved.

Fraudulent Charges

When billing third-party payers, the PT's medical records will be examined to determine whether the interventions provided match the billing for those interventions. If the PT charges for something that was not done or not supported by documentation, legal action can be taken on the part of the third-party payer. It is critical that the PT's documentation supports the reporting of the *Current Procedural Terminology* codes by the provider (see Chapter 5). Furthermore, for payment by third parties (particularly Medicare), the physical therapy notes must justify that the services provided were skilled and *medically necessary*. The essential elements to demonstrate medical necessity can be third-party payer specific. Reviewing these requirements on the payers' websites or in current manuals can be very helpful in successfully navigating payer audits of medical records. If the treatments proposed or performed are not deemed to be medically necessary and the therapist attempts to bill an insurance company or Medicare for these services, the therapist may be vulnerable to audit recoupment and/or legal action by that payer.

Preventive Actions

A therapy practice or facility can take several actions to minimize the risk of an audit by a third-party payer or government agency or other legal action. Most importantly, a practice should have a systematic plan to stay up to date and in compliance with current rules related to coding, billing, documentation, and requirements for documenting medical necessity and skilled therapy services (Fearon et al., 2009).

The following is a list of strategies that facilities or private practices can use to minimize their risk for an audit or investigation:

- Minimize errors and prevent potential penalties for improper billing and documentation before they occur by performing self-audits, with proper communication and feedback to therapists of the results.
- Set up controls to counter risks by reviewing pertinent policies of the most relevant third-party payers being billed for services.
- Perform preaudit self-examination of compliance activities to identify and address vulnerabilities.
- Hire compliance experts through legal counsel (attorney client privilege established).
- Develop and train staff in compliance plans; such plans can limit your liability by providing standards of conduct for your practice or facility.
- Develop corrective action plans; such plans can be used to fix any areas of weakness or vulnerability that may have been determined after a risk assessment.

▌ SUMMARY

- Documentation in a medical record by PTs or PTAs is considered a legal document.
- Documentation must comply with individual state practice acts, to which therapists should refer for information related to authentication and other specific requirements.
- Documentation of informed consent is recommended to ensure that the patient was given all necessary information pertaining to his or her condition and evaluation results and

to demonstrate that the patient consented to the proposed plan of care prior to treatment.
- Understanding the Privacy Act as part of the HIPAA legislation is important to PTs who are providing care as "covered entities."
- Although PTs and other health care professionals are vulnerable to legal actions, complete and accurate documentation practices can help to minimize legal risks.

RECOMMENDED RESOURCES

Important resources pertaining to legal aspects of documentation follow.

Websites

- APTA Guidelines for Documentation, Appendix A
  https://www.apta.org/your-practice/documentation
- APTA Guide for Professional Conduct
  http://www.apta.org/uploadedFiles/APTAorg/Practice_
    and_Patient_Care/Ethics/GuideforProfessionalConduct.
    pdf
- APTA Directory of Physical Therapy State Practice Acts
  http://www.apta.org/Licensure/StatePracticeActs/

- The Federation of State Boards of Physical Therapy
  http://www.fsbpt.org/Licensees.aspx
- Centers for Medicare and Medicaid Services
  http://www.cms.gov
- Health Insurance Portability and Accountability Act
  http://www.hhs.gov/ocr/privacy

Books and Articles

- Scott RW. *Legal, Ethical, And Practical Aspects of Patient Care Documentation: A Guide for Rehabilitation Professionals.* 4th ed. Boston: Jones and Bartlett Publishers; 2013.
- Purtilo R. Consent to Patient Care Legal and Ethical Considerations for Physical Therapy. *Phys Therapy.* 1984;64(6): 934–937.

Standardized Outcome Measures

Julie Fineman and Lori Quinn

LEARNING OBJECTIVES

After reading this chapter, the reader will be able to:

1. Describe the four levels of measurement used in outcome measures.
2. Define different types of reliability, validity, and responsiveness and discuss their importance in choosing evaluation tools.
3. Describe effect sizes and typical statistics used to report them.
4. Describe how measurement error is evaluated, including minimal detectable change and minimal clinically important difference.
5. Discuss considerations for selecting appropriate outcome measures for a patient population.
6. Discuss the pros and cons of performance-based versus self-report measures.

The use of standardized outcome measures has become an integral part of physical therapy documentation, and over the past 20+ years there has been a significant increase in their use in most clinical settings. Standardized outcome measures are measures that have been determined to be reliable and validated in specific patient populations. Third-party payers often recommend and can even dictate the use of standardized measures to inform eligibility for continued services. They can be useful in quantifying patient performance and demonstrating the value of therapy services, both to patients and third-party payers.

Most rehabilitation outcome measures are designed to be evaluative, which means they can be used to effectively measure change between two or more time points. This enables the therapist to accurately monitor a client's progress during rehabilitation or to determine the effectiveness of a given intervention. Hundreds of outcome measures are available to therapists measuring all levels of disablement, and choosing the right outcome measure is an important part of clinical assessment. In this chapter, we provide an overview of the critical features of selecting and interpreting outcome measures that are used as part of evaluations, reevaluations, progress notes, session notes, and discharge summaries. Table 4.1 provides a list of some of the most commonly used rehabilitation outcome measures. In Chapters 8-10, tables are also provided that list additional measures that specifically evaluate levels of participation, activities, and impairments. For additional information and access to a wide range of assessment tools, the reader is referred to the Recommended Resources at the end of this chapter.

LEVELS OF MEASUREMENT

Standardized measures typically use numbers to assign value to a specific construct. For example, time is measured in seconds, range of motion is measured in degrees, and distance walked is measured in length. Each measurement can be categorized into one of four levels: nominal, ordinal, interval, and ratio. A description of these different levels and examples of measures in each category can be found in Table 4.2.

These four levels of measurement are typically ranked in order of hierarchy, as shown in Table 4.2. Nominal and ordinal are both categorical; nominal measures are sufficient to measure the proportion or frequency of a population achieving a particular outcome, whereas ordinal measures have a distinctive relationship or order between the categories. Interval and ratio measures are both quantitative, with equal values between levels. Ratio measures provide the most flexibility in terms of analysis and comparison; ordinal data, which are very commonly used in rehabilitation rating scales, have more limitations, and statistical comparisons should be approached cautiously (Roach, 2006).

PSYCHOMETRIC PROPERTIES

Reliability

Therapists must have knowledge of the reliability and validity of an outcome measure and understand the purpose for which the measure was designed. In addition, therapists should consider the sensitivity of a measure: Was it designed to adequately capture changes in a patient's status that may occur as a result of intervention? It is therefore important for therapists to perform due diligence in properly researching assessment tools and ensure they are properly trained in their use. Table 4.3 provides descriptions of commonly used terminology to describe the psychometric properties of different measures. Understanding the reliability of a measure is one of the first components of determining its

TABLE 4.1   Some Commonly Used Outcome Measures at Different Levels of the ICF Framework[a]

Outcome Measures	Description	ICF Level	Performance or Self-Report
Participation-Level Measurements			
Disability of the Arm, Shoulder and Hand Questionnaire (DASH) (Hudak et al., 1996) and Quick DASH. (Gummesson et al., 2006)	A 30-item, 5-level ordinal scale (0, 1, 2, 3, 4), measuring functional difficulty and symptoms resulting from upper extremity dysfunction. Quick DASH is a shortened version that uses 11 items.	Participation/ activity/ impairment	Self-report
Lower Extremity Functional Scale (Binkley et al., 1999)	A 20-item, 5-level ordinal scale (0, 1, 2, 3, 4). Used to evaluate the functional impairment of a patient with a disorder of one or both lower extremities.	Participation/ activity	Self-report
Oswestry Disability Index (Fairbank et al., 2000)	Used for evaluation of disability in people with low back pain. Assesses disability/participation in 10 functional areas with 6-item responses (0-5) each.	Participation/ activity	Self-report
36-Item Short Form Health Survey Questionnaire (SF-36) (Stewart et al., 1988)	Measure that includes 36 items pertaining to general well-being and quality of life and frequency and degree of participation in daily living, social, and recreational activities. Role and social functioning subscale measure at level of participation.	Participation	Self-report
Activity-Level Measurements			
5 Time Sit to Stand Test (Whitney et al., 2005)	Measures one aspect of transfer skill. This test provides a method to quantify functional lower extremity strength and opportunity to identify a patient's movement strategies during this transitional movement.	Activities	Performance based
Patient-Specific Functional Scale (Stratford et al., 1995)	Individualized measure that asks patients to list three activities that they are unable to do or have difficulty with and to rate the level of difficulty on a 0-10 scale.	Activities	Self-report
6-Minute Walk Test (Guyatt et al., 1985)	Measures the distance a patient can quickly walk on a flat surface in 6 min.	Activities	Performance based
Timed Up and Go (Podsiadlo & Richardson, 1991)	Measures time to stand up from a chair, walk 10 ft, turn around, walk back, and sit down.	Activities	Performance based
Impairment-Level Measurements			
Berg Balance Test (Berg et al., 1992)	Measures balance ability on 14 balance items, such as standing with eyes closed, turning in place, and standing on one leg.	Activities/ impairment	Performance based
Fugl-Meyer (Fugl-Meyer et al., 1975)	Measures recovery after a stroke. Most items scored on a 3-point scale (0, 1, 2); includes motor function, balance, sensory function, range of motion, and pain.	Impairment	Performance based
Numeric Pain Rating Scale (McCaffery & Beebe, 1989)	Measures the intensity of pain experienced by a patient in the past 24 hr on a 0 (no pain) to 10 (worst imaginable pain) scale.	Impairment	Self-report
Short Physical Performance Battery (Guralnik et al., 1994)	Evaluates balance, gait, strength, and endurance by evaluating a patient's ability to perform various balance and walking tasks.	Activities/ Impairment	Performance based

[a] A more comprehensive list of standardized measures can be found in Tables 8.4, 9.2, and 10.1.
Notes: Some measures evaluate across two or more levels of the ICF. *ICF,* International Classification of Functioning, Disability and Health.

acceptability for use in clinical settings. Reliability is typically measured by correlation coefficients, such as intraclass correlation coefficients (ICC), which provides a statistical rating of how well a measure holds up under repeated observations or performances in unchanged patients. If a measure does not have an acceptable level of reliability (typically >0.75), then it may have limitations as a useful outcome measure (Portney & Watkins, 2007). Often the ICC alone is not sufficient to truly evaluate the reliability of a test, and researchers can use other methods, such

as analyzing mean differences, standard error, and confidence intervals, to determine how reliable a tool is and uncover any systematic biases (see the following section on measurement error).

Validity

Validity refers to the ability of an assessment to measure what it purports to measure. Validity of a specific outcome measure can be determined only in relation to a particular question as it pertains to a defined population (Roach, 2006). There are also

TABLE 4.2 Outcome Measure Examples at Different Levels of Measurement

Levels of Measurement	Properties	Measurement Examples
Nominal	Classification is based on name only, including common characteristics or identity	• Gender • Ethnicity
Ordinal	Categories are determined based on a certain order or rank, but the difference between the categories is not known to be equal.	• PD Hoehn & Yahr Scale • Gross Motor Functional Classification System (GMFCS) • Manual Muscle Testing (MMT) • Berg Balance Test • Numeric Rating Scale or Verbal Rating Scale for Pain (NRS)* • Verbal Rating Scale for Pain • Satisfaction level (e.g. very dissatisfied, dissatisfied, neutral, satisfied, very satisfied) • Agreement level (e.g. strongly disagree, disagree, neutral, agree, strongly agree)
Interval	Data are measured along a scale that have an equal distance between numbers but there is no absolute zero	• Temperature (F) • Body Mass Index
Ratio	Data are measured along a scale that have an equal distance between numbers which includes an absolute zero value	• 6-Minute Walk Test • Weight • Visual Analog Scale for pain (VAS)*

*Numeric and Verbal Rating Scales for Pain are considered ordinal because the interval because the numbers (e.g. 1, 2, 3) are not known to be equal; Visual Analog Scale for pain has a true zero and has equal distance between points.
Adapted from Dittmar & Gresham, 1997.

TABLE 4.3 Psychometric Properties of Rehabilitation Outcome Measures

Measurement Property	Component	Description
Reliability	Test/retest	Reliability gives us an indication of the amount of random error that exists in the outcome measure. Test/retest measures the agreement of the same test for repeated administrations. Reliability is typically reported as correlation coefficients (e.g., ICC), % agreement, or kappa coefficients.
	Intrarater	The agreement between the same rater administering the same test.
	Interrater	The agreement between different raters administering the same test.
	Internal consistency	The relationship between the individual items in an outcome measure and the overall score. Typically reported as Cronbach's alpha. Internal consistency provides an indication of the homogeneity of an outcome measure.
Validity	Construct Convergent Discriminant	The degree that an outcome measures what it purports to measure. The developer proposes ideas or constructs about the measure and evaluates the constructs. Constructs could be that the outcome measure evaluates one or more domains (convergent) or that it differentiates groups of patients and others (discriminant validity).
	Criterion validity	Evaluates the degree to which an outcome correlates with other measures or outcomes that are already known to be valid.
	Concurrent validity	The ability of a measure to estimate another measure taken at the same time point.
	Predictive validity	The ability of a measure to predict a future outcome.
Responsiveness	Internal responsiveness	The ability of a measure to evaluate change over time; it is often assessed before and after an intervention.
	External responsiveness	The extent to which change in a measure is related to changes in other measures.
Measurement error	Standard error of measurement (SEM)	Estimates the standard error resulting from inherent unreliability in the measurement in a set of repeated scores. Any change in scores from one test period to another (e.g., before and after an intervention) that is smaller than the SEM is likely a result of measurement error, rather than a truly valid change.
	Minimal detectable change (MDC)	The amount of change that needs to take place to be more than measurement error. Measured in same units as the outcome measure (e.g., meters for the 6-Minute Walk Test). Both 90% and 95% confidence intervals can be expressed.
	Minimal clinically important difference (MCID)	Smallest difference in a measured variable that signifies an important, rather than a trivial, difference in the patient's condition. The MCID should exceed the MDC.

Adapted from Stokes E. *Rehabilitation Outcome Measures*. Elsevier; 2010.

different types of validity, such as construct validity and criterion validity (see Table 4.3). *Construct validity* refers to the degree that an outcome measures what it purports to measure. One aspect of construct validity is discriminative validity. A discriminative measure is one that has been developed to "distinguish between individuals or groups on an underlying dimension (test score) when no external criterion or gold standard is available for validating these measures" (Law, 2001, p. 287). A test is said to have discriminative validity if it is able to distinguish between known groups. An example of a measure with discriminative validity is the Functional Gait Assessment, which has been shown to classify falls risk in elderly populations (Wrisley & Kumar, 2010).

Criterion validity refers to the degree to which one test or measure is able to estimate or predict the values of another measure. There are two types of criterion validity: concurrent and predictive. *Concurrent validity* refers to the ability of a measure to estimate another measure taken at the same time point; *predictive validity* is the ability of a measure to predict a specific outcome in the future (Adams, 2002). An example of a predictive test is the Test of Infant Motor Performance, administered in infants, which has been shown to predict preschool motor development (Kolobe et al., 2004).

Responsiveness

Responsiveness refers to the ability of a measure to evaluate change over time and is, in fact, a type of validity. For a measure to be responsive, it must be reliable and include a range of items that are likely to change over a given period. Furthermore, the design of the scoring system must allow for improvement (Roach, 2006). There are two types of responsiveness. *Internal responsiveness* is the ability of a tool to measure change in a certain time frame; it is often assessed before and after an intervention. *External responsiveness*, on the other hand, evaluates the extent to which change in a measurement tool is related to changes in other related measures (Roach, 2006). The responsiveness of a measure is important for physical therapists when evaluating changes before and after interventions. If a tool is highly responsive, it will likely be able to identify true changes in a patient's clinical status. Alternatively, if a measurement tool has low responsiveness because of problems with reliability or measurement design, then it will likely not be useful as an outcome measure in clinical settings.

Measurement Error

Several statistics can be used to estimate the amount of measurement error in a given outcome measure or tool. *Standard error of measurement* (SEM) is one that is commonly used, and it estimates the standard error, resulting from inherent unreliability in the measurement, in a set of repeated scores. Any change in scores from one test period to another (e.g., before and after an intervention) that is smaller than the SEM is likely a result of measurement error, rather than a truly valid change.

Two additional psychometric properties of outcome measures related to measurement error are *minimal detectable change* (MDC) and *minimal clinically important difference* (MCID). The MDC refers to the minimal amount of change that is required to go above and beyond that which might be attributable to error alone. For example, the MDC of the Quick Disability of the Arm,

Shoulder and Hand Questionnaire (DASH) has been reported to be 12.85 for a cohort receiving physical therapy treatment (Franchignoni et al., 2014). The MCID, on the other hand, is the smallest difference that signifies an important, rather than a trivial, difference in a patient's condition. The MCID is a patient-derived score, usually based on a patient's perception of improvement, which reflects changes that are meaningful for a patient. The MCID for the Quick DASH, for example, has been reported to be 15.91, which is larger than the MDC. Therapists may use the known values of both the MDC and MCID for a given patient population to determine whether changes in outcomes are not due to error alone and are likely to be meaningful changes.

Effect Sizes

Effect sizes are used to estimate the magnitude and the direction of a treatment effect and are being used with increasing frequency in rehabilitation research. In a randomized controlled trial, the effect size would report the difference between two treatment groups on a certain outcome measure or measures. Although standardized effect sizes are dimensionless measures (they have no measurement units), they are influenced by the study design and random and measurement error (McGough & Faraone, 2009); therefore comparing effect sizes across different studies should be done with caution. Standardized effects sizes, using Cohen's d, typically have a value between 0 and 1 and are typically interpreted as follows (Sullivan & Feinn, 2012):
- 0.20 minimal effect size
- 0.50 moderate effect size
- 0.80 large effect size

Other measures of effect sizes include odds ratio or relative risk or risk ratio.

INSTRUMENT SELECTION: CHOOSING APPROPRIATE OUTCOME MEASURES

With the large number of outcome measures available to therapists, it can be quite daunting to determine which outcome measure to select for a given patient or patient population. There continues to be a considerable effort to develop databases and recommendations for outcome measures in different patient groups. Developing consensus for use of outcome measures in patient groups is critical to compare patient outcomes and to accurately assess intervention effectiveness. The American Physical Therapy Association (APTA) along with other organizations have developed several resources for cataloging outcome measures used by physical therapists. These include the APTA's Patient Care: Tests and Measures database (apta.org/patient-care/evidence-based-practice-resources/test-measures), the Academy of Neurologic Physical Therapy's (ANPT) outcome measures recommendations developed by the Evidence Database to Guide Effectiveness (Edge) Task Forces (https://www.neuropt.org/practice-resources/neurology-section-outcome-measures-recommendations), and the Shirley Ryan Abilities Lab's Rehabilitation Measures Database (https://www.sralab.org/rehabilitation-measures). Table 4.4 provides a list of some key factors to consider and questions to ask when choosing a clinical outcome measure.

TABLE 4.4 Selecting an Outcome Measure

Review Areas	Review Questions
Purpose of the outcome measure	• What does the instrument plan to measure, and was it originally designed for that purpose? • What are the domains or categories that the assessment focuses on? • How adequately does the instrument measure domain(s) being sampled? • What type of scoring system is used? • How long does the instrument take to complete?
User-centeredness	• Are the outcomes meaningful to the patient/client, the health care professional, the caregiver, and/or the service provider? • Is the measure an observation of performance, a measure of opinions/attitudes, or a self-reported measure of impact or performance?
Psychometric properties	• What evidence is there about reliability with this population/setting? • What evidence is there about validity with this population/setting? • Is there information about the minimal detectable change and minimal clinically important difference? • What evidence is there that it is responsive to change?
Feasibility	• Is there training required for administration? • What is the amount of equipment/space needed to administer the test? • Is the data easy to analyze, and will reports be meaningful to both patients/clients and other interested parties? • Is there a cost associated with the use of the test?
Utility	• How acceptable (e.g., time to complete, difficulty) is it for the clinician and/or the patients? • Will gathering the information be useful to the patient/client? • Can it be used to facilitate clinical decision-making? • Does it provide unique information not available elsewhere? • Will it capture the impact of service?

Adapted from Greenhalgh J, Long AF, Brettle AJ, Grant MJ. Reviewing and selecting outcome measures for use in routine practice. *J Eval Clin Pract*. 1998;4(4):339–350; O'Sullivan SB, Schmidt TJ, Fulk G. *Physical Rehabilitation*. Elsevier; 2013.

Performance Versus Self-Report Measures

Two types of instruments available for use in the clinic include performance-based and self-report measures. A performance-based test involves the therapist observing the patient perform a given activity. A performance-based test can be used to identify a patient's current level of functioning. The patient will be given a specific set of instructions and will proceed to carry out the task without additional assistance from the therapist unless they are unsure of what to do or unable to complete the task. As always with therapy assessment and intervention, safety precautions should be taken into consideration. Performance-based tests may examine the patient at the participation, activity, or impairment level, or they may be a combination of all three. They may capture what a patient can accomplish independently or may measure the level of assistance needed for task completion. Examples of performance-based measures are the 6-Minute Walk Test (Guyatt et al., 1985) and the Timed Up and Go (Podsiadlo & Richardson, 1991). Such measures require direct observation of performance of tasks such as walking and balance.

In contrast to performance-based outcome measures using a method of direct observation, self-report measures gather information regarding a patient's functional level of ability through interviewer report or self-administered report format. An example of a self-report measure is the Lower Extremity Functional Scale (Binkley et al., 1999), which asks patients to rate the degree of difficulty they have performing various tasks, such as walking, sitting, and running. Thus the ratings for self-report measures are based on patient's perceptions, not on their actual performance. They may be administered either in person or over the phone, via survey link or telehealth. Therapists or trained interviewers gather data by asking questions to the patient or caregiver. Clear and consistent question wording must be present to elicit appropriate responses and reliable outcomes. A self-report instrument must identify a time frame for the performance: For example, are you asking about the past 24 hours, the last week, or the last year? Self-report measures also need to be able to differentiate between the patient reporting what they are actually capable of performing versus what the person perceives their abilities to be.

Participation Outcome Measures

As the International Classification of Functioning, Disability and Health (ICF) has been used more frequently by health care professionals, new research efforts have been undertaken to identify outcome measures that distinctly measure the levels of participation, activities, and body structures and function. Outcome measures at the level of participation typically encompass general health status. For example, the Euro Quality of Life Dimension Scale (Brazier et al., 1992) is a brief, standardized assessment that provides a general measure of health status. This measure is used frequently in rehabilitation settings in Europe.

Most measures of participation, indeed probably all, do not measure only participation but also some aspects of activity and body structures and function (Perenboom & Chorus, 2003). Those instruments that most closely measure only participation are the Craig Handicap Assessment and Reporting Technique (Walker et al., 2003) and the London Handicap Scale (Perenboom & Chorus, 2003). In fact, participation and activities may not be able to be truly differentiated into distinct domains (Jette et al., 2007). Measures at the level of participation also encompass a construct known as *quality of life*. Quality of life is the degree of well-being felt by an individual or group of people. Although quality of life itself cannot be directly measured, a patient's perception of their quality of life can be via self-report measures. The 36-Item Short-Form Health Survey Questionnaire (SF-36) (Ware & Sherbourne, 1992) is a commonly used quality of life measure in the general population. There are many disease-specific quality of life measures that have been developed, such as the Multiple Sclerosis Quality of Life Instrument-54 (Vickery et al., 1995) for multiple sclerosis and the Parkinson's Disease Questionnaire-39 (Bushnell & Martin, 1999), and these measures, or similar disease-specific ones, should be considered for these populations.

Activity Limitations and Impairment-Based Outcome Measures

Many different standardized tests and measures are useful in assessing activities and functional skills, as well as impairments in body structure and function (see Tables 9.2 and 10.1). Several books and resources provide detailed information on the many functional assessment tools in current use, including their intended purpose (see Recommended Resources at the end of this chapter). Many standardized assessment tools measure across more than one level of the ICF model, and this frequently occurs with functional measures that also measure some degree of impairment in body structure or function. An example of such a test is the Berg Balance Scale (Berg et al., 1992). This scale measures standing balance at the impairment level, as in standing with eyes closed or with a narrowed base of support, and at the functional level, as in picking up an object from the floor.

Standardized activity and impairment-based measures are an important aspect of physical therapy documentation; however they should never be used *in place of* an evaluation tailored to the specific activities pertinent to a patient. If a standardized test is conducted as part of an evaluation, the therapist should report summary scores and their clinical significance in the evaluation report and attach the scoring form to the report. Reporting results of the entire test as part of the body of an evaluation report is too cumbersome, but therapists may choose to highlight specific components or provide a brief summary of the patient's performance on the test.

SUMMARY

Standardized outcome measures are an integral part of physical therapy documentation and are being required for use by most third-party payers. However, outcome measures are important not just for reimbursement purposes but also to be able to compare outcomes of rehabilitation interventions for both individual patients and across patient groups. This will ultimately lead to better care and patient management.

Therapists should familiarize themselves with the psychometric properties of any measure they choose to use for a given patient, most importantly, the purpose, the patient population it was designed for, and the reliability and validity of the measure. Therapists should carefully consider the psychometric properties and the design of the measure when deciding whether it is appropriate in a clinical setting. Standardized measures of participation, activities, and impairments in body structures and function provide different sources of information but should never replace a comprehensive evaluation.

RECOMMENDED RESOURCES

Websites to Access Information About Outcome Measures, Including Purpose, Content, and Psychometric Properties

APTA's Patient Care: Tests and Measures database (apta.org/patient-care/evidence-based-practice-resources/test-measures).

Academy of Neurologic Physical Therapy's outcome measures recommendations developed by the Evidence Database to Guide Effectiveness (Edge) Task Forces (https://www.neuropt.org/practice-resources/neurology-section-outcome-measures-recommendations).

Shirley Ryan Abilities Lab's Rehabilitation Measures Database (https://www.sralab.org/rehabilitation-measures).

Texts

Enderby P, John A, Petheram B. *Therapy Outcome Measures for Rehabilitation Professionals: Speech and Language Therapy, Physiotherapy, Occupational Therapy.* 2nd ed. Wiley; 2013.

Portney LG, Watkins MP. *Foundations of Clinical Research: Application to Practice.* 4th ed. Pearson/Prentice Hall; 2020.

Stokes E. *Rehabilitation Outcome Measures.* Churchill Livingstone; 2010.

5

Payment Policy and Coding

John G. Wallace

LEARNING OBJECTIVES

After reading this chapter, the reader will be able to:
1. Provide a brief overview of health care reform and its impact on physical therapy and third-party payers in the context of reform environment.
2. Describe Medicare settings that outpatient services are provided in, as well as the characteristic policies and key compliance elements required by Medicare and other third-party payers.
3. Outline Medicare guidelines for documenting skilled therapy services.
4. List the components of documentation for Medicare, including initial evaluations (including plan of care),

progress notes, session notes, reevaluations, and discharge summaries.

5. Understand the basics of the Centers for Medicare and Medicaid Services Quality Payment Program, diagnosis coding (International Classification of Diseases, 10th Revision), and Current Procedural Terminology (CPT) coding for billing and payment purposes.
6. Summarize guidelines for CPT coding that may facilitate payment for services and minimize payment delays and denials.

THE BIG PICTURE OF HEALTH CARE REFORM AND PHYSICAL THERAPY

The topic of health care reform in the United States usually includes a discussion of changes in the way health care services are financed and the various service delivery models that have emerged. In the years following the passage of the Affordable Care Act, which contained the major provisions for health care reform for the country, more than 20 million Americans have gained health care coverage (https://www.cbpp.org/research/health/chart-book-accomplishments-of-affordable-care-act). With this large of a transition in how Americans attain and maintain their health insurance, there are bound to be positives and negatives from the effort. On the positive side, approximately 30 million young adults cannot be denied coverage based on pre-existing conditions, more than 100 million Americans no longer have a lifetime limit on their health coverage, and 76 million are benefitting from preventive health coverage. On the negative side, approximately 28 million Americans remain uninsured. The law has extended affordable insurance to 40 million people, facilitated the implementation of a number of consumer protections and reforms, and improved the quality of health care for many Americans. (https://www.cbpp.org/research/health/chart-book-accomplishments-of-affordable-care-act)

The American Physical Therapy Association has been addressing payment reform for several years from the perspective of achieving a reformed payment system that incentivizes efforts

to improve quality of care, recognizes and promotes the clinical judgment of the physical therapist (PT), and provides policymakers and payers with an accurate payment system that ensures the integrity of medically necessary services. Part of this effort includes reforming payment for outpatient (OP) physical therapy services by transitioning from the current fee-for-service, procedural-based payment system to other systems that would better incorporate elements of reporting that would reflect the key characteristics of clinical decision-making and achievement of functional outcomes through effective patient management. These efforts have included ongoing work updating how PTs describe their services in current and evolving payment systems. Ongoing review of the present *Current Procedural Terminology* (CPT) codes used by therapists to report their services under a procedure-based system is regularly done in the context of these reform efforts.

Reform initiatives also include legislative provisions that have a significant impact on how health care insurance is structured and therefore have an inevitable effect on what is required for medical record documentation. The purpose of this chapter is to provide an overview of current payment policies in the United States and understand their effect on documentation by therapists. Because of the dynamics involved in the health care reform environment, information presented here is likely to change, so readers are encouraged to use this chapter as an overview of payment policies and to consult current health care policy manuals, websites, and other related resources for the most up-to-date information.

THIRD-PARTY PAYERS

A third-party payer is an organization or entity that finances health care services for a patient or client. The patient is considered the first party, and the health care provider is considered the second party. In the United States third-party payers are typically either insurance companies, third-party administrators (which are private entities), or the Centers for Medicare and Medicaid Services (CMS). CMS oversees Medicare, Medicaid, and other government health care programs.

For all third-party payers, it is necessary from the outset for therapists to justify the necessity of the services they are providing. The main way this is achieved is through appropriate documentation of therapy services because this is the crucial method for payers to obtain information about the appropriateness of the services for which they are providing payment. One of the primary roles of third-party payers is cost containment. The United States currently has the highest per-capita health care expenditure in the world at over $10,000 (https://data.oecd.org/healthres/health-spending.htm). This is in part because of the rising and unsustainable costs of health care. Reviews and audits of rehabilitation services commonly demonstrate that services are provided without the evidence to support their effectiveness or relation to positive health and functional outcomes. Documentation often does not justify the necessity of services based on the patient's clinical presentation. Both government agencies and insurance companies are under pressure to find methods to reduce health care costs, especially for services that may not be necessary. Therefore the importance of communicating the medical necessity for services, as defined by the third party responsible for payment of health care claims, has never been greater.

Third-party payers set standards or policies regarding the method and amount of payment for health care services they cover. These policies affect PTs and other providers of rehabilitation services and, moreover, are often developed specifically for rehabilitation services because of concerns of overutilization and unwarranted variation in treatment provided. For example, an insurance company may set a policy that limits the number of physical therapy visits in a calendar year or may determine that only certain types of interventions will be covered for a particular diagnosis. Each third-party payer typically has its own requirements for what is considered appropriate documentation to support what is billed and uses that information to scrutinize providers' compliance with their policies. As discussed in Chapter 2, physical therapy documentation has many different purposes, one of which is to provide justification for payment by third-party payers. Although therapists must become familiar with the policies and requirements of each of their patient's third-party payers, many—if not most—payers look to Medicare to set the standard for payment policy, including documentation requirements. Therefore the focus of much of this chapter is on current Medicare requirements; therapists who are familiar with and incorporate these guidelines for documentation and coding will, in most instances, meet the requirements of most other third-party payers. One of the challenges of attending to Medicare and third-party payers' policies is keeping up with policy changes resulting from the progression of

the standard care and documenting that care. Virtually all Medicare administrative contractors and third-party payers provide email policy updates. Therapists, administrators, and billers can subscribe to these updates on the payers' websites. It is the responsibility of the therapist to remain current.

Medicaid

Medicaid provides health care benefits to people (1) who meet certain financial requirements or (2) have a permanent disability. It is a joint federal and state program offering some benefits not normally covered by Medicare, such as nursing home care and personal care services. Medicaid is administered by individual states, which set guidelines regarding individual eligibility as well as application processes for both providers and patients. CMS, a government agency, provides recommended guidelines for documentation purposes related to patients who receive Medicare or Medicaid benefits. Box 5.1 provides some commonly used abbreviations related to payment policy and third-party payers. Because Medicaid guidelines are updated frequently and are state driven, an in-depth discussion is beyond the scope of this book. For additional information specific to your state, https://www.medicaid.gov/state-overviews/index.html, or for general information, see http://medicaid.gov.

Medicare

Medicare is the federal health insurance program for people who are 65 or older, some individuals with a permanent disability, and people with end-stage renal disease (permanent kidney failure requiring dialysis or a transplant, sometimes called ESRD). Because Medicare is the largest source of funding for medical and health services for people in the United States without private health insurance, its guidelines and regulatory features are of particular concern to PTs and rehabilitation professionals. Table 5.1 describes the OP Part B Rehabilitation Service Settings in which a Medicare physician fee schedule (MPFS) is applicable. There are four "parts" to the Medicare program, which are briefly described in the following sections.

Medicare Part A (Hospital Insurance)

Part A covers inpatient hospital stays, care in a skilled nursing facility, hospice care, and some aspects of home health care (individuals discharged from the hospital, who are considered homebound). Payment is made based on diagnostic-related groups for these inpatient services.

BOX 5.1	**Key Abbreviations Related to Payment Policy and Coding**
BPM	Benefit Policy Manual
CMS	Centers for Medicare and Medicaid Services
EOC	Episode of care
LCD	Local coverage determinations
MACs	Medicare administrative contractors
MPFS	Medicare physician fee schedule
POC	Plan of care
PQRS	Physician quality reporting system

TABLE 5.1 Outpatient Part B Rehabilitation Service Settings

Therapists participate in the delivery of physical therapy services to Medicare beneficiaries through various outpatient settings and structures. Their key characteristics are summarized as follows, and all of these settings at this time are paid under the Medicare physician fee schedule.[a]

Comprehensive Outpatient Rehabilitation Facilities (CORF) (Part B)	Requires at a minimum physician, physical therapy, and psycho/social services. Allows for PT/OT/SLP to be provided offsite as well as a single home visit for evaluation purposes. Requires a medical director and a signed plan of care (POC) for each patient describing durations for up to 60 days. General supervision of PTAs (PT available through telecommunications) with any stricter state law rules applied. Claims submitted on UB-04 claim forms with CORF provider number, not by individual enrollment number. Chapter 12 of the CMS Benefit Policy Manual offers additional guidance.
Home Health (Part B)	PT/OT/SLP services allowed to be provided with no minimum requirement for those beneficiaries not under a HH POC or homebound. The Medicare Benefit Policy Manual (BPM, Chapter 15) guidance is applicable for documentation and claims benefit manual (CBM, Chapter 5) helpful for guidance with claims submission. POC required to be signed within 30 days of initial evaluation developed for up to a 90-day duration. CMS-1500 claim form used with place of service code 12. If providing services outside of the 97000 family of codes, may need to contact your MAC.
Outpatient Hospital	PT/OT/SLP services can be provided with no minimum service requirement. Medicare's BPM used for documentation guidance and CBM for guidance with claims submission using UB-04 forms. POC required to be signed within 30 days of initial visit and can be developed for up to a 90-day duration.
Physical Therapist in Private Practice (PTPP)	PT/OT/SLP services can be provided with PT required at a minimum. If either OT or speech services are the primary service, then those are handled in a similar manner through OT in private practice or speech pathologist in private practice. PTAs require direct (onsite) supervision. Medicare's BPM used for documentation guidance and CBM for guidance with claims submission using CMS-1500 forms. POC required to be signed within 30 days of initial visit and can be developed for up to a 90-day duration. Therapists providing services in this setting must enroll as Part B providers with their MACs and also attain a National Provider Identification Number before billing for their https://nppes.cms.hhs.gov/#/. Also they may be required to report under one of the Medicare Part B Quality Payment Program (QPP). Please refer to further information on CMS QUALITY PAYMENT PROGRAM section later in this chapter.
Physician Offices	PT/OT/SLP services provided as incident to the physician's professional services (must be directly supervised by physician or other qualified provider) or provided by an enrolled PT, OT, or SLP with payment reassigned to physician practice. All other aspects of this setting are similar to PTPP.
Outpatient Rehabilitation Facility (Rehab Agency) (Part B)	PT/OT/SLP services provided with a minimum of PT or SLP required. PTAs require general supervision, but, if providing offsite services, a supervisory visit required every 30 days. State law is followed if requirements are stricter than Medicare guidance. Claims submitted on UB-04 under rehabilitation agencies certification number. Otherwise Medicare's manuals provide guidance for documentation and claims submission in addition to the required state survey process. For more information, follow this link to the CMS website https://pecos.cms.hhs.gov/pecos/login.do#headingLv1.
Skilled Nursing (Part B)	If resident's comprehensive plan includes the requirement of specialized rehabilitative care (PT, OT, and SLP), then these services must be offered. Also can provide services to patients residing outside of a skilled nursing facility. Requires a medical director and the same provisions as other settings previously described in regard to POC signatures and duration. References regarding guidance with documentation and billing can be found in the CMS online manuals.

[a]For more information about these specific settings where therapists provide their services to Medicare beneficiaries, visit the Medicare website specific to therapy issues at http://www.cms.gov/Medicare/Billing/TherapyServices.
Mac, Medicare administrative contractors; *OT*, occupational therapy; *PT*, physical therapy; *PTA*, physical therapist assistant; *SLP*, speech-language pathology.

Medicare Part B (Medical Insurance)

Part B covers certain physician and nonphysician medically necessary OP services, medical supplies, and specified preventive services. Individuals pay a premium to access this coverage and, specific to rehabilitation, can receive covered services when evaluated and treated by a PT, occupational therapists, and speech-language pathologists. Payment is made under a fee-for-service methodology based on the CPT codes reported. The MPFS is the basis for payment under the OP rehab benefit for services received in any OP setting.

Medicare Part C (Medicare Advantage Plans)

Part C includes types of Medicare health plans that are offered by private insurance companies and other private companies that contract with Medicare to provide both Part A and Part B benefits. These Medicare Advantage Plans include health maintenance organizations, preferred provider organizations, private fee-for-service plans (FFS), special needs plans, as well as Medicare medical savings account plans (MSAs). When a person is enrolled in a Medicare Advantage Plan, many of the services covered by Medicare are not paid for under traditional (or Original) Medicare. The MPFS is also the basis for payment methodology under these advantage plans, with the beneficiary paying a co-pay as designated by the plan.

Medicare Part D (Prescription Drug Coverage)

Part D Medicare adds prescription drug coverage to Original Medicare, some Medicare private FFS plans, MSAs, and other special needs plans. Insurance companies and other private companies approved by Medicare offer these plans. Medicare Advantage Plans may also offer prescription drug coverage that follows the same rules as Medicare Prescription Drug Plans.

Medicare is often looked to as a standard from which other insurance companies design their own coverage and payment decisions. Other private third-party payers often incorporate payment policies adopted by Medicare. Understanding Medicare payment policy is a good place to start when navigating other payers' policies, giving the provider a way in which to understand how the private payer may differ from these policy standards.

The discussion in this text focuses on Medicare Part B requirements for documentation because OP practice comprises the majority of physical therapy practice. Although some components and requirements for documentation of Medicare Part A and B differ, the general principles, especially the requirement to demonstrate medical necessity, are the same. Efforts continue to eliminate discrepancies in documentation requirements between inpatient and OP settings.

For Medicare services, the CMS contracts with different insurance companies, called Medicare Administrative Contractors (MACs), to manage and implement Medicare benefits. Section 911 of the Medicare Prescription Drug Improvement and Modernization Act of 2003 mandated that the Secretary of Health and Human Services replace Part A FIs (fiscal intermediaries) and Part B carriers with MACs. This effort to reform the contracting structure was intended to improve Medicare's administrative services to beneficiaries and health care providers through the use of new contracting tools, including competition and performance and quality incentives. According to the CMS website, a network of MACs processes Medicare claims, and MACs serve as the primary operational contact between the Medicare FFS program and approximately 1.5 million health care providers enrolled in the program. MACs enroll health care providers in the Medicare program and educate providers on Medicare billing requirements, in addition to answering provider and patient inquiries. To get updated on the current status of the MAC jurisdictions and contract awards, visit https://www.cms.gov/Medicare/Medicare-Contracting/Medicare-Administrative-Contractors/Who-are-the-MACs.

The current consolidated MACs require specific documentation to justify payment under the Medicare benefit. Title XVIII of the Social Security Act, Section 1833(e), prohibits Medicare payment for any claim that lacks the necessary information to process the claim. Section 1862(a)(1)(A) of the Act allows payment to be made only for those services considered medically reasonable and necessary. Each MAC has a website that clearly identifies those coverage policies that Medicare leaves up to the MAC to determine and audit. These are called local coverage determinations or LCDs. LCDs are defined in Section 1869(f)(2)(B) of the Social Security Act (the Act). This section states: For purposes of this section, the term local coverage determination means a determination by a fiscal intermediary or a carrier under part A or part B, as applicable, respecting whether or not a particular item or service is covered on an MAC basis under such parts, in accordance with section 1862(a)(1)(A).

In addition, as a result of the Benefits Improvement and Protection Act of 2000 (BIPA, 2000), all local medical review policies (LMRPs) were converted to LCDs. The difference between LCDs and previously written LMRPs is that LCDs contain only reasonable and necessary conditions of coverage as allowed under Section 1862(a)(1)(A) of the Act. LMRPs may have also contained information related to coding and

payment guidelines. Coding and payment information that is not related to Section 1862(a)(1)(A) is not contained in an LCD, with the MACs communicating this type of information in their newsletters and provider communication tools.

To access information about LCDs that may have an impact on a provider's delivery of services to their Medicare patients, visit http://www.cms.gov/Medicare/Coverage/DeterminationProcess/LCDs.html.

Key Features of Medicare Documentation

The Benefit Policy Manual (CMS), Chapter 15, Section 220.3.A, states:

To be payable, the medical record and the information on the claim form must consistently and accurately report covered therapy services, as documented in the medical record. Documentation must be legible, relevant and sufficient to justify the services billed. In general, services must be covered therapy services provided according to Medicare requirements. Medicare requires that the services billed be supported by documentation that justifies payment. Documentation must comply with all requirements applicable to Medicare claims.

If records are requested for review and those records are not deemed sufficient to justify medical necessity, or not submitted at all, this will result in complete or partial denial of payment for services. For a service to be covered under the Medicare program, all of the following must be true:

- It must have a benefit category in the statute (therapy services are a benefit under Section 1861 of the Social Security Act).
- It must not be excluded.
- It must be reasonable and necessary.

In addition to the coverage requirements previously listed, the following additional Conditions of Payment must exist for therapy services to be paid under Medicare's Part B Benefit:

- The individual needs therapy services.
- A plan for furnishing such services has been established by a physician or nonphysician provider or by the therapist providing such services and is periodically reviewed by a physician or nonphysician provider.
- Services are or were furnished while the individual is or was under the care of a physician on an OP basis.

In certifying an OP plan of care (POC) for therapy, a physician/notice of privacy practice (NPP) is certifying that these three conditions are met [42 CFR 424.24(c)]. Certification is required for coverage and payment of a therapy claim.

Since October 2012 claims submitted for OP and Comprehensive Outpatient Rehabilitation Facility (CORF) physical therapy, occupational therapy, and speech-language pathology (SLP) services must contain the National Provider Identification Number (NPI) of the certifying physician identified for a PT, OT, and SLP POC. (Reference for this requirement is Publication 100-04, Medicare Claims Processing Manual, Chapter 5, Section 10.3.)

Medicare provides guidance to its requirements in its Benefit Policy Manual (BPM), 100-02, Chapter 15, Section 220. This manual and the one previously referenced are published online and can be found on the CMS website at http://cms.gov/Regulations-and-Guidance/Guidance/Manuals/Internet-Only-Manuals-IOMs.html.

Following are the key elements of Medicare documentation excerpted from the BPM, which must exist to support payment for therapy services under Medicare and which must be evident in the providers' documentation throughout the therapy episode of care (EOC):

1. **Medical necessity**. Medicare refers to the concept of medical necessity using the phrase *reasonable and necessary* in its benefit policy language. Many PTs wrongly believe the physician's order or referral establishes medical necessity for physical therapy services. Although a physician's order or referral (sometimes referred to as a prescription, although the most appropriate professional terminology is *referral*) is not required by Medicare, the Medicare benefit for therapy services does require that the patient be under the care of a physician for some diagnoses (which may or may not be related to the diagnosis for which the therapist is treating the patient) for therapy services to meet coverage guidelines. However, simply because the patient is under a physician's care and a referral to physical therapy has been made, this does not automatically justify the medical necessity of therapy services. Medical necessity for therapy services is determined by the evaluating PT, and there must be clear evidence of this medical necessity demonstrated in the PT's documentation. It is critical that PTs understand that documentation of the initial evaluation is the baseline from which medical necessity for therapy services is established, progress toward identified functional goals is measured, and payment for services are justified.

2. **Reasonable and necessary**. The BPM clarifies that, to be considered reasonable and necessary, each of the following conditions must be met:
   - The services shall be considered under accepted standards of medical practice to be a specific and effective treatment for the patient's condition. Acceptable practices for therapy services are found in the following locations:
     - Medicare manuals (such as Publications 100-02, 100-03, and 100-04)
     - Contractor LCDs (described earlier in this chapter) and CMS National Coverage Determinations, which are available on the Medicare Coverage Database at http://www.cms.gov/medicare-coverage-database/overview-and-quick-search.aspx
     - Guidelines and literature of the professions of physical therapy, occupational therapy, and SLP
   - Services provided are at such a level of complexity and sophistication or the condition of the patient shall be such that the services required can be safely and effectively performed only by a therapist or under the supervision of a therapist. Medicare coverage does not turn on the presence or absence of a patient's potential for improvement from the therapy but rather on the patient's need for skilled care. (Maintenance Programs guidance is addressed later in this chapter.)
   - A Medicare patient's diagnosis or medical condition is a valid factor in making decisions related to the need for skilled therapy but cannot be the sole factor in making decisions as to whether a service is skilled or not skilled. Key to this decision are the need for the skills of a therapist to treat the illness, injury, or disease process and whether the services needed could be provided by other nonskilled personnel.
   - The amount, frequency, and duration of therapy services must be reasonable according to accepted standards of practice in regard to utilization, as described by and through resources provided by the various professional associations representing PT, OT, and SLP professionals.

   Although the BPM provides broad identification of the requirements for coverage under Medicare, CMS provides significant discretion in determining the specific services to be considered reasonable and necessary to its MACs. The MACs do this through establishment of LCDs, which are described earlier in this chapter.

3. **Skilled services**. For therapy services to be considered medically necessary or reasonable and necessary under the Medicare benefit (as well as most other third-party payers), they must also be of a skilled nature. The BPM identifies that services are considered skilled when the knowledge, abilities, and clinical judgment of a therapist are necessary to safely and effectively furnish a recognized therapy service whose goal is one of the following:
   1. Improvement of an impairment or functional limitation
   2. Maintenance of functional status
   3. Prevention or slowing further deterioration in function

   Services must not only be provided by the qualified professional (the therapist) or qualified personnel (the therapy assistant), they must also require the expertise, knowledge, clinical judgment, decision-making, and abilities of a therapist that assistants, qualified personnel, caretakers, or the patient cannot provide independently. Also, a therapist may not merely supervise any care being provided by a therapy assistant; the therapist must also apply his or her skills regularly during the EOC by actively participating in the treatment of the patient. This involvement must be evident in the documentation.

   Examples of coverage policies that apply to all OP therapy claims are in this chapter (Publication 100-04, Chapter 5, and Publication 100-08, Chapter 13). Some policies in other manuals are repeated here for emphasis and clarification. Further details on documenting reasonable and necessary services are found in Section 220.3 of this chapter.

   A therapist's skill also may be required for safety reasons if a particular condition or status of the patient requires the skill of a therapist to perform an activity that might otherwise be done independently by the patient at home. Once the patient is judged safe for independent performance of the activity, the skill of a therapist is not required, and the reasonable and necessary requirements are not met under Medicare.

   Services provided by professionals or personnel who do not meet CMS qualification standards and services provided by qualified people who are not appropriate to the setting or conditions are not considered skilled services. In addition, services that are repetitive or reinforce previously learned skills or maintain function after a maintenance program has been developed are considered unskilled services and do not meet the requirements for covered therapy services in Medicare manuals.

They are therefore not payable using codes and descriptions for therapy services.

Some examples of how a therapist's skills may be documented in the medical record include the following:

- Through the clinician's descriptions of his or her skilled treatment techniques
- By identifying the changes made to the treatment from a clinician's assessment of the patient's needs on a particular treatment day
- By identifying the changes attributable to progress the clinician judged sufficient to modify the treatment toward the next more complex or difficult task
- By identifying any safety issues that were addressed by the clinician in order to effectively treat them

In summary, the deciding factors regarding whether services are considered skilled and medically necessary are always whether the services are considered reasonable and effective treatments for the patient's condition and require the skills of a therapist or whether they can be safely and effectively carried out by nonskilled personnel without the supervision of qualified professionals. If at any point in the therapy treatment it is determined by the treating therapist, or through review of the documentation by an MAC (or other third party), that the treatment does not legitimately require the services of a qualified professional, the services will no longer be considered reasonable and necessary and therefore are not considered for payment under the Medicare benefit. Box 5.2 provides general suggestions for improved documentation for Medicare and other third-party payers.

BOX 5.2 Suggestions for Improved Documentation for Medicare and Other Third-Party Payers

1. Initial evaluations should consider three important components:
   - The services are considered part of the covered benefit for therapy services.
   - Medical necessity is established through documentation of the most appropriate treating diagnosis, objective measures, and clinical decision-making that guides the development of the plan of care, including functional goals.
   - Skilled intervention of a physical therapist is required to provide the services to achieve functional outcomes.
2. Focus treatment on functional return and with measured outcomes:
   - The initial evaluation should include measures of participation restrictions and activity limitations in addition to impairment measures.
   - Goals should be measurable and relate to patient-centered functional activities.
   - Quantifiable outcome measures should be used to evaluate progress whenever possible.
3. Avoid vague terminology:
   - Instead of "Patient is improving," document "Patient's ambulation distance has improved from 250 to 500 ft (avg. gait speed increased from 0.6 to 0.8 m/sec)."
   - Instead of "Patient is tolerating treatment well," write "Patient demonstrates increased lumbar spine mobility by 20° flexion and is able to maintain pain-free sitting position for 15 min after manual therapy treatment."

Initial Evaluation

Medicare identifies specific documentation components necessary to meet minimal documentation requirements, which include the initial evaluation and POC, certification (and recertification) of the POC, session notes, progress notes, and a discharge report. The initial evaluation is the most critical component of documentation because it establishes the medical necessity for therapy interventions, identifying the necessity for a course of therapy through documented objective findings and subjective patient self-reporting. In addition to clearly identifying these findings, documentation of the initial evaluation should list any complexities that are present and, where not obvious, describe the impact of these complexities on the prognosis and/or the plan for treatment such that it is clear upon reviewing the documentation that the services planned are appropriate for the individual.

Medicare provides guidance for including areas that should be clearly documented in the initial evaluation. These include but are not limited to the following:

- A therapy diagnosis and the reported medical diagnosis from the referral or other communications and description of the specific problem(s) to be evaluated and/or treated
- Support for illness, disease, or injuries
- Identification of any medical care before the current episode, if any
- Indication of the patient's social support, including where the patient lives (e.g., private home, private apartment, rented room, group home, board and care apartment, assisted living, skilled nursing facility) and whom they live with (e.g., lives alone, spouse or significant other, child or children, other relative, unrelated person(s), personal care attendant)
- Provision of objective, measurable, physical function, including the following:
  - Functional assessment scores from commercially available therapy outcomes instruments
  - Functional assessment scores from tests and measurements validated in the professional literature that are appropriate for the condition/function being measured
  - Other measurable progress toward identified goals for functioning in the home environment at the conclusion of the therapy EOC
- Communication/consultation with other providers (e.g., supervising clinician, attending physician, nurse, another therapist)

As indicated in the beginning of this chapter, many, if not most, third-party payers look to Medicare to set the standard for documentation of therapy services. Therefore therapists are strongly encouraged to develop consistent documentation standards based on an understanding of these Medicare requirements. In addition to the previously noted concepts, Medicare identifies the following elements as key factors that should be documented by the PT for the initial evaluation. Each of the following elements has been explained in detail in other chapters:

- Demographic information, such as patient's age, date of birth, primary diagnosis (*International Classification of Diseases*, 10th Revision; ICD-10), facility, and patient identification numbers

- Date of onset of symptoms or any exacerbation of a chronic condition that warrants a new EOC
- Medical history, which should include the likely impact of any unrelated conditions on the anticipated POC
- Reason for therapy intervention
- Current status—subjective and objective evaluation of impairments and functional activities, including the relation between impairments and functional activities
- Signature (including professional designation) and date

Furthermore, Medicare requires that therapy services must relate directly and specifically to a written treatment plan (POC), which shall contain, at minimum, the following:

- Diagnoses for which therapy is being provided
- Long-term treatment goals, which should be measurable, pertain to identified activity limitations, and be developed for the entire EOC (any impairment goals should be linked to a functional activity)
- Type of treatment (e.g., physical therapy, occupational therapy) and the anticipated frequency and duration of therapy services

Recent CPT coding revisions have impacted how PTs and OTs report their evaluation services. In the context of documenting the evaluation, it is important to thoroughly document aspects of the patient's presentation that communicate his or her previous medical and functional history, any impact that existing comorbidities will have on the condition and complaints that bring them to a PT for an evaluation. It will also likely be a requirement in the future to use an assessment tool to be able to objectively describe the patient's functional status at the time of their initial evaluation, periodically through the EOC and at discharge of the EOC. Documentation and communication between the evaluating therapist and other health care providers involved with the patient's care is also an important element of the evaluation documentation.

Certification and Recertification of the Plan of Care

Medicare requires certification of the POC for each interval of treatment. In the OP setting, this initial certification period can typically be up to, but cannot exceed, 90 calendar days from the initial therapy evaluation and treatment. Certification requires that the POC, including the minimally required elements, be signed and dated by the physician or nonphysician provider (including MD, doctor of osteopathy, nurse practitioner, certified nurse specialist, physician's assistant, and a doctor of podiatric medicine or optometrist as appropriate) and provides evidence in the medical record that the patient is under the care of a physician or qualified NPP as noted. Certification of the POC by the physician/NPP must occur within 30 days of the initial evaluation.

Medicare payment and coverage conditions require that the POC be recertified according to the duration documented in the POC by the clinician (up to 90-day certified periods are allowed) if medically necessary treatment continues to be required for an extended period or whenever a significant change in the patient status or POC occurs. Examples provided by Medicare of a significant change include a change in diagnosis, an extension of the duration of care previously certified, or changes in the

long-term functional goals. Changes in the interventions provided or frequency of treatment appropriate to a change in the patient status as therapy progresses are not considered significant changes and would not require recertification of the POC but should be documented in the record. It is not required that the same physician or nonphysician provider who participated initially in recommending or planning the patient's care certify or recertify the plans. Recertifications of a POC do not require a reevaluation of the patient.

Session Notes

Third-party payment (including Medicare) relies on documentation as its primary (if not only) source of determining whether a claim is paid or denied. Therefore although therapists may be providing excellent patient care and obtaining clinical results reflecting positive functional outcomes, if this information is not evident in the medical record the care provided may go uncompensated by third-party payers. Thus therapists must be diligent in ensuring that their documentation appropriately reflects the skilled care the patient is receiving as well as the patient's current objective functional status.

Therapists have historically focused their documentation on recording the specific activities or exercises that the patient is performing, typically listing exercises on flow sheets or within the session notes that appear to be of a repetitive nature or reinforcing previously learned activities, without focusing on the interaction between the therapist and patient. Typically, exercise documented solely in this fashion will not be considered for payment. Skilled care is best documented in the medical record by focusing documentation on what expertise, knowledge, clinical judgment, or decision-making abilities the therapist or assistant is providing to the patient during the visit, in addition to recording the specific procedural interventions or techniques being performed by, or provided to, the patient.

With the exception of a few areas in which Medicare requirements are different than other third-party requirements, such as the requirement of the physician certification of the POC, therapists are best served if they are payer blind with regard to ensuring documentation adequately justifies payment for therapy services and focus on documenting consistently for all patients regardless of third-party payer. Current Medicare guidelines state that the purpose of the session note is to serve as a record of the skilled interventions that were provided to the patient and document the time of the services to justify use of CPT codes used to bill therapy services (see the Billing and Coding section). This is critical because, in the event of a medical record review, a reviewer can determine whether specific interventions should be paid only if the appropriate treatment documentation is present. Reviewers look for evidence that the intervention could have been provided independently or by other nonskilled personnel, so documentation of provision of skilled intervention by the PT is a key component evaluated by Medicare and other third-party reviewers.

There are some elements of documentation that would be included in the clinician's session notes based on their relevance to the outcome of the session that day. If not included in the session note, then these elements should be included in any documentation of progress and/or at the end of the EOC. These documentation elements include the following:

- Patient self-report
- Adverse reaction to intervention
- Additional or continued communication/consultation with other providers (e.g., supervising clinician, attending physician, nurse, another therapist)
- Significant, unusual, or unexpected changes in clinical status
- Equipment provided; instruction in use or applications

Medicare or its contractors do not specify the exact format of the session note. Although many therapists have transitioned to the use of an electronic medical record, many also continue to use paper and pen and often use a grid format or flow sheet covering several days of interventions. These formats are often deficient in providing the required elements of documentation of a session note. The session note, in whatever format it takes, should include information indicating the skilled intervention that was performed, including treatment techniques, therapist interaction with patient, significant changes in the patient's condition or progress toward stated functional goals, in objective and measurable terms. Time is an important element of the session notes as well because the CPT codes being reported to a third party are primarily timed codes, typically described in 15-minute units. Medicare requires the documentation of two elements of time spent with the patient, total treatment time, and the amount of time spent in direct contact with the patient (supporting the reporting of the time-based CPT procedure codes). In Table 5.3, the CPT codes found in the Physical Medicine and Rehabilitation (PM&R) (97000) section of the American Medical Association's (AMA) CPT book will be discussed in more detail.

Progress Reports

Third-party payers require that progress toward established functional goals be evident in the therapy documentation to help reviewers and auditors determine whether the services provided continue to be payable under defined benefit categories. If progress toward stated goals is documented within the routine documentation of session notes so that such progress is clearly evident and objective in nature, then a separate progress report is not required as long as the key components of a progress report are included and obvious to the reader.

If the session notes do not identify objective and measurable progress, then the current Medicare Part B policy requires a progress note to be documented in the OP setting at least once every 10 treatment days. For Medicare payment purposes, information required in progress reports shall be written by a clinician, that is, either the physician or nonphysician provider who provides or supervises the services or by the therapist who provides the services and supervises an assistant. It is not appropriate for physical therapist assistants (PTAs) to document progress reports, although assistants can document data that they have collected and that can be used by the therapist to document the progress report.

The progress report should address many of the same components of the initial evaluation, but it should do so in the context of progress made toward stated goals or lack of progress and the reasons for that result of treatment. Justification of the need for continued skilled therapy or discharge, if appropriate, could also be noted in this document. Reports of the patient's subjective statements, if relevant, should be included in addition to the objective measurements or description of changes in status relative to each goal currently being addressed with the various treatment techniques. The progress report should clearly include the extent of progress toward stated goals and an assessment of continued improvement in context of anticipated discharge of the episode.... Plans for continuing treatment, reference to additional evaluation results, and/or treatment plan revisions as well as any communication or collaboration with other caregivers involved with the patient's care should also be documented in the progress report. Medicare does not require that any progress note be signed by a physician or other qualified nonphysician provider, unless the progress note is included as part of the recertification process where the therapist is describing progress made and also extending the certification for an additional described duration.

Reevaluation

Continuous assessment of the patient's progress is a component of ongoing therapy services and is not separately payable as a reevaluation. A reevaluation is not a routine, recurring service but is focused on evaluating progress toward current goals, documenting objective measures in a comparative fashion, making a professional judgment about continued care, modifying goals and/or treatment, or making a decision to discharge the EOC. A formal reevaluation is covered only if the documentation supports the need for further tests and measurements to revise the POC after the initial evaluation.

Indications for a reevaluation include the following:
- New clinical findings
- A significant change in the patient's condition
- Failure to respond to the therapeutic interventions outlined in the POC, with a documented change in plan for treatment to support ongoing care
- Before planned discharge for the purposes of determining whether goals have been met and revising goals in order to progress to discharge of the episode

It is important to note that a recertification of a POC and reevaluation are very different. A **reevaluation** can be a billable service if the requirements for performing it are met, but, as noted, it is not necessarily a routine component of an EOC. **Recertification** is a document that is required under Medicare policy in order to be compliant with Part B physician oversight of treatment under a certified POC that must be performed at least every 90 days. The recertification process does not necessarily require that a reevaluation be performed.

Discharge Note

A PT should document the discharge of his or her patient from the EOC. Not only is this typically a documentation requirement under the various practice acts around the country, it is a Medicare requirement and part of the guidance in Chapter 15, Section 220.3D, of the BPM.

The discharge note (or discharge summary) is required for each episode of OP treatment. In provider settings where the physician/NPP writes a discharge summary and the discharge documentation meets the requirements of the provider setting, a separate discharge note written by a therapist is not required. The discharge note shall be a progress report written by a clinician and shall cover the reporting period from the last progress report to the date of discharge. In the case of a discharge unanticipated in the plan or previous progress report, the clinician may base any judgments required to write the report on the session notes and verbal reports of the assistant or qualified personnel.

Documentation at the time the patient is discharged from his or her EOC should effectively summarize the treatment, progress toward goals, as well as final disposition of goals, and, importantly, outline any recommendations or plans for the patient moving forward (after care, other clinical, provider services, etc.). At the discretion of the clinician, the discharge note may include additional information. For example, it may summarize the entire episode of treatment and therefore justify services that may have extended beyond those usually expected for the patient's condition. Therapists should consider the discharge note as the last opportunity to justify the medical necessity of the entire treatment episode in case the record is reviewed. (See Chapter 15 for more information on writing discharge summaries.)

Maintenance Programs

In January 2013 the US District Court for the District of Vermont approved a settlement agreement in the case of *Jimmo v. Sebelius*, in which the plaintiffs alleged that Medicare contractors (MACs) were inappropriately applying an Improvement Standard in making claims determinations for Medicare coverage involving skilled care (e.g., OP therapy benefits). The settlement agreement describes a series of specific steps for the CMS to undertake, including issuing clarifications to existing program guidance and new educational material on this subject. The goal of this settlement agreement is to ensure that claims are correctly adjudicated in accordance with existing Medicare policy, so that Medicare beneficiaries receive the full coverage to which they are entitled.

The key to the settlement agreement is that there was no expansion of Medicare coverage through this lawsuit. Specifically, the settlement agreement states: Nothing in this Settlement Agreement modifies, contracts, or expands the existing eligibility requirements for receiving Medicare coverage. What was agreed upon and clarified through this process is that when skilled services are required in order to provide care that is reasonable and necessary to prevent or slow further deterioration, coverage cannot be denied based on the absence of potential for improvement or restoration. As such, any actions undertaken in connection with this settlement do not represent an expansion of coverage, but rather, serve to clarify existing policy so that Medicare claims will be adjudicated consistently and appropriately.

To describe some of the impacts of this decision, skilled therapy services that do not meet the criteria for progress toward functional goals may be covered under certain circumstances as a maintenance program. Goals under such a program could describe the maintenance of an achieved level of function or describe the manner in which further deterioration of functional abilities can be slowed or prevented.

Services that include the design and establishment of a maintenance program to provide for stability of an achieved level of function or slow or prevent deterioration of that achieved functional level would be covered under the Part B benefit if they demonstrate that they required the skill, knowledge, and clinical judgment of a therapist to provide the content and also instruct the patient and/or caregiver. In addition, if skilled therapy services are needed for periodic reevaluation of the patient's functional status, these would also be covered. Once a maintenance program has been established, the coverage of the actual therapy services to be carried out is decided by the patient's need for that level of skilled care. As stated in Medicare guidance on the topic: …skilled therapy services are covered when an individualized assessment of the patient's clinical condition demonstrates that the specialized judgment, knowledge, and skills of a qualified therapist are necessary for the performance of safe and effective services in a maintenance program. Such skilled care is necessary for the performance of a safe and effective maintenance program only when (1) the therapy procedures required to maintain the patient's current function or to prevent or slow further deterioration are of such complexity and sophistication that the skills of a qualified therapist are required to furnish the therapy procedure or (2) the particular patient's special medical complications require the skills of a qualified therapist to furnish a therapy service required to maintain the patient's current function or to prevent or slow further deterioration, even if the skills of a therapist are not ordinarily needed to perform such therapy procedures.

The Medicare BPM (Chapter 15, Section 220) provides several examples, including patient scenarios that illustrate the appropriate application of this area of the Medicare benefit. Additional information and guidance can be found at http://www.cms.gov/Medicare/Medicare-Fee-for-Service-Payment/SNFPPS/Downloads/Jimmo-FactSheet.pdf.

PROSPECTIVE PAYMENT, BILLING, AND CODING

Prospective Payment

Prospective payment systems are used in Medicare Part A inpatient settings, including home health agencies, skilled nursing facilities, and rehabilitation hospitals, as a means to manage escalating Medicare costs. A prospective payment system is a means of payment for health care services in which Medicare payment is made based on a predetermined, fixed amount associated with a patient's diagnosis or classification. CMS has developed different patient classification systems for different inpatient health care settings. These classifications are determined by specialized documentation completed by medical personnel to categorize the patient's condition/status according to various functional and medical factors, depending on the setting.

TABLE 5.2 Examples of Required Forms in Settings Under Prospective Pay Methods

Form	Setting or Population	Description
Inpatient Rehabilitation Facility-Patient Assessment Instrument (IRF-PAI)	Inpatient rehabilitation	Uses data items from the Quality Indicators Section of the IRF-PAI Case Mix Groups to establish payment categories
Minimum Data Set—Patient-Driven Payment Model	Nursing home: skilled nursing facilities	Comprehensive assessment of patient's functional status and medical condition; used to categorize patients into case mix groupings to determine the amount of payment
Outcome and Assessment and Information Set—Patient-Driven Groupings Model	Home health agencies	Measures outcomes in home health care and determines case mix groupings for payment of services

The minimum data set, outcome and assessment and information set, and the inpatient rehabilitation facility-patient assessment instrument are the assessment instruments used in skilled nursing facilities, home health agencies, and inpatient rehabilitation, respectively. Table 5.2 describes each of these tools.

The primary purpose of these tools is to provide a method for patient classification for prospective payment. In addition, these standardized tools provide methods for quality control and outcomes assessment across a wide range of patient populations. The involvement of therapists in completing these tools varies depending on the institution or agency. Some institutions require PTs to complete portions of these tools, such as the mobility section, and others require nursing staff to complete the entire assessment. These tools use numerical ratings rather than narrative reporting, and extensive training is typically provided. If electronic documentation is used in a practice setting, these forms can be completed more easily and integrated into institution-specific documentation formats.

Billing and Coding

To bill a third-party payer for services rendered, for the purposes of being paid under a stated benefit, PTs need to document their clinical services and also provide the reason for the need for their services (medical necessity) and describe procedures performed that reflect their interaction with the patient. Third-party payers each have their own billing requirements, but most, if not all, incorporate the reporting of standard terminology for diagnosis (ICD-10) and treatment procedures (CPT-4). Medicare requires mandatory claims submission. Providers in office-based settings must submit a claim form, the CMS-1500, to their MAC. For those providers in facility

environments and rehabilitation agencies, the UB-04 claim form is submitted to the MAC. Commercial auto liability and workers' compensation payers also accept the CMS-1500 claim form. For Medicare, most providers or facilities are required to submit their bills through an electronic payment system. The paper versions of the CMS-1500 and UB-04 also have electronic equivalents that allow for electronic submission of claims to Medicare and other third-party payers. Eventually paper claim submission will become limited. Fig. 5.1 shows the CMS-1500 claim form, which is the standard claim form used by a noninstitutional provider or supplier to bill for services. As seen in the figure, the claim form typically requires therapists to document demographic information about the patient as well as diagnosis codes and CPT procedure codes.

When considering the billing and payment process, it is a reasonable goal for therapists to strive for the most appropriate coding, which will then result in the most appropriate payment on the first attempt to receive payment on a claim. Following the guidelines listed here and frequently consulting with current CMS and other third-party payer guidelines can help therapists minimize denial of payment. If payment is denied, therapists typically have recourse by way of appeal. The appeals process requires further documentation by the therapist and thus can be very time consuming, with an administrative burden that increases the cost of the claims process.

Coding of Diagnosis

An important component of documentation for billing purposes involves assigning a diagnosis or diagnoses to the patient's condition. (*Note:* The diagnosis the patient is referred with is typically a medical diagnosis, but the therapist needs to identify a treatment diagnosis for billing purposes, which often may be different than the referring medical diagnosis.) In 1967 the World Health Assembly adopted the WHO Nomenclature Regulations, which required member states to use the ICD in its most current form for mortality and morbidity statistics. Thus ICD is the international standard for classifying diagnoses for a variety of purposes. The United States officially adopted ICD-10-CM on October 1, 2015, whereas various other countries, including Canada and the United Kingdom, have been using ICD-10 terminology for years. The change to ICD-10-CM allows for greater specificity in coding and requires a greater level of detail in patient care as well as an enhanced standard in documentation.

ICD-10 code sets are contained in manuals that provide numerical listings of more than 70,000 diagnoses, ranging from medical to psychiatric conditions. Table 5.3 provides examples of ICD-10 codes used in physical therapy practice. For billing purposes, a therapist must decide which ICD code or codes are appropriate for each patient. Therapists should first choose a primary code—a diagnosis that best fits the reason that the patient will be receiving physical therapy services. This may be, and often is, different from the medical diagnosis that accompanies the patient to physical therapy. The therapist can also choose other diagnoses as secondary. Secondary codes are used to provide more detail in terms of the medical necessity for the interventions included as part of the POC. Secondary diagnosis

BCBS
P O BOX 890179
CAMP HILL PA 17089

CARRIER

HEALTH INSURANCE CLAIM FORM

APPROVED BY NATIONAL UNIFORM CLAIM COMMITTEE (NUCC) 02/12

| PICA | | PICA |

1. MEDICARE (Medicare #) **MEDICAID** (Medicaid #) **TRICARE** (ID#/DoD#) **CHAMPVA** (Member ID#) **GROUP HEALTH PLAN** [X] (ID#) **FECA BLK LUNG** (ID#) **OTHER** (ID#)

1a. INSURED'S I.D. NUMBER (For Program in Item 1)
123456789

2. PATIENT'S NAME (Last Name, First Name, Middle Initial)
ALBANESE, JANET

3. PATIENT'S BIRTH DATE 10 MM 15 DD 1958 YY **SEX** M ☐ F [X]

4. INSURED'S NAME (Last Name, First Name, Middle Initial)
ALBANESE, JANET

5. PATIENT'S ADDRESS (No., Street)
123 BRISTOL DR

6. PATIENT RELATIONSHIP TO INSURED
Self ☐ Spouse ☐ Child ☐ Other ☐

7. INSURED'S ADDRESS (No., Street)
123 BRISTOL DR

CITY MIDDLETOWN **STATE** NY

8. RESERVED FOR NUCC USE

CITY MIDDLETOWN **STATE** NY

ZIP CODE 10941 **TELEPHONE** (Include Area Code) (845) 457 0694

ZIP CODE 10941 **TELEPHONE** (Include Area Code) (845) 457 0694

9. OTHER INSURED'S NAME (Last Name, First Name, Middle Initial)

10. IS PATIENT'S CONDITION RELATED TO:

11. INSURED'S POLICY GROUP OR FECA NUMBER
NONE

a. OTHER INSURED'S POLICY OR GROUP NUMBER

a. EMPLOYMENT? (Current or Previous) ☐ YES [X] NO

a. INSURED'S DATE OF BIRTH 10 MM 25 DD 1947 YY **SEX** M ☐ F [X]

b. RESERVED FOR NUCC USE

b. AUTO ACCIDENT? [X] YES ☐ NO **PLACE (State)** PA

b. OTHER CLAIM ID (Designated by NUCC)

c. RESERVED FOR NUCC USE

c. OTHER ACCIDENT? ☐ YES [X] NO

c. INSURANCE PLAN NAME OR PROGRAM NAME

d. INSURANCE PLAN NAME OR PROGRAM NAME

10d. CLAIM CODES (Designated by NUCC)

d. IS THERE ANOTHER HEALTH BENEFIT PLAN? ☐ YES [X] NO *If yes, complete items 9, 9a and 9d.*

READ BACK OF FORM BEFORE COMPLETING & SIGNING THIS FORM.
12. PATIENT'S OR AUTHORIZED PERSON'S SIGNATURE I authorize the release of any medical or other information necessary to process this claim. I also request payment of government benefits either to myself or to the party who accepts assignment below.
SIGNED SIGNATURE ON FILE DATE 06 03 2015

13. INSURED'S OR AUTHORIZED PERSON'S SIGNATURE I authorize payment of medical benefits to the undersigned physician or supplier for services described below.
SIGNED SIGNATURE ON FILE

PATIENT AND INSURED INFORMATION

14. DATE OF CURRENT ILLNESS, INJURY, or PREGNANCY (LMP) 06 MM 15 DD 2013 YY QUAL. 431

15. OTHER DATE QUAL. MM DD YY

16. DATES PATIENT UNABLE TO WORK IN CURRENT OCCUPATION FROM MM DD YY TO MM DD YY

17. NAME OF REFERRING PROVIDER OR OTHER SOURCE DN DANIEL TOMLINSON MD **17a.** **17b. NPI** 1760600431

18. HOSPITALIZATION DATES RELATED TO CURRENT SERVICES FROM MM DD YY TO MM DD YY

19. ADDITIONAL CLAIM INFORMATION (Designated by NUCC)

20. OUTSIDE LAB? ☐ YES [X] NO **$ CHARGES**

21. DIAGNOSIS OR NATURE OF ILLNESS OR INJURY. Relate A-L to service line below (24E) ICD Ind. 10

A. M25.51 B. M75.41 C. S46.01 D.
E. F. G. H.
I. J. K. L.

22. RESUBMISSION CODE **ORIGINAL REF. NO.**

23. PRIOR AUTHORIZATION NUMBER

24. A. DATE(S) OF SERVICE From / To					B. PLACE OF SERVICE	C. EMG	D. PROCEDURES, SERVICES, OR SUPPLIES (Explain Unusual Circumstances) CPT/HCPCS / MODIFIER	E. DIAGNOSIS POINTER	F. $ CHARGES	G. DAYS OR UNITS	H. EPSDT Family Plan	I. ID. QUAL.	J. RENDERING PROVIDER ID. #
MM	DD	YY	MM	DD	YY								
1	01 07 15	01 07 15			11		97110	ABC	120 00	2		NPI	1003845918
2	01 07 15	01 07 15			11		97140	ABC	55 00	1		NPI	1003845918
3	01 07 15	01 07 15			11		G0283	ABC	25 00	1		NPI	1003845918
4												NPI	
5												NPI	
6												NPI	

PHYSICIAN OR SUPPLIER INFORMATION

25. FEDERAL TAX I.D. NUMBER 03 0509743 **SSN EIN** [X]

26. PATIENT'S ACCOUNT NO. 0001007

27. ACCEPT ASSIGNMENT? (For govt. claims, see back) [X] YES ☐ NO

28. TOTAL CHARGE $ 200 00

29. AMOUNT PAID $ 0 00

30. Rsvd for NUCC use

31. SIGNATURE OF PHYSICIAN OR SUPPLIER INCLUDING DEGREES OR CREDENTIALS (I certify that the statements on the reverse apply to this bill and are made a part thereof.)
JANET ALBANESE PT
SIGNED 06 03 DATE 2015

32. SERVICE FACILITY LOCATION INFORMATION
ACCESS PT & WELLNESS POM
14 THIELLS MOUNT IVY ROAD
POMONA NY 10970 3021
a. 1831539493 b.

33. BILLING PROVIDER INFO & PH. # (845) 636 4344
ACCESS PT & WELLNESS POMONA
16 MAYBROOK RD SUITE L
CAMPBELL HALL NY 10916 2713
a. 1942239850 b.

NUCC Instruction Manual available at: www.nucc.org **PLEASE PRINT OR TYPE** APPROVED OMB 0938-1197 FORM 1500 (02-12)

WCMS-1500CS-12

Fig. 5.1 CMS-1500 (Centers for Medicare and Medicaid Services-1500) form. This is the standard claim form to bill Medicare Fee-For-Service contractors. CPT (Current Procedural Terminology) codes are included in this form following dates of service. In this example, codes 97110, 97140, and G0283 are used. It is important for therapists to include more than one code if it can be supported in their documentation and helps to substantiate the plan of care.

TABLE 5.3 Examples of ICD-10 Codes Used in Physical Therapist Practice

Problem	ICD-10 Code
Abnormal gait	R26.0 Ataxic gait
	R26.1 Paralytic gait
	R26.9 Unspecified abnormalities of gait and mobility
	R26.81 Unsteadiness on feet
Difficulty walking	R26 Abnormalities of gait and mobility
	R26.3 Immobility (bedfast, chairfast)
	R26.2 Difficulty in walking (not elsewhere classified)
	R26.8 Other unspecified abnorm of gait and mobility, unsteadiness on feet nos
Low back dysfunction	M51.15 Intervertebral disk disorders with radiculopathy, lumbar region
	S39.012 Strain of muscle, fascia, and tendon of lower back
Knee pain	M22.40 Chondromalacia patellae, unspecified knee
Shoulder injury	M75.100 Unspecified rotator cuff tear or rupture of unspecified shoulder, not specified as traumatic

ICD-10, International Classification of Diseases, 10th Revision.

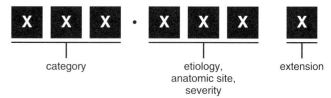

Fig. 5.2 The International Classification of Diseases, 10th Revision (ICD-10) includes 22 chapters indicated in code structure by alpha character: ICD-10 CHAPTER → CATEGORY → SUB-CATEGORY → ICD-10 CODE. Chapters XIII (M) and XIX (S) are typically accessed by physical therapists. Some chapters may need seven characters reported (e.g., XIII, XIX), indicating type of encounter. Codes will be denied if the required number of characters is not included. If necessary, a placeholder "X" may be used in the fifth and sixth character places.

codes can be descriptive of complicating diagnoses. An example would be another condition currently being treated by another provider that could affect the therapy POC. It is important to recognize that ICD codes are a therapist's first step toward demonstrating medical necessity: What is the patient's diagnosis, and is that diagnosis appropriate to be evaluated and treated by a PT? The ICD diagnosis codes are not equivalent to a movement-system diagnosis, which is critical for treatment planning (see Chapter 11). Rather, third-party payers use ICD codes to have a common language for understanding the nature of the patient's disease, illness, disorder, or injury to make judgments about prognosis and POC.

Structurally, ICD-10 codes are three to seven digits in length with the first digit alpha, the second digit numeric, and digits three to seven being either alpha or numeric (Fig. 5.2). A decimal is placed after the third character, and a placeholder X is used in certain cases to allow providers to code to the highest level of specificity. CMS recommends that providers always use the most specific code available (e.g., if a five-digit code is applicable, use that over a four-digit code). ICD-10 has greater specificity built into the code sets, allowing for laterality and severity to be captured in the code. Combination codes are also available that may better capture the patient's presentation. Documentation must clearly support the selection of the codes chosen.

Medicare provides the following guidance in regard to the most recently updated CMS BPM, Chapter 15, Section 220. A diagnosis (where allowed by state and local law) and description of the specific problem(s) to be evaluated and/or treated should be provided. The diagnosis should be specific and as relevant to the problem to be treated as possible. In many cases, both a medical diagnosis (obtained from a physician/NPP) and an

impairment-based treatment diagnosis related to treatment are relevant. The treatment diagnosis may or may not be identified by the therapist, depending on their scope of practice. Where a diagnosis is not allowed, use a condition description similar to the appropriate ICD code. For example, the medical diagnosis made by the physician is CVA; however, the treatment diagnosis or condition description for PT may be abnormality of gait; for OT, it may be hemiparesis; and for SLP, it may be dysphagia. For PT and OT, be sure to include body part evaluated. Include all conditions and complexities that may affect the treatment. A description might include, for example, the premorbid function, date of onset, and current function.

Furthermore, current policies state that the most relevant diagnosis should be billed (CMS Claims Policy Manual, Chapter 5, Section 10.3, B2). As always, when billing for therapy services, the diagnosis code that best relates to the reason for the treatment shall be on the claim, unless there is a compelling reason to report another diagnosis code. For example, when a patient with diabetes is being treated with therapy for gait training due to amputation, the preferred diagnosis is abnormality of gait (which characterizes the treatment). Where it is possible in accordance with state and local laws and the contractors' LCDs, avoid using vague or general diagnoses. When a claim includes several types of services or where the physician/NPP must supply the diagnosis, it may not be possible to use the most relevant therapy diagnosis code in the primary position. In that case the relevant diagnosis code should, if possible, be on the claim in another position.

Codes representing the medical condition that initiated the treatment are used when there is no code representing the treatment. Complicating conditions are preferably used in nonprimary positions on the claim and are billed in the primary position only in the rare circumstance that there is no more relevant code.

Current Procedural Terminology

The CPT coding system was developed and is maintained by the AMA. CPT offers physicians and nonphysicians across the country a uniform process for coding their medical services that allows for an administratively streamlined reporting mechanism. CPT strives to increase accuracy and efficiency of the reporting of provider services as well as to positively affect the third-party payment process. The first CPT code set was published in 1966 and since then, through its rigorous editorial process, has provided physicians and qualified health care professionals a communication tool used with colleagues, patients, hospitals, and insurers about the services and procedures they have provided to their AMA patients.

The CPT Editorial Panel, which is made up of physicians, nonphysicians, payers, and regulators, is tasked with ensuring that CPT codes remain up to date and reflect the latest medical care provided to patients. To accomplish this, the panel maintains an open process, and their meetings occur three times per year to solicit input of practicing physicians and nonphysicians, including PTs, medical device manufacturers, developers of the latest diagnostic tests, and advisors from more than 100 societies/associations representing physicians and other qualified health care professionals.

There are three categories of CPT codes, with category I being codes that describe procedures and services provided by physician and nonphysician providers. Numbers are assigned to services that physicians and other qualified health care professionals provide to a patient. CPT codes are not provider specific, and there are many codes that describe the scope of practice of a PT. Although the majority of codes describing physical therapy practice are found in the Medicine section of the code set, under the heading Physical Medicine and Rehabilitation (PM&R), CPT guidance recognizes that a provider can bill any code as long as the provider can legally render that service according to state licensure laws. Therefore it is necessary for PTs to become familiar with codes outside of the 97000 series of PM&R codes, because many codes appropriately describe services provided by PTs. Therapists assign codes to the interventions they have provided and documented as part of their POC for a patient, which is a requirement for the third-party payer in order to process claims submitted by providers for payment of their services. Medicare, Medicaid, as well as workers' compensation, local, regional, and national private payers use CPT codes to adjudicate claims for payment for medical procedures. Payment for the service described by the code is based on the specifics of a patient's covered benefits under his or her insurance policy and the contract between the provider and the payer to pay for these benefits. CPT codes are technology neutral and include no brand names in their nomenclature.

CPT includes important guidance related to reporting and use of the codes throughout the CPT manual. There is an entire chapter that provides instructions along with an additional introductory language before each family of codes. CPT codes are not a payment system and therefore do not set payment rates nor instruct payers in coverage of services. The majority of the CPT codes in the 97000 family of codes are time based, with a descriptor that includes "each 15 minutes" as part of the descriptor. This is also often described as a unit of time for that particular procedure. AMA CPT guidance (AMA CPT Professional Edition, 2020) includes the following in the introduction to CPT regarding CPT codes that include time in their descriptor: A unit of time is attained when the midpoint is passed. As part of the introduction to the PM&R family of codes, it is stated this way: For the purpose of determining the total time

of a service, incremental intervals of treatment at the same visit may be accumulated. As part of the billing process, and to support those procedures that include a time descriptor, therapists should document the time involved in delivering the service to their patient.

Some payers include a policy to pay timed codes based on total treatment time and how much of that time is spent in direct contact with the patient. This, in fact, is the basis for how Medicare policy addresses the payment of time-based codes. According to Medicare policy, the total treatment time incorporates only time spent in the delivery of skilled interventions by PTs and properly supervised PTAs; time for other aspects of service delivery (e.g., preparing patient, documentation, other communications) is not separately reported but is considered in how the services are described and valued for payment. Under Medicare policy, the time is totaled and then reported with the correct number of units to reflect the direct contact time and the correct codes reflecting the clinical service(s) provided for that time. If a therapist provides more than one type of service in a visit, the codes reported should reflect the intervention(s) and the number of units associated with the time spent. Under Medicare payment policy, the total number of units that can be billed is therefore constrained by the total amount of treatment time. For additional information specific to this topic of reporting timed codes under Medicare's therapy benefit, visit the following website: http://www.cms.gov/Medicare/Billing/TherapyServices.

Determining the correct coding of interventions is critical to ensuring appropriate payment and avoiding claim denials. It is also important for legal reasons. If a therapist submits a CPT code for a procedure but it is not documented to reflect that the procedure was performed or the documentation describes a different procedure being provided, this could be a reflection of a false claim on review and audit. Such an error, although potentially innocent, may open up a therapist to additional audit, potential fines, or possibly litigation. AMA CPT includes the option for reporting an unlisted code if there is no published code that the provider feels describes the clinical service that they provided to their patient. The unlisted codes in the PM&R 97000 code set should be clearly documented to allow the third party to understand what the provider is communicating regarding their services.

Table 5.4 provides a summary of the listing of CPT codes commonly reported by PTs. CPT codes are continually under review, and the AMA CPT manual is published annually each fall for the next calendar year, to reflect code deletions, additions, and modifications. To access the full CPT code instruction and nomenclature, for the current year in which you are reporting services, contact AMA at https://www.ama-assn.org/practice-management/cpt.

It is important to note that simply because a procedure has a valid CPT code does not mean that that service is reimbursable. That determination is made by the third-party payers, including payers contracted with Medicare as part of the MACs, Medicaid payer guidelines, or the many private-pay and managed care organizations. Therapists should be familiar with the various CPT codes applicable to physical therapy practice, even though

TABLE 5.4	**CPT Codes Commonly Reported by Physical Therapists (PTs)**	
Action	**Code**	**Description**
Evaluation, tests, and measures	97161	PT evaluation: low complexity
	97162	PT evaluation; moderate complexity
	97163	PT evaluation: high complexity
	97164	PT reevaluation of physical therapy-established plan of care
	97750	Physical performance test or measurement (e.g., musculoskeletal, functional capacity), each 15 min
	95851-95852	Range of motion measurements
	96000	Motion analysis, video
	96001	Motion test with foot pressure measurement
	96002	Dynamic surface electromyography (EMG)
	96003	Dynamic fine-wire EMG
	96004	Review and interpretation by qualified health care professional of computer-based motion analysis, pressure measurements and surface EMG during walking and fine-wire EMG
Therapeutic procedures	97110	Therapeutic exercise to develop strength, ROM, flexibility, and endurance, with direct (one-on-one) contact, each 15 min
	97112	Neuromuscular reeducation, with direct (one-on-one) contact, each 15 min
	97113	Aquatic therapy with therapeutic exercises, with direct (one-on-one) contact, each 15 min
	97150	Group therapeutic procedures, requiring direct contact of provider with group
	97116	Gait training, with direct (one-on-one) contact, each 15 min
	97124	Massage, therapeutic, with direct (one-on-one) contact, each 15 min
	97140	Manual therapy techniques, with direct (one-on-one) contact, each 15 min
	97530	Therapeutic activities, use of dynamic activities to improve functional performance, with direct (one-on-one) contact, each 15 min
	97532	Cognitive skills development, each 15 min
	97535	Self-care/Home management training, each 15 min
	97537	Community/Work-reintegration training, each 15 min
	97542	Wheelchair management (e.g., assessment, fitting, training), each 15 min
	97545	Work hardening/work conditioning, each 2 hr
	97546	Work hardening/work conditioning, each additional hour
	97533	Sensory integration, each 15 min
Modalities	97010	Hot/cold packs, one or more areas
	97012	Mechanical traction, one or more areas
	97014	Electrical stimulation, unattended, one or more areas
	97016	Vasopneumatic device therapy, one or more areas
	97018	Paraffin bath, one or more areas
	97022	Whirlpool therapy (non-Hubbard tank)
	97024	Diathermy, one or more areas
	97026	Infrared therapy, one or more areas
	97028	Ultraviolet therapy, one or more areas
	97032	Electrical stimulation, direct one-on-one contact, manual, each 15 min
	97033	Electrical current therapy/iontophoresis, direct one-on-one contact, each 15 min
	97034	Contrast bath, direct one-on-one contact, each 15 min
	97035	Ultrasound, direct one-on-one contact, each 15 min
	97036	Hubbard tank, direct one-on-one contact, each 15 min

TABLE 5.4 CPT Codes Commonly Reported by Physical Therapists (PTs) —cont'd

Action	Code	Description
Active wound care management	97597	Selective debridement, first 20 cm² or less
	97598	Selective debridement, >20 cm²
	97602	Nonselective debridement
	97605	Negative pressure wound therapy, less than or equal to 50 cm²
	97606	Negative pressure wound therapy, greater than 50 cm²
	97607	Negative pressure wound therapy, using durable, nondurable medical equipment, less than or equal to ≤50 cm²
	97608	Negative pressure wound therapy, using durable, nondurable medical equipment, greater than >50 cm²
	97610	Low-frequency, noncontact, nonthermal ultrasound, per day
Orthotics and prosthetics management	97760	Orthotic(s) management and training (including assessment and fitting when not otherwise reported), upper extremity(ies), lower extremity(ies) and/or trunk, initial orthotic(s) encounter, each 15 min
	97761	Prosthetic training, upper and/or lower extremities, initial encounter, each 15 min
	97763	Orthotic(s)/Prosthetics management and/or training, upper extremity(ies), lower extremity(ies), and/or trunk, subsequent orthotic(s)/prosthetic(s) encounter, each 15 min
Patient education in disease management	98960	Education and training for patient self-management by a qualified, nonphysician health care professional using a standardized curriculum
	98961	As above, for 2-4 patients
	98962	As above, for 5-8 patients
Biofeedback	90901	Biofeedback training
	90912	Biofeedback training, peri/uro/rect, initial 15 min
	90913	Biofeedback training, peri/uro/rect, each additional 15 min
Vestibular	95992	Canalith repositioning procedure(s) (e.g., Epley maneuver, Semont maneuver), per day
Patient management: a. Remote b. Patient conferences	98966	Telephone assessment and management service, 5-10 min
	98967	Telephone assessment and management services, 11-12 min
	98968	Telephone assessment and management services, 21-30 min
	G2010	Brief virtual check-in with provider via telephone or other telecommunication device, 5-10 min
	G2012	A remote evaluation of recorded video or images submitted by an established patient, reviewed with patient, 5-10 min
	G2061	Qualified nonphysician health care professional online digital assessment and management service, for established patient, 5-10 min
	G2062	Qualified nonphysician health care professional online digital assessment and management service, for established patient, 11-20 min
	G2063	Qualified nonphysician health care professional online digital assessment and management service, for established patient, 21 or more min
	99366	Medical team conference with interdisciplinary team of health care professionals, patient, and/or family present
	99368	Medical team conference with interdisciplinary team of health care professionals, patient, and/or family not present

Notes: Current Procedural Terminology (CPT) codes are published annually and therefore are frequently modified. Please refer to American Medical Association (AMA) CPT Manual for annual updates to CPT codes. To access information regarding the Official AMA CPT code set, please visit http://www.ama-assn.org/. *ROM,* Range of motion.

the degree to which a therapist may be involved in the actual billing of CPT codes differs for each hospital, facility-based organization, and private practice.

A frequently asked question when considering the reporting of CPT codes is, "Do I need to follow the same rules for CPT coding related to direct contact and the provision of one-on-one services to non-Medicare patients that are required under the Medicare program?"

Providers of physical therapy services who bill non-Medicare payers and report their services using the CPT codes are bound by the definition of the CPT codes as published and copyrighted by the AMA. Although Medicare utilizes CPT codes in its fee schedule and has policies guiding providers in their use, the CPT code nomenclature is also applicable to other payers' use in their payment methodology. A payer could be more specific (i.e., how timed codes will be paid based on its reporting), but the code nomenclature that states a procedure is provided in a direct one-to-one contact manner is attached to that procedure whether billed to Medicare or another private payer.

It is important to keep in mind that coding for a service is separate from payment for a service. A common misperception is that therapists should code their services describing their treatment to Medicare patients one way while coding for services provided to non-Medicare patients in another way.

Putting this misperception into practice can place PTs that do so in a position of risk related to the possible submission of a false claim or adverse effects of a payer audit.

As an example, the description for the CPT code Therapeutic Exercise, 97110, states: Therapeutic procedure, one or more areas, each 15 minutes; therapeutic exercises to develop strength, endurance, range of motion, and flexibility. Although a PT or PTA may read this and interpret that the service descriptor does not include any reference to the need for direct (one-on-one) contact in order to support the reporting of this code, providers need to be aware of how to read, interpret, and apply the CPT codes in order to be compliant with any specific payer policy. The preamble of the Therapeutic Procedures section of the 97000 series includes the following language related to the codes listed in this section of CPT:

A manner of effecting change through the application of clinical skills and/or services that attempt to improve function. Physician or other qualified health care professional (i.e., therapist) required to have direct (one-on-one) patient contact.

This preamble applies to the codes printed beneath it in the CPT manual. CPT code 97110, describing Therapeutic Exercise, therefore includes the requirement for direct (one-on-one) patient contact.

There are currently no CPT codes in the PM&R section to describe supervised exercises in which the PT or PTA is overseeing the service but not providing direct, one-on-one contact with one patient at a time. This inability to code for supervised services has no relationship to the ability to have one or more patients in the facility during any part of the day and clinic's hours of service. Coding should all be done from the perspective of the therapist and the services they are providing to patients—not from the perspective of the patient or those sharing the clinic's services. Specifically, the PT or PTA should be coding for the skilled intervention they are providing to the patient that requires a PT or PTA's knowledge and expertise and not coding and billing for situations in which the patient is performing exercises on their own or with only occasional supervision by the provider. Most important, therapists should be aware that this coding advice is based on the correct interpretation of the CPT codes and applying the codes accurately when describing clinical services. CPT code 97110 has been an example used to help convey this information, but there are other CPT codes that also require direct (one-on-one) contact with the patient, regardless of whether the services are being submitted to Medicare or non-Medicare payers. State law and third-party payers may provide for additional requirements and a specific payment policy related to the reporting of CPT codes, and providers should be certain to follow those requirements, in addition to all applicable CPT rules.

Suggestions for Improving CPT Coding by Physical Therapists

- The reporting of a CPT code must be supported by appropriate documentation of the service provided.
- The reporting of any code should be supported in the objective documentation through a clear relation to the functional activity goals included in the POC, and medical necessity should be evident from the documentation.
- Therapists can report codes for both group therapy and individual therapy provided on a date of service, but documentation must support both the group treatment and the individual (one-on-one) treatment being provided as separately identifiable skilled interventions. Typically, a billing modifier is required when these two services are billed on the same date of service.
- The number of timed units that can be reported and billed for is constrained by the amount of direct contact time provided to the patient and payer policy regarding the reporting of timed codes.

CMS QUALITY PAYMENT PROGRAM

Before the establishment of the Quality Payment Program (QPP), health care provider payment for services in most Medicare programs were based on the volume of services performed. Maximum expenditures for Medicare, and increases in payments, were established by the Sustained Growth Rate (SGR) law. The SGR law was designed to cap total spending in the Medicare program. This would hold the expenditures for Medicare constant from year to year.

As clinicians increased their utilization of services, and more people became eligible for Medicare, the payment for each unit of service had to be adjusted downward to hold costs constant. The SGR law would have resulted in substantial decreases in the Physician Fee Schedule. These potential drastic decreases in provider payments forced Congress to pass new legislation each year. All these elements resulted in significant increases in the overall cost of the Medicare program and were unsustainable in the long term.

The Medicare Access and CHIP Reauthorization Act of 2015 (MACRA) did away with the SGR. CMS developed methodology to reward high-value, high-quality clinicians with payment increases while at the same time reducing payments to those clinicians who do not meet the quality performance standards of the QPP.

For PTs in the Medicare program, the Merit-based Incentive Payment Program (MIPS) involves participation in two categories, Quality Measures and Improvement Activities. Together, successful participation in these two categories determine whether a PT or practice receives an incentive payment or a penalty for the year.

The Quality Measures category evaluates the quality of a PT's or practice's care using performance measures. Therapists select the performance measures most applicable to the care of their patients from a CMS-approved list of quality measures and submit them for analysis at the conclusion of the performance year. In MIPS, therapists earn points toward a total score that determines their incentive or penalty for the performance year. Quality Measure performance accounts for 85% of the total score.

The remaining 15% of the total score is determined by performance in the Improvement Activities category of the MIPS program. This category assesses the ways in which therapists and practices are engaging in quality improvement efforts in their clinical practice. Improvement activities must be performed for 90 days or more during the performance year and are weighted either "medium" or "high" depending on the demands of the activity, for example, by enhancing care coordination, expanding patient access to care, and improving patient–clinician decision-making.

CMS has developed a list of Improvement Activities. Scoring is determined by choosing one of a combination of medium and high Improvement Activities from the Medicare list and reporting on implementing these activities within the therapist's or practice's clinical activities for 90 or more days over the reporting year. Points are assigned based on the consistency of performance. For each participation year, the points total earned from the Quality Measures Reporting and Improvement Activities

determine whether the therapist or practice earns an incentive payment or a penalty for that participation year. For example, in 2020, the required success point total to receive an incentive payment was 45 points. The QPP requirements, point levels, and incentive/penalty adjustments change yearly.

The QPP is part of Medicare's value-based payment initiatives. These initiatives drive value-based payment principles into all of Medicare's many health care programs, including hospitals, long-term care/skilled nursing facilities, home health care, and OP services. These programs went into effect in 2017 and significant changes are introduced into these programs every year. The readers can keep up with these changes by visiting the Medicare Value–Based Programs webpage https://www.cms.gov/Medicare/Quality-Initiatives-Patient-Assessment-Instruments/Value-Based-Programs/Value-Based-Programs.

SUMMARY

- This chapter provides an overview of current policies, regulations, and guidelines related to payment, documentation, coding, billing, and compliance for PTs practicing in or administrating programs in OP facilities and private practices throughout the United States.
- PTs are required to follow policies, regulations, and guidelines developed by third-party payers, including Medicare, to facilitate payment for services provided to the beneficiaries of these payers' programs.

- An important component of participating in the Medicare program and any other third-party payer program as a provider is to ensure that documentation reflects the services provided were medically necessary, skilled, and focused on return of function.
- Although formats and requirements for third-party payers may change regularly, the principles related to functional outcomes documentation provide a consistent framework for all types of documentation.

RECOMMENDED RESOURCES

General Information: Health Care Reform

- Centers for Medicare and Medicaid Services
  http://www.cms.gov
- American Physical Therapy Association
  http://www.apta.org
- Kaiser Family Foundation
  http://www.kff.org
- ICD-10
  http://cms.gov/Medicare/Coding/ICD10/index.html
  http://apps.who.int/classifications/apps/icd/ICD10Training/
  http://www.cdc.gov/nchs/icd/icd10.htm
  Merit-based Incentive Payment Program and Quality Payment Program

- https://qpp.cms.gov/
- https://qpp.cms.gov/mips/overview
- https://www.cms.gov/Medicare/Quality-Initiatives-Patient-Assessment-Instruments/Value-Based-Programs/Value-Based-Programs

Documentation, Coding, Billing, and Compliance

- American Medical Association
  http://www.ama-assn.org/ama/pub/physician-resources/solutions-managing-your-practice/coding-billing-insurance/cpt.page
- Centers for Medicare and Medicaid Services
  https://www.cms.gov/Medicare/Billing/TherapyServices
- American Physical Therapy Association
  http://www.apta.org/DefensibleDocumentation/

6

Electronic Medical Records

John G. Wallace

LEARNING OBJECTIVES

After reading this chapter, the reader will be able to:
1. Understand electronic medical record (EMR) application development and design.
2. Identify what elements of the documentation process the EMR deals with effectively as well as the potential shortfalls of electronic documentation.
3. Describe the importance of including patient-specific data, clinical judgment, and establishing medical necessity for physical therapy treatment.

Computerized health records can be broad-based applications that include all the facilities and providers within a health system. These are usually referred to as electronic health records (EHRs). They can also be specialty-specific such as behavioral health, pediatrics, and physical rehabilitation specialties like physical therapist (PT). In these cases, the electronic documentation applications are referred to as electronic medical records (EMRs). These can be specific to practice settings like acute inpatient rehabilitation facilities, skilled nursing, and outpatient physical therapy.

The Health Information Technology for Economic and Clinical Health Act of 2009 was passed to promote the adoption of EHRs. CMS reports the adoption of EHRs throughout the US health care system is very high with over 95% of hospitals and over 80% of physician and other health care provider practices having adopted EHRs (https://www.healthit.gov/topic/health-it-basics/benefits-ehrs). As part of this act, incentive payments were available for early adopters, and, eventually, penalties for those nonconforming with the adoption standards. This large-scale adoption of electronic documentation has driven significant changes in the ways in which patient health information is managed and in how population health and chronic disease management are analyzed and deployed.

PTs, regardless of the setting in which they work, are key members of the patient care team. The success of the patient episode of care often depends on the communication among multidisciplinary members. Communication between practitioners in the health care environment has often been a challenge. Government regulations, through the use of incentives and penalties, are moving health care institutions and providers toward effective, real-time sharing of patient health care history and treatment. Patients are also able to access their electronic health information. Efficiencies in care can increase dramatically as interoperability between EHRs and consolidation of personalized health records allow for e-prescribing, electronic authorizations, real-time access to laboratory results and test reports, and better care coordination.

The move from paper to electronic documentation began in earnest in the mid-2000s. Interestingly, for PTs, outpatient settings have seen the highest conversions to EMRs. This is largely due to the heavily compliance-driven administrative burden of government and third-party payers. Hospital outpatient departments, step-down units, and acute rehabilitation have lagged in the move to electronic documentation because the hospital EMR systems are physician and nursing oriented and have historically been less developed for the particular needs of physical therapy.

Health care today faces constant pressure to decrease costs, reduce waste, and provide care in a safe environment using the best-known practices of medicine. A paper-based documentation environment includes inherent barriers to improving efficiency, safety, and quality. Making patient information immediately accessible and easily transferable between patient-practitioner encounters is one of the most important initiatives of 21st century health care. Box 6.1 lists many of the advantages of electronic documentation over handwritten documentation.

DEVELOPING AND PRODUCING A PT EMR

EMRs are developed by software engineers working closely with PT documentation experts to define the functionality requirements of the application. In essence, this is the process of incorporating legal/regulatory requirements, payer policy, and the standards of the practice of PT into a list of well-defined elements and workflows that define what is captured in the EMR and how it is displayed in the medical record. It is the transformation of the "community standard" of the practice of physical therapy into a computer application to create the patient's medical record.

Payers, attorneys, and health care stakeholders rely on "community standard" when evaluating medical record completeness. The community standard is established by the policies and regulations of government agencies like CMS and state workers' compensation authorities, professional organizations like the American Physical Therapy Association, and the medical policies of payers like the Medicare Administrative Contractors, Blue Cross Blue Shield, United Healthcare, and so on.

Application development is an iterative process that involves taking complex functional requirements and producing a software that is capable of accurately reflecting the presentation and care of the patient while assuring that the regulatory and community standard of care is maintained. This process involves many people and relies on communication from the PT professional experts to the software engineers. The extent to which this is done successfully determines the quality and usability of a particular application. Add in concepts like clinical guidance and customizability of the user interface, and readers can understand how the number of different applications just in PT can evolve over time.

This iterative process is complicated. It starts with assumptions about the community standard of care being turned into system functionality that has to be transformed into development requirements and finally into programming code. Readers should keep in mind that the application is a set of data collection and manipulation tools. What you enter and see on the screen is not the actual EMR. The real EMR in its final form is the result of the output created by the application, usually in the form of PDF documents. Reading the output before you finalize your entry is a critical element of producing high-quality documentation.

HOW ELECTRONIC DOCUMENTATION IMPROVES PRACTICE

Aggregating and Manipulating Data

EMRs excel at managing information and tracking. There are a number of required elements in the PT medical records. For Medicare, this would include a Plan of Care generated by the PT and certified (signed) by the physician, a Progress Report every 10 visits, a daily treatment note for each patient visit, and a Discharge Progress Report (see Chapter 2 for more on these documents). EMRs can be programmed to track that these required elements have been completed and signed on a timely

basis. EMRs can track authorizations for treatment, remind therapists of updates due to the referring physician, flag expiring physician referrals, and provide alerts about a payer's policy that may affect the patient's coverage of services.

Aggregating data and reporting are other critical features that EMRs provide. These would include reports of diagnoses seen, new patients per month, patient visits per episode, physician referrals, patients seen per therapist per week or per location per week, and Current Procedural Terminology (CPT) codes used. From a patient management perspective, being able to run a report that identifies patients with ongoing Plans of Care but who do not have additional PT visits scheduled allows a practice to provide outreach and positively affect patient outcomes. EMRs will typically have a lengthy list of reports and queries that can be run to improve clinical performance and administrate the practice. As therapists join a practice, getting thorough training in the EMR is critical to being able to take full advantage of these functions.

Standardization of Data Elements

A computerized system creates standard data collection formats for the initial evaluation, session notes, reevaluations, and discharge assessments. Therapists can use a variety of devices to access and document in the EMR. Laptops and handheld devices allow clinicians to document their services during the patient evaluation and treatment encounters when the patient is present. Therapists naturally become faster and more efficient note writers through repetition and practice. In addition, training of new staff is made easier and more consistent throughout the organization. Computerized documentation allows for consistent collection of data within a patient diagnostic type, in which the same information can be captured in the same order for all patients with similar diagnoses. This helps those reading the documentation as they become familiar with the format, allowing them to locate pertinent information quickly and easily. Automation also can eliminate the use of abbreviations and reduce the need for interpretation when the written documentation is unclear and unknown.

Interoperability and Reducing Data Errors

Most hospitals and facilities already have computerized registration, financial services, and/or scheduling systems where basic patient demographic and financial information is entered and stored. Through the use of interfaces and connectivity, patient demographic, and clinical data can be imported into an electronic documentation system by simply selecting the patient's name and verifying an account or medical record number. This interoperability of sharing information between systems through interfaces will significantly reduce the documentation time normally required to reenter information into other systems. It also reduces the human error that is associated with multiple data reentry.

Just as information can be received *into* an electronic documentation system, it also can be forwarded *out* to another system. This is the case with the interface into a billing or outcomes data collection system. Such an interface allows billing/charging elements to be forwarded or interfaced into the financial system, again reducing potential billing errors and discrepancies by eliminating an extra step in the documentation and billing workflow processes. Payment policy regulations require a perfect match between CPT codes billed and treatment rendered. Inconsistencies in documentation and billing could result in payment denials. The practice of assuring a match between documentation with billing helps to alleviate those issues, thereby reducing potential denials.

Interoperability and the ability to share discreet information allow e-prescribing and electronic authorization to be sent from a referring physician or health center directly to the PT practice. It allows automated appointment requests and response to facilitate patient management. EMRs in different systems can share large varieties of information directly through Health Information Exchange companies allowing for requests and exchange of important patient medical records like progress reports to physicians, operative reports, and test results.

Accessing Outcome Measures and Other Clinical Tools

With electronic documentation, data collection from outcomes, tests, and other measures can be captured during routine patient encounters and flow simultaneously into systems designed to score and track this information. Without electronic documentation, outcome measures such as the Lower Extremity Functional Scale and the Minimum Data Set (MDS)-Patient Driven Payment Model items need to be documented or entered twice: within the physical therapy EMR evaluation and the outcomes application. Automated documentation systems allow for the information to be embedded into a documentation template and transferred to a freestanding electronic documentation such as an MDS or Inpatient Rehabilitation Facility-Patient Assessment Instrument report. This direct routing of clinical information into regulatory reporting systems for outcome analysis is another example of a more efficient system in which redundancies and errors are reduced.

An electronic documentation template incorporates outcome measures within the documentation templates. Standardized outcome measure scores can easily be incorporated into a template. With EMR systems, a patient's functional or activity status can be assessed and can incorporate standardized assessment tools that capture a picture of the patient at different intervals during rehabilitation. Such assessments can be used to determine progress and eventually the outcome of a patient's total rehabilitation encounter.

Case Mix Indexing

At a facility level, case mix indexing and other management-level information can provide information regarding patient acuity, which may translate to reimbursement measures in a prospective payment environment such as a skilled nursing facility, home care, or inpatient rehabilitation setting. The *case mix index* is an economic indicator that describes the average patient's morbidity in a hospital. It is calculated by determining the total cost of all inpatients for a specified period divided by the number of admissions (Kuster et al., 2008).

Clinical Research

Clinical research efforts can be simplified when data are collected and retrieved from an EMR. During this important time of promoting and using evidence-based practice, documentation of clinical research at all levels—whether a case study, descriptive analysis, or randomized controlled trial—is an important role of the physical therapy community. For example, Herbold et al. (2014) conducted a randomized controlled trial analyzing the outcomes of patients who used a continuous passive motion after total knee replacement using electronic documentation, which readily allowed analysis of outcomes data.

POTENTIAL PITFALLS WHEN USING ELECTRONIC DOCUMENTATION

Decision Support

The first two generations of physical therapy-specific EMRs have not been user-friendly in supplying clinical decision support. Historically, they have not provided any support to the PT in their clinical decision-making or they provided a fairly rigid approach based on established clinical guidelines. On the one hand, no decision support gives the therapist full control of the intervention and treatment strategies. On the other hand, a rigid decision support tool may not allow enough leeway for patient comorbidities or other personal factors that need to be taken into account for a successful conclusion to the episode of care. Therapists would be well served to look at the EMR they will be using before accepting a position as well as talk to other therapists with experience in the EMR they will be using.

One of the potential benefits and pitfalls of electronic documentation is decision support around payer regulatory compliance. This aids the therapist in determining whether particular documentation is out of date like a Plan of Care expiring or when a 10th-visit Progress Report is due. It could also include authorization and referral tracking, completion, and return of the physician-certified Plan of Care. At the time this functionality was first built, it likely worked to meet the regulatory requirements. However, over time, these requirements inevitably change. It is incumbent on the EMR vendor to monitor these changes, interpret them correctly, and keep their application up to date. This type of issue underscores the importance of therapists and practices staying current on documentation requirements promulgated by government regulators and payment policy members. As the signatory of the medical record, the therapist, not the EMR vendor, is ultimately responsible for the content of their records and any penalties that could occur for noncompliance.

Similarly, decision support around diagnostic code and CPT code selection and other payer policy guidance can be subject to programming shortcuts and development cost consideration by EMR vendors. Again, as with regulator guidance, the codes and rules can be updated annually, such as International Classification of Diseases, 10th Revision and CPT codes, or, in the case of payer PT policies, can be updated at any time. Both practices and vendors have significant administrative burdens to stay current. Therapists would do well to keep this in mind.

Excessive Use of Templates and Automated Phrase Generation

Born of the pressure to spend less time documenting and to increase treatment productivity, therapists can over-rely on the EMR application to help them write documentation. This is generally done via templates based on documentation type (e.g., evaluation and Plan of Care) or by diagnostic group or body part (e.g., hemiplegia, shoulder, and amputation). The standardization that comes from the following best-evidence guidelines is very good and helps therapists to be consistent. However, when informational elements that should be patient specific are written in nonpatient-specific formats, the documentation generated by the EMR will not be adequate to demonstrate medical necessity. As an example, patient problems should be specific to the patient and their unique collection of impairments, work, and avocational requirements, and not be vague representations that could apply to any patient (e.g., pain, decreased range of motion, and weakness). Figure 6.1 provides an example of a therapist's view of an EMR template for documenting a balance assessment. This template demonstrates how an EMR can be used to prompt the therapist to conduct a comprehensive evaluation, including measures of time, support needed, and movement analysis..

Some EMRs use automated phrase generation to speed up the documentation of patient care. Certainly, automated and context-specific phrase generation can be very helpful when used correctly. Figure 6.2 provides the print view of the balance assessment shown in Fig. 6.1. The EMR system automatically generated a narrative output from the therapist responses. Many EMR systems allow the therapist to generate and store a library of phrases, sentences, and even entire paragraphs or more to make the automated completion tools more effective. As long as these phrases, sentences, and paragraphs are diagnostic or impairment specific and are applied judiciously, they can significantly speed up documentation writing. The danger comes when these stored phrases are too nonspecific and used too often that medical record reviews can have negative outcomes and result in payment denials and even sanctions against the therapist. See Table 6.1 for contrasting examples of phrasing. This combination of nonpatient-specific application aids can create notes that do not adequately support skilled care based on individual patient-specific needs.

Documentation Cloning

Note or documentation cloning usually occurs inadvertently because the therapist is trying to save time. EMR developers use two primary ways to make previous treatment entries available to the PT. First, they use a tab or link to previously completed documentation entries. Second, within a daily session note, the application will reproduce the immediately previous note entry from the same section of the note. For example, in a section titled Patient Subjective Comments, the application will carry over the entry from the last visit. The therapist has the option of leaving the previous note entry word-for-word for the current visit, editing that entry and adding to it, or deleting that entry from the current visit note and adding entirely new patient comments. If the therapist does not delete or edit the previous visit patient comment, that same comment can appear in the documentation visit note after visit note.

Widespread practice of not editing or replacing previously referenced entries can unintentionally make the treatment notes look "cloned"—as if each note was copy and pasted to create the new note. Of course, in the case of fraudulent practice when

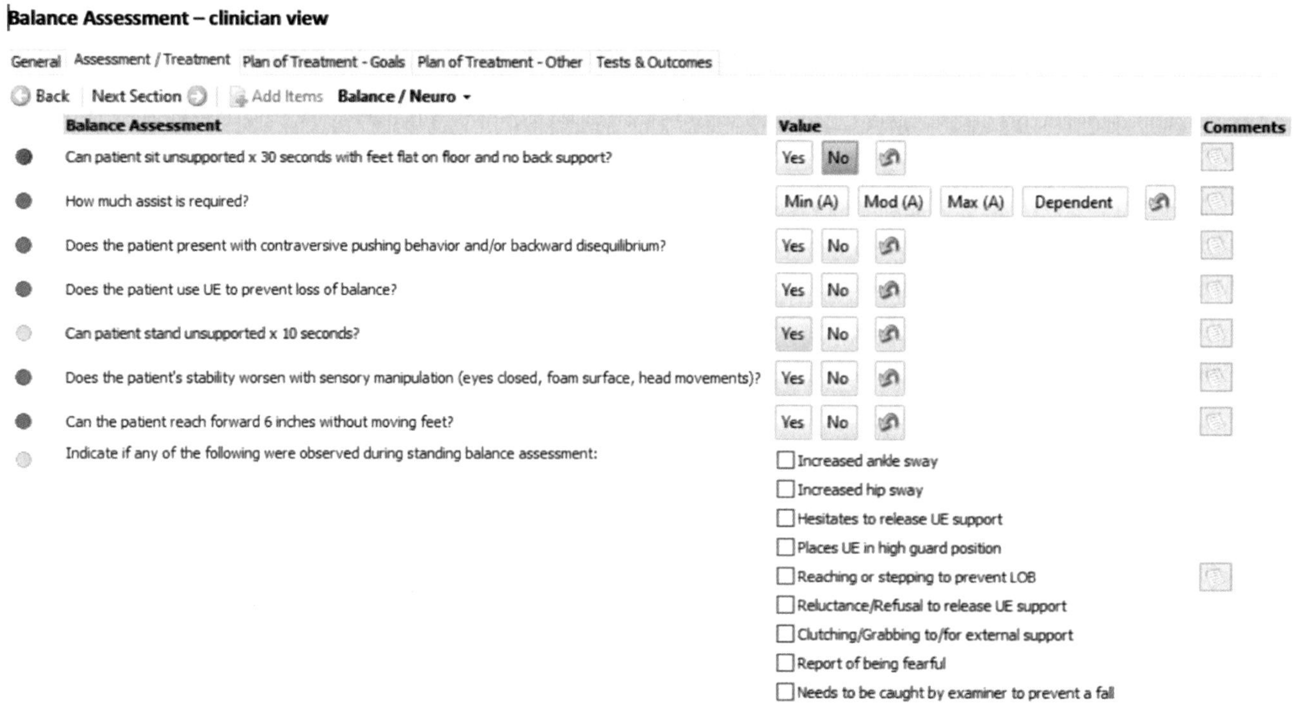

Fig. 6.1 An example of a therapist's view of an EMR template for documenting a balance assessment. The EMR can be used to prompt the therapist to evaluate specific aspects with forced responses/checklists. Courtesy of Patricia Scheets, PT, DPT, Infinity Rehab.

Balance Assessment – Print Result

Sitting Balance	Patient = can sit unsupported for at least 30 seconds indicating at least a base level of steady-state postural control; patient = cannot reach forward with trunk displacement at least 14 inches without loss of balance; patient = uses upper extremities to prevent loss of balance in sitting.
Standing Balance	Patient = can stand without use of UE for at least 10 seconds; patient's stability = worsens with sensory manipulation (i.e. eyes closed, foam, head movements); patient = cannot reach forward at least 6 inches without moving feet; The following additional observations were made during the standing balance assessment = increased ankle sway, hesitates to release UE support, clutching/grabbing to/for external support, needs to be caught by examiner to prevent a fall

Fig. 6.2 EMR output of a balance assessment. Based on data provided by the PT (see Figure 6.1), the EMR generated a narrative response that can be easily interpreted by third—party payers and other healthcare professionals. (Courtesy of Patricia Scheets, PT, DPT, Infinity Rehab.)

TABLE 6.1 Contrasting Examples of Less Ideal (e.g., Stored Phrases) and More Ideal Phrasing Using Computerized Documentation

Daily Note Section: Less Ideal	Daily Note Section: More Ideal
Patient input (S): Patient states they are having less pain posttreatment.	Patient states they are having less pain when carrying and lifting groceries.
Intervention documentation (O): Patient with frozen shoulder should receive manual therapy.	Manual therapy to R glenohumeral (GH) joint consisting of soft tissue mobilization to supraspinatus insertion, post glides R GH joint grade 2 progressed to grade 4, long-axis traction grade 4, manual shoulder elevation with guided GH head movement to pain limit for 4 min.
Assessment/clinical reasoning: Patient is tolerating treatment well with less sharp pain on movement.	Patient is experiencing improvement as evidenced by improved functional levels of I-ADLs of lifting and carrying. This reflects improvement in joint arthrokinematics and right shoulder cuff/scapular stabilizer endurance. Patient will be able to tolerate more challenging exercises.
Treatment planning: Continue to progress with shoulder treatment as the patient tolerates.	With the patient's continued improvement, the plan is to decrease manual therapy on next visit and add overhead resistance training and lifting mechanics training along with adding scapular stabilizer isometrics to home program.

I-ADLs, Instrumental activities of daily living.

treatments are not carried out by licensed physical therapy personnel or not performed at all, note cloning can be purposely used to create medical records for the purpose of billing third-party payers.

WHAT PAYERS AND OTHER STAKEHOLDERS WANT FROM THE MEDICAL RECORD

There are basically four questions the medical record of your patient episode of care should answer:
1. What did you do to the patient? The answer represents the interventions you used to treat the patient clearly traceable to the CPT codes and the number of units that were billed.
2. Why did you choose these particular interventions and progress them the way you did? The answer to this question describes your clinical reasoning and rationale for your treatment of the patient.
3. How did/is your treatment approach helping and how do you know? This question gets to the completion of the goals for your patient. What patient problems did you try to solve, what outcome tests and measures did you choose and what results can you measure?
4. How much longer or how much more do you need to do to achieve your outcomes-based goals? When your patient is still on mid-episode, how accurate and specific can you be when forecasting successful completion of the goals for the episode of care? The therapist's ability to do this relies on the experience achieved over time and the appropriate application of tests and measures to the patient.

SUMMARY

The benefits of an automated documentation system used in a physical therapy setting—either freestanding or as a part of an integrated delivery system—are numerous. Automation allows for legible, consistent, standardized documentation that can be completed at the point of care or when the patient is present. Additional benefits include accessibility of clinical information by all members of the medical team, data retrieval for outcomes management, and clinically defined best practice (clinical decision-making) in an environment that reduces redundancy and error.

Readers should note, however, that without purposeful activity, therapists can write nearly identical notes treatment after treatment for a single patient or multiple patients via overused picklists, phrase libraries, and templates. It is easy for therapists to rely on an EMR to make the case for skilled care by relying on volumes of impairment data and the completion of required document types rather than considering the elements of skilled care that are specific to each patient.

Clinical Decision-Making and the Initial Evaluation Format

LEARNING OBJECTIVES

After reading this chapter and completing the exercises, the reader will be able to:

1. Outline a model for organizing an initial evaluation based on a functional outcomes approach.
2. Identify the basic elements for each section of the initial evaluation format.
3. Describe the relationship between the American Physical Therapy Association's *Guide to Physical Therapist Practice* Management Process and the sections of the initial evaluation format.
4. Categorize components of an initial evaluation for physical therapy documentation.

This chapter presents a format for organizing physical therapy documentation that is based on two important models: the International Classification of Functioning, Disability and Health (ICF) framework and the Physical Therapist Management Process from the American Physical Therapy Association's (APTA) *Guide to Physical Therapist Practice* (the *Guide*) (APTA *Guide to Physical Therapist Practice 4.0*). The format is based on three fundamental assumptions presented in Chapter 1:

1. Documentation both shapes and reflects clinical problem-solving strategies.
2. An enablement model of disablement provides a useful framework for clinical problem solving and thus documentation.
3. Documentation should be organized around functional outcomes.

The format presented here is intended to provide a set of general guidelines for organizing documentation that can be adapted to different practice settings. It is not intended to be a rigidly applied procedure for writing documentation. Physical therapists (PTs) practice in a variety of settings, encounter many different types of patients and clients, and write documentation for many different reasons. No single format could be applicable to all these situations. Nevertheless, the general principles of functional outcomes documentation can be captured in a generic format and adapted to different purposes and contexts.

Two main formats for documentation are presented in this book: (1) a format for writing the initial evaluation of a patient and (2) a format for writing progress and session notes. Other types of documentation, such as discharge summaries, letters to referral sources, and others, can easily be constructed from these

two main types. (Examples of such forms of documentation can be found in Case Examples provided in Chapter 15) The major focus of this book is on the initial evaluation format because it is the most critical to establishing a framework for clinical decision-making. The sections of the initial evaluation format are further detailed in separate chapters (see Chapters 8-13). The format for progress and session notes is a modified form of the SOAP note and is presented in Chapter 14. Practice exercises in categorizing statements into the different sections of the initial evaluation format are provided at the end of this chapter.

THE INITIAL EVALUATION FORMAT AND THE PHYSICAL THERAPIST MANAGEMENT PROCESS

The format for an initial evaluation is based on the enablement model presented in Chapter 1. There are six main sections (Table 7.1). The first three sections include information related to the ICF framework: health condition and participation (Reason for Referral section), activities (Activities section), and body structures and functions (Impairments section). The next three sections present the Assessment, including diagnosis; Goals; and Plan of Care.

One of the important contributions of the *Guide* is the Physical Therapist Management Model. This model describes the process by which a PT determines the critical problems that require intervention and develops an intervention plan to address those problems. The model defines six integrated elements of the process: examination, evaluation, diagnosis,

TABLE 7.1 **Six Sections of the Initial Evaluation Format, incorporating tests and measures recommended by the Guide to Physical Therapist Practice 4.0**	
Section	**Information Included**
Reason for Referral	Current condition
	Patient demographics
	Past medical history
	Medications
	Social history/participation
	Prior level of functioning
Activities	Adaptive and Assistive technology
	Community, Social and Civic Life
	Education Life
	Environmental Factors
	Mobility (e.g. locomotion)
	Self-care and Domestic Life
	Work and Community Integration
Impairments	Systems review
	Can include any of following as appropriate:
	Aerobic capacity/endurance
	Anthropometric characteristics
	Balance
	Circulation (Arterial, Venous, Lymphatic)
	Cognitive and Mental Function
	Cranial and peripheral nerve integrity
	Gait
	Integumentary integrity
	Joint integrity and mobility
	Motor function
	Muscle performance (including strength, power, endurance, and length)
	Neuromotor development and sensory processing
	Pain
	Posture
	Range of motion
	Reflex integrity
	Sensory integrity
	Skeletal integrity
	Ventilation and respiration
Assessment	Summary of evaluation including prognosis and diagnosis
Goals	Goals (focusing on activities or participation) with time frames
Plan of Care	Education interventions
	Procedural interventions

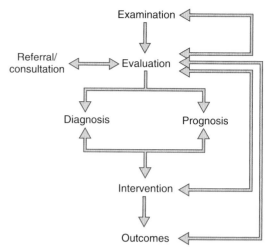

Fig. 7.1 The Physical Therapist Management Model. (From *APTA Guide to Physical Therapist Practice 4.0. American Physical Therapy Association, 2023.*)

for data collection is the Reason for Referral section, which establishes both the primary reasons for referral and the patient's participation restrictions. This then leads to specific examination procedures to determine which activities are related to the participation restriction and which impairments are leading to activity limitations. Thus the functional outcomes format applies a logical sequence to the reporting of the data that were collected.

A critical step in clinical reasoning is establishing both a diagnosis and an expected prognosis. The diagnosis establishes the causes of specific problems that the PT or physical therapist assistant (PTA) will address in the intervention strategy. Usually, the diagnosis will include a statement about the nature, location, and etiology of the health condition that is causing the problem. In addition, the diagnosis will delineate the causal links between impairments and activity limitations. Diagnosis is considered in more detail in Chapter 11. Establishing a prognosis is important to determine the expected outcomes, based on the history, examination, and other factors. Goals are then written to document these expected outcomes.

In the last section of the initial evaluation, the PT plans a strategy for intervention. As noted in the *Guide*, this typically involves educational interventions and procedural interventions. Again, each is given a separate subsection in the initial evaluation format to encourage explicit documentation of these categories.

DESCRIPTION OF COMPONENTS OF THE INITIAL EVALUATION

The following sections explain the main purposes of each of the main components of the initial evaluation format. Each component is further detailed in Chapters 8-13, and Case Examples of complete initial evaluations can be found at the end of this chapter.

Ideally, the format of the initial evaluation should guide the PT's clinical decision-making. Table 7.3 summarizes the evaluation process, emphasizing clinical decision-making. This process uses an *enablement model*. After obtaining patient history and pertinent medical information, therapists ask patients about their *participation restrictions* and then ascertain which

prognosis, intervention, and outcomes. The process of PT patient/client management is illustrated in Fig. 7.1 and each of the elements is defined in Table 7.2.

The initial evaluation format fits very closely with the patient/client management model (Table 7.2). As is emphasized in Fig. 7.1, evaluation is a dynamic process—not something that is initiated only after all data have been collected. Therefore, there is an interplay between examination and evaluation. Data are collected and evaluated, and then decisions are made about what additional data to collect. This process may involve hypothesis testing. In the functional outcomes approach the starting point

---

TABLE 7.2   Relationship of the Guide's Physical Therapist Management Process to the Documentation Format

Physical Therapist Management Process	Components of the Initial Evaluation	Process
Examination/evaluation	Reason for Referral	Explain medical and health conditions that are pertinent to patient's current problems, and determine current level of participation in work and personal roles.
	Activities	Measure patient performance on the activities that the individual needs to perform to overcome or prevent participation restrictions.
	Impairments	Identify and measure the impairments that contribute to the observed functional activities.
Diagnosis	Assessment	Establish a diagnosis and justify necessity of physical therapy intervention.
Prognosis	Goals	Develop a set of goals in consultation with the patient.
Intervention	Plan of Care	Plan an intervention strategy that will facilitate achievement of goals.

TABLE 7.3   Process Used to Evaluate a Patient and Develop a Plan for Intervention

Main Sections of Initial Evaluation	Questions the Physical Therapist Asks
Reason for Referral	What is the primary health condition? What other medical conditions may affect the primary health condition? What was the individual's prior level of functioning? What is the individual's current life situation—home environment, work, social support? How is the current condition affecting the individual's life and life roles?
Activities	What specific activities (or functional skills) does the individual need to learn (or relearn) to be able to accomplish patient's life roles? How does inadequate performance in specific activities prevent the individual from fulfilling life roles?
Impairments	How are/why are the individual's movements dysfunctional? What neuromuscular, sensorimotor, or cardiovascular mechanisms are inadequate (e.g., range of motion, strength, sensation, pulmonary function)?
Assessment	What is the patient's diagnosis, or can the current diagnosis be modified? What is the justification for physical therapy intervention? What are the causal links between activity limitations and participation restrictions? Between impairments and activity limitations? Between health condition and impairments?
Goals	What goals have the therapist and patient agreed on? What level of participation does the patient need/want to achieve? What activities will be used to benchmark the patient's progress toward accomplishing the overall goals? Are there any impairment goals that are critical to be achieved and would have a significant impact on function?
Plan of Care	What musculoskeletal, neuromotor, and physiological resources must be enhanced to enable the individual to relearn the specified functional skills? What sequence of tasks will optimally challenge the patient? What should be done to promote tissue healing or prevent damage? What other health care professionals or family members need to be involved to optimize patient care? What patient-related instructions are needed to educate the patient and/or family members? How long and how often is therapy required for optimal response?

---

activities are limited and whether *impairments* exist in body structures and functions that contribute to these activity limitations and participation restrictions. This leads to a process of developing an *assessment*, which includes a diagnosis and prognosis; setting of *goals*; and developing a *plan of care*.

Reason for Referral

The Reason for Referral section typically entails a short narrative summary of the reason for evaluating a particular patient in physical therapy (see Chapter 8). This includes defining any previously established diagnoses and pertinent medical history, as well as the patient's social history and current level of participation. This information is linked together in this one section as it provides the rationale for why the patient was referred for evaluation. The following subcategories are therefore included in the Reason for Referral.

- *Current condition*: Current condition includes information such as patient demographic information (e.g., name, age, and gender) and background information pertaining to the patient's medical diagnosis.

- *Past medical history*: Information documented in past medical history (PMH) should include any medical history that may be relevant (even indirectly) to the current condition. This typically includes any prior surgeries, other diagnoses, or preexisting conditions.
- *Medications*: Therapists should document medications the patient is taking for the current condition, as well as any medications taken for other medical conditions.
- *Social history/participation*: Social history includes information about a person's living environment and situation (e.g., where the person lives and with whom) and current work or employment situation. This section typically incorporates participation-based information: The PT describes a patient's desired or required personal, social, or occupational roles and reports any restrictions in the patient's ability to fulfill those roles.
- *Prior level of function*: This refers to the degree of functional skill of a patient in self-care, leisure, and social activities before the onset of the current medical diagnosis or health condition. This section also incorporates participation information, for example, current and prior work status. It provides a minimal benchmark for the level of functioning that the patient might expect to achieve.

Activities

Information in the Activities section is intended to identify the critical activity limitations that contribute to participation restrictions (see Chapter 9). Which functional skills are needed to fulfill the individual's goals and required roles? In which of these does the individual demonstrate deficits in performance? Limitations in performance should be reported concretely and completely and should be quantified to the degree possible. This can be done by use of objective measurements (e.g., walking speed or distance walked) or by use of standardized tests that measure activity level.

Impairments

This section of the initial evaluation identifies those impairments, such as range of motion limitations or strength deficits, that have a causal relationship to the observed activity limitations or that might cause activity limitations in the future if not addressed (see Chapter 10). This information should be documented using objective measures, such as degrees of range of motion or manual muscle testing grade, whenever possible.

Assessment

The Assessment section typically begins with an overall impression: a brief statement summarizing the patient's reason for being referred for physical therapy. The PT then outlines a diagnosis that includes three components: differential diagnosis, classification based on etiology or movement system (if pertinent), and the relationships among impairments, activity limitations, and participation restrictions (see Chapter 11). APTA *Guidelines for Physical Therapy Documentation* state that a physical therapy diagnosis is required for all initial evaluations. The assessment concludes with a statement summarizing

the PT's recommendations and the necessity of physical therapy intervention.

Goals

The Goals section identifies the expected outcomes of physical therapy intervention, the ends toward which physical therapy intervention is directed (see Chapter 12). Specific goals are written that are related to these outcomes. All goals must be measurable and must include a time frame. The goals can have several levels:

- *Participation goals*: Typically, one or two participation goals are useful to highlight the overall level of participation in work, social, recreational, and home activities that a patient is expected to achieve.
- *Activity goals*: Activity goals state the predicted functional performance at the end of therapy. These goals must be related to a specific activity, skill, or task that can serve as a benchmark for an individual's progress.
- *Impairment goals*: Impairment goals document expected improvements or changes in impairments that will result at the end of therapy. Impairment goals should be written sparingly, because the focus of goals should be on the functions or activities that the patient will achieve. When impairment goals are included in documentation, they should be written with a clear relationship to the stated activity goals.

Plan of Care

The Plan of Care outlines the specific interventions that will be utilized to achieve the goals listed in the previous section and presents a concise rationale for the intervention strategy chosen (see Chapter 13). It is useful to begin with the proposed frequency and duration of treatments, as well as a tentative date for reevaluation. Many institutions and third-party payers mandate this approach. The intervention plan should then be documented in the following two categories:

- *Educational interventions*: The PT should document specific instruction or teaching of the patient, caregivers/family members, or other health care professionals.
- *Procedural interventions:* These are the interventions that will be performed by the PT or PTA (e.g., therapeutic exercise, functional training, manual therapy techniques).

CASE EXAMPLES

Five examples are included here to illustrate how the initial evaluation format might be used in actual practice. Readers, especially beginning students, should not see this format as a rigid blueprint to be copied exactly in other situations. Rather, this format should be perceived as a starting point, a set of guidelines to be used for designing effective physical therapy documentation.

Case Examples 7.1 to 7.5 show the variability in how the same format can be applied in different settings and for different patient populations. Some evaluations are shorter; some longer. Each includes different evaluative information (particularly in the Activities and Impairments sections) as is pertinent for the specific case.

CONCLUSION

This chapter has outlined the initial evaluation format for physical therapy documentation. This format is designed so that documentation reflects the evaluative, diagnostic, and planning processes that PTs use in contemporary clinical practice. Indeed, as evident in the *Guide to Physical Therapist Practice*, practice has moved from a format based on medical models to a more patient-centered, top-down approach. The format outlined in this chapter attempts to capture both of these aspects of physical therapy practice.

▌ SUMMARY

- The format for writing functional outcomes reports is based on (1) clinical problem-solving strategies, (2) an enablement model, and (3) organization around functional outcomes.
- The format provides a set of general guidelines that can be adapted to different practice settings.
- The format has six main sections: Reason for Referral, Activities, Impairments, Assessment, Goals, and Plan of Care (see Table 7.1).

- The critical step in the evaluation process and clinical reasoning is establishing an assessment and diagnosis. The diagnosis states the causal links among impairments, activities, and participation and justifies the need for intervention. The diagnosis therefore establishes the specific problems that the PT or PTA will address in the Plan of Care.

CASE EXAMPLE 7.1 Physical Therapy Initial Evaluation   Setting: Outpatient

Name: Smith, Herbert   **D.O.B.:** 6/4/63   **Gender**: Male   **Date of Eval.:** 07/29/22

REASON FOR REFERRAL
Current Condition
Mr. Smith is a 59 y.o. male s/p L TKA on 7/21/22. Pt. reports an insidious onset with gradually increasing pain in B knees over the last 2-3 yr, c̄ L knee becoming severe within the last 6 mo.

PMH
OA B knees diagnosed 3 yr ago via x-rays; controlled HTN.

Medications
Lopressor—100 mg 2×/day by mouth for high blood pressure, Coumadin—2 mg 1×/day by mouth (blood thinner postsurgery), Percocet—2.5 mg/325 mg 1-2 tablets q6h by mouth as needed for pain.

Social History
Pt. lives c̄ wife in two-storey home with 5 steps to enter and 12 steps between floors. Pt. is employed as a surgeon.

Prior Level of Function
Before surgery pt. was unable to stand s̄ UE support for >30 min and reported walking "very slowly" with "sharp" L knee pain when putting weight on L leg. Pt. required A from wife when walking long distances. Prior to this surgery, pt. worked FT, up to 12 hr/day, and was required to stand for up to 2 hr at a time. Pt. has not returned to work 2° to standing and walking limitations postsurgery. Pt. reports that for many years they enjoyed playing golf 2×/wk but had been unable to do so for the last 4 mo before surgery 2° to pain and walking limitations. At present, pt. is unable to perform household tasks such as cleaning and assisting with house maintenance. Pt.'s wife assists c̄ ADLs as needed. No reported falls or history of falls in the past year.

ACTIVITIES
Standardized Tests
Optimal Instrument Baseline Scores: Difficulty 57/105 demonstrates 43% impairment in function; self-confidence 62/105 demonstrates 49% impairment. *Lower Extremity Functional Scale (LEFS):* Preop = 39/80 demonstrating 51% impairment, current = 28/80 demonstrating 65% impairment.

Ambulation
Pt. is allowed WBAT and walks c̄ RW and 3-point gait pattern c̄ S for indoor distances; can amb. 50 ft in 60 sec before needing to sit 2° to pain. Pt. demonstrates ↓ L stance time and antalgic gait pattern. Has not attempted outdoor ambulation.

Stair-Climbing
↑↓ 12 steps of 8-in height using arm railing and 1 str cane c̄ step-to-step pattern c̄ S within 2 min; unable to negotiate stairs using a reciprocal pattern.

Self-Care
Pt. reports they are I in dressing x̄ requires min A to don/doff L sock and shoe. Pt. reports they shower in a stall shower holding onto grab bar; needs min A of wife (to reach LEs and occasionally to maintain balance).

Standing Tasks
Able to stand for 10 min at countertop while reaching c̄ either hand, using other hand for support, limited 2° to pain (6/10). Able to reach for objects above shoulder height c̄ UE support. Unable to reach for objects below knee height to either side.

IMPAIRMENTS
Systems Review
Resting vitals: HR 76 beats per minute; BP 128/84 mm Hg; RR 16. Vitals postambulation (50 ft): HR 84 beats per minute; BP 132/84 mm Hg; RR 22. Normal peripheral pulses and capillary refill in distal L LE. No evidence of cognitive or neurological impairments; able to communicate effectively.

AROM	Left	Right
Knee ext	−18°	−10°
Knee flex	18°-68°	10°-100°
Ankle DF	−5°	0°-5°

MMT	Left	Right
Knee ext	3+/5	4/5
Knee flex	3+/5	4/5

(Continued)

CASE EXAMPLE 7.1   Physical Therapy Initial Evaluation   Setting: Outpatient—cont'd

Name: Smith, Herbert   **D.O.B.:** 6/4/63   **Gender**: Male   **Date of Eval.:** 07/29/22

Anthropometric Characteristics

Height 5′8″, weight 220 lb; BMI: 33.4 kg/m²; circumferential measurements: mid-patella L > R by 1.5 cm, mid-malleoli L > R by 0.75 cm.

Pain

Pt. has experienced pain around entire L knee joint since surgery 8 days ago; gradually improving. Pain at rest is described as "aching" (3/10 on pain scale), c̄ occasional "sharp" pain c̄ WB (6/10), and at end ROM (8/10). Pain in R knee 2/10 described as "constant, dull pain."

Integumentary

Observation reveals L knee is edematous c̄ significant erythema; surgical site is clean, dry, and intact c̄ Steri-Strips in place. No observable exudate present nor signs of infection.

ASSESSMENT

Pt. is a 59 y.o. moderately obese male, s/p L TKA who presents c̄ limitations in L knee ROM, weakness, and postsurgical edema. This has resulted in an inability to ambulate and climb stairs independently c̄ reduced speed and limited distance, as well as limited independence in dressing and bathing. Edema, pain, and ↓ L knee strength have also resulted in reduced ability to bear weight on L side, which is evident by pt.'s impaired gait pattern and standing tolerance. Pain and ↓ R knee strength 2° to OA may additionally limit pt.'s functional recovery. Based on pt.'s preop LEFS and relatively young age, pt. is expected to achieve >60 points on LEFS and at least 600 m on 6-min walk test within 6 mo postop.[1] Pt. requires outpatient PT to address the above impairments and activity limitations to facilitate functional independence and return to work and previous recreational activities.

GOALS

Participation Goals

1. Pt. will return to work at the same capacity as 6 mo ago, within 3 mo.
2. Pt. will be able to participate in household chores and moderate-intensity home maintenance within 3 mo.

Long-Term Goals

1. Pt. will be able to ambulate independently without an assistive device on all surfaces safely at a pace of 1.2 m/sec or better within 8 wk.
2. Pt. will report the ability to stand unsupported for greater than 60 min, pain 1/10 or less within 8 wk to facilitate return to work.
3. Pt. will independently ascend/descend 4 flights of stairs (48 stairs; 8″ height) step-over-step without the use of railings within 8 wk to facilitate safety and independence in home.

4. Pt. will be independent in all ADLs, including showering and assisting in household tasks within 8 wk.

Short-Term Goals

1. Pt. will be able to don/doff shoes and socks independently 3/3 days within 1 wk.
2. Pt. will be able to ambulate 500 ft inside clinic corridors, gait speed at least 1.0 m/sec s̄ an assistive device independently within 2 wk.
3. Pt. will stand s̄ UE support for up to 30 min, pain <2/10 within 4 wk.
4. Pt. will ambulate outside on varied terrain using str cane within 4 wk.

PLAN OF CARE

Pt. will be seen 2-3×/wk for 12 wk. Pt. will be reevaluated in 4 wk.
  Order will be placed through medical supplier for a straight cane.

Educational Interventions

Pt. instructed in pain/edema management activities c̄ elevation and ice, ther ex emphasizing quadriceps and hamstring flexibility, strength and function in both open and closed kinetic chains (supine, seated, and standing). Patient also instructed in safety precautions on stairs and uneven surfaces. Patient verbalized understanding of all instructions. Will continue to progress pt. c̄ HEP, and instruct pt. in importance of proper diet and long-term exercise.

Procedural Interventions

1. Therapeutic exercise for quadriceps/hamstring/calf stretching and A/PROM activities in supine, sitting, and standing to B knees.
2. Gait training indoors and outdoors on a variety of surfaces and inclines to improve safety, endurance, speed, and ↓ need for A device.
3. Stair-climbing training to improve safety, endurance, and independence.
4. Therapeutic activities and functional training in variety of activities incorporating UEs in standing (including kitchen tasks, self-care activities, and golf swings) to improve standing tolerance, knee strength, and stability.
5. Cryotherapy as needed to reduce edema and pain for improved activity tolerance.
  The findings of this evaluation were discussed c̄ the patient, and they consented to the above intervention plan.

_____   _____

Jen L., Therapist   Date: 7/29/2022

[1]Kennedy DM, Stratford PW, Riddle DL, et al. Assessing recovery and establishing prognosis following total knee arthroplasty. *Phys Ther.* 2008;88:22.

CASE EXAMPLE 7.2   Physical Therapy Initial Evaluation   Setting: Inpatient Rehabilitation

Name: Rizzo, Rachel   **D.O.B.:** 2/7/76   **Gender**: Male   **Date of Eval.:** 07/10/22

REASON FOR REFERRAL
Current Condition
Pt. is a 46 y.o. male, assigned sex at birth-female, admitted to County Rehabilitation Center on 7/9/22 $\bar{c}$ dx of exacerbation of RRMS (initial diagnosis 2002). Pt. admitted to County Hospital 7/4/22 for IV steroid treatment. Referral by primary MD requests gait training 2° to recent exacerbation leading to difficulty walking.

PMH
R ACL repair 15 yr ago.

Medications
Avonex, Copaxone, methylprednisolone, Lioresal (10-mg tablets b.i.d. for spasticity), Amantadine (for fatigue), Prozac (for depression).

Social History/Participation
Pt. lives $\bar{c}$ 21 y.o. son in ground floor apartment $\bar{c}$ no steps to enter; responsible for light housekeeping and some cooking. His son assisted $\bar{c}$ some housekeeping and daily chores; son states he is available to assist $\bar{c}$ other tasks as needed when his dad returns home. Pt. has not been employed for past year 2° to disability. Pt. reports fatigue is 1° limiting factor.

Prior Level of Function
Prior to admission, pt. I with ADLs and ambulated community distances with SC. Volunteers 1 day/wk for 4 hr at local library sorting books and assisting $\bar{c}$ computer searches.

Kurtzke Expanded Disability Status Scale[1]
6.5

ACTIVITIES
Bed Mobility
Pt. positions self in bed and rolls B independently using bilateral side rails. Supine ↔ sitting on bed $\bar{c}$ min A for single LE management.

Transfers
Pt. transfers from sit ↔ stand @ bed $\bar{c}$ min A. Uses B arms to assist $\bar{c}$ push off but needs min A to stand. W/C ↔ bed $\bar{c}$ min A $\bar{c}$ RW; CG $\bar{c}$ use of sliding board.

ADLs
Bathing requires mod A from nurse's aide for tub transfers and for hard to reach places; remains seated 2° to fatigue and balance deficits. Dressing $\bar{c}$ mod A.

Sitting Ability
Sitting balance on edge of bed with supervision for 5 min $\bar{s}$ UE support (time limitation due to fatigue). ***Tolerance:*** Can sit I in W/C for >30 min.

Standing Ability
Pt. can stand for up to 3 min at bathroom sink and perform simple one-handed self-care activities using R UE for support with $\bar{c}$ⓢ. Can stand 3 min $\bar{c}$ S using RW.

Mobility
Pt. ambulates 75 ft $\bar{c}$ rolling walker and min A on a smooth floor hospital corridor in 2.25 min. Min A provided to facilitate weight shift M/L, allowing improved limb clearance and advancement. HR increased to 130 beats per minute. Pt. can propel W/C for distances in hospital corridor up to 100 ft limited by fatigue.

Section: GG Mobility

	Independent —06	Setup/ Cleanup Assist —05	Supervision/ Touch Assist—04	Partial/ Mod Assist—03	Substantial /Max Assist—02	Dependent —01	Refused —07	NA—Not Performed Prior—09	NA—Envir. Limits—10	NA— Medical/ Safety—88
Roll left and right	X									
Lying to sitting on side of bed			X							
Sit to lying			X							
Sit to stand			X							
Chair, bed to chair transfer			X							
Car transfer										
Picking up object										
Walk 10 ft			X							
Walk 50 ft with 2 turns			X							
Walk 150 ft										
Walking 10 ft on uneven surfaces										
1 Step (curb)										
4 Steps										
12 Steps										

(Continued)

CASE EXAMPLE 7.2   Physical Therapy Initial Evaluation   Setting: Inpatient Rehabilitation—cont'd

Name: Rizzo, Rachel   **D.O.B.:** 2/7/76   **Gender**: Male   **Date of Eval.:** 07/10/22

IMPAIRMENTS

Systems Review
HR 72 beats per minute; BP 130/84 mm Hg, RR 20 at rest. Pt. reports STM loss, mild deficit noted during interview and evaluation. Pt. able to communicate effectively via appropriate verbal expression. Increased reports of fatigue impacting activity tolerance with all functional mobility.

Aerobic Capacity/Endurance
Fatigue measured on Modified Fatigue Impact Scale: 52/84. Fatigue has worsened since recent exacerbation.

Reflex Integrity
Modified Ashworth Scale (muscle tone) 2/4 B hip adductors and ankle plantar flexors.

Sensory Integrity
Impaired sensation to light touch (5/8 correct responses) and pin prick (4/8 correct responses) below knees B.

MMT	Left	Right
Hip flexion	2/5	3/5
Hip extension	2/5	3/5
Hip abduction	2/5	3/5
Hip adduction	3/5	3/5
Knee extension	3/5	3/5
Knee flexion	3/5	3/5
Ankle dorsiflexion	2/5	3/5
Ankle plantar flexion	2/5	3/5

PROM
B LE PROM WNL except the following:
Hip abd: L 0°-25°; R 0°-30°
Ankle DF L 0°; R 0°-5°

Gait
Has difficulty advancing L leg during swing $\bar{c}$ ↓ hip and knee flexion and foot drop noted; pt. requires min A to advance L LE 25% of the time. Trendelenburg gait to compensate for L abd weakness during L stance.

Balance
Berg Balance Score: 7/56

Sitting
Able to reach 5 in. beyond arm's length in forward and bilateral directions. Able to maintain balance to mod external perturbations $\bar{c}$ recovery in all directions (5/5 trials).

Standing
Able to reach 3 in. outside arm's length to front and both sides. Pt. able to maintain bal $\bar{c}$ mod ant. and post. perturbations 3/5 trials; stepping strategy used 2/3 trials to post. perturbation. Able to stand 10 sec $\bar{s}$ walker with shoulder-width BOS; reports fear of falling.

Integumentary Integrity
Edema B ankles, L < R (28 cm circumference L malleoli, 26 cm R).

Pain
Pt. reports no pain at time of eval.

ASSESSMENT
Pt. is a 46 y.o. male who presents $\bar{c}$ symptoms of an acute exacerbation of multiple sclerosis. Pt. presents $\bar{c}$ LE weakness (L>R), impaired balance, fatigue, and limited PROM B hip abd and ankle DF, which have led to limitations in performing bed mobility, self-care, and amb. Limited activity tolerance and LE weakness have led to limitations in pt. using ambulation as his primary means of mobility. Pt. is at increased risk for falls 2° to decreased symmetry and rhythmicity of gait. Pt. requires inpatient rehabilitation to address this recent decline in functional abilities and to assist patient in returning to prior functional level.

GOALS
Long-Term Goals
1. Pt. will carry out self-care activities and mobility within the home $\bar{c}$ supervision of an HHA aide. (1 mo).
2. Pt. will stand for 10 min at bathroom sink I while performing self-care tasks (2 wk).
3. Pt. will walk 200 ft within 2 min, in hospital hallway $\bar{c}$ supervision using a rollator, $\bar{c}$ HR <110 beats per minute (2 wk).

Short-Term Goals
1. Pt. will rise from supine → sitting on edge of flat bed I 5/5 trials within 20 sec (1 wk).
2. Pt. will maintain sitting on edge of bed without BUE support, for 10 min I (1 wk).
3. Pt. will transfer sitting on bed → standing ($\bar{c}$ walker) I, 5/5 trials (1 wk).

PLAN OF CARE
Pt. will be seen b.i.d. 7 days/wk for 4 wk during IP rehab stay. Full reeval. in 2 wk. PT should continue on daily basis s/p DC.

Training in bathing and other self-care activities will be coordinated $\bar{c}$ OT. Will request compression stockings from MD and training in proper use via Nursing. Consider referral to orthotic clinic within 1-2 wk for possible L AFO. D/C planning to coordinate OPPT upon discharge.

Educational Interventions
Pt. and nursing aides will be instructed in optimal strategies for performing functional activities, esp. transfers. Pt. and family will be instructed in p.m. and weekend exercises to increase PROM hip abd and ankle DF, and for guarding during transfers and amb. Fatigue management and energy conservation techniques discussed $\bar{c}$ pt. and will continue to be incorporated t/o PT sessions.

Procedural Interventions
ROM and strengthening exercises are needed to optimize walking and transfer abilities. Ther ex to ↑ PROM hip abd and ankle DF. AROM and strengthening exercises in supine and standing for B LE musculature, focusing on hip flex and abd, knee flex/ext, and ankle PF/DF. Training in bed mobility, transfers, and sitting (to increase endurance). Standing bal training to address standing bal limitations and improve activity tolerance. Gait training in different environments to improve speed, safety stability, and endurance, and decrease need for assist. Progress pt. with AD to use of a 4-wheeled rollator, to consider for home use.

The findings of this evaluation were discussed $\bar{c}$ the patient, and she consented to the above intervention plan.

_____   _____
Jen L., Therapist   Date: 7/10/22

---

[2]KURTZKE EDSS is a standardized measure that evaluates disability status in people with multiple sclerosis. It provides a total score from 0 to 10, with lower scores referring to higher functioning.

CASE EXAMPLE 7.3 Physical Therapy Initial Evaluation Setting: Outpatient

Name: Jones, Susan   **D.O.B.:** 6/17/80   **Gender:** Female   **Date of Eval.:** 1/19/23

REASON FOR REFERRAL
Current Condition
Ms. Jones is a 42 y.o. female $\overline{c}$ dx of whiplash associated disorder s/p MVA on 1/3/23. Pt. reports cervical pain radiating into L shoulder since the accident, with increasing intensity during the last week.

PMH
C-section 2005; otherwise insignificant.

Medications
Cyclobenzaprine (5-mg t.i.d. by mouth); ibuprofen (600 mg t.i.d. by mouth).

Social History/Participation
Pt. lives with husband and 10 y.o. daughter in two-storey home. Pt. is limited in performing household tasks such as cleaning and cooking due to L hand dominance and limited endurance with any task >20 min. Pt. is employed as an administrative assistant at a marketing firm with a normal schedule of 30 hr/wk. The pt. is currently limited to working 15 hr/wk due to limited tolerance $\overline{c}$ computer tasks, phone calls, and other administrative duties. Pt. sits with computer positioned to the R and is not equipped with a headset for the phone.

Prior Level of Function
I in all functional tasks without pain; worked 30 hr/wk; enjoyed running and skiing as recreational activities. Patient reports their goal is to be pain free so they can return to normal activities and work to help take care of and support their family.

Neck Disability Index
28/50 = severe impairment.

ACTIVITIES
Ambulation and Stair-Climbing
Unaffected.

Self-Care
Pt. reports increased time necessary to complete dressing, from 5 to 10 min 2° to pain. Pt. with limitations in reaching above shoulder height on L side.

Driving
Pt. reports difficulty driving and limits most car rides to <30 min 2° to pain.

IMPAIRMENTS
Systems Review
HR 60 beats per minute; BP 120/72. Height: 5'6"; weight: 125 pounds; BMI: 20.2—within normal range. Pt. reports being a visual learner. No reported history of falls in the past year.

AROM
Cervical flexion 50°
Cervical extension 30°
L cervical sidebend 15°
R cervical sidebend 25°
B cervical rotation 45°

Muscle Performance
B C1-4 myotomes: 5/5
R C5-T1 myotomes: 5/5
L C5-T1 myotomes: 4/5
B scapular musculature grossly 3+/5 with lower traps 3/5 B

Circulation
Negative vertebral artery test; negative Roos test B, and negative Adson test B.

Pain
Central post. c-spine, C5-6 spinous processes tender upon palpation (4/10 on pain scale) with occasional radiation into L upper trap. Pain at rest rated as 3/10 on pain scale with ↑ to 6/10 $\overline{c}$ attempted L sidebend and L rotation.

Joint Integrity and Mobility
Hypomobility noted with passive accessory intervertebral motion at C2-3 and hypermobility noted at C5-6 and C6-7 segments.

Posture
Forward head and ↑ thoracic kyphosis noted with static and dynamic sitting and standing postures.

Reflex Integrity
Biceps, brachioradialis, and triceps 2+ B.

Sensory Integrity
Dermatomes C1-T1 intact B to light touch.

ASSESSMENT
Pt. is a 42 y.o. female who presents with pain and limitations in cervical ROM, weakness of cervical and scapular musculature, altered static and dynamic postures, and joint hyper- and hypomobility consistent with a whiplash associated disorder following at MVA. This has resulted in reduced capacity to perform computer and phone activities related to work, as well as self-care limitations and decreased ability in performing household tasks. Pt. requires outpatient PT to address these impairments and activity limitations to facilitate functional independence and return to work full capacity.

GOALS
1. Pt. will return to working 30 hr/wk schedule in 6 wk.
2. Pt. will perform household tasks, including cleaning and cooking, $\overline{s}$ pain in 6 wk.
3. Pt. will be I in self-posture correction $\overline{s}$ cues in 6 wk.

PLAN OF CARE
Pt. will be seen 3×/wk for 6 wk. Pt. will be reevaluated in 3 wk.
   Ergonomic assessment will be performed at pt.'s work site.

Educational Interventions
Pt. instructed in postural exercises, pain management with cryotherapy and heat as needed, ther ex for cervical and scapular musculature, and AROM exercises. Pt. also instructed in general ergonomic concepts and given pt. education pamphlet with pictures and online video links of proper postures and techniques. Pt. verbalized understanding of all instructions. Will continue to progress pt. with exercises and HEP as tolerated.

Procedural Interventions
- Postural instruction to increase overall endurance with static and dynamic postures.
- Prone and sitting exercises to target scapular and cervical musculature.
- AROM exercises to increase mobility and increase flexibility to the c-spine.
- Cryotherapy to c-spine to reduce pain and heat as needed to facilitate active movement.

The findings of this evaluation were discussed with the pt., and they consented to the above intervention plan.

_____   _____
Mark O., Therapist   Date: 1/19/23

CASE EXAMPLE 7.4   **Physical Therapy Initial Evaluation**   **Setting: Acute Care**

Name: Robert LaGrange   **D.O.B.:** 5/16/50   **Gender:** Male   **Date of Eval.:** 6/9/22

REASON FOR REFERRAL
Current Condition
Pt. was admitted to ICU following CABG ×4 6/4/22. Pt. had renal failure and contracted pneumonia following surgery and on day 4 was still intubated. PT eval and Rx ordered 6/8/22.

PMH
Angioplasty (March 2017) and type 2 diabetes (×12 yr)

Medications
Cephalosporin infusion with 0.9% sodium chloride 20 mg/mL

Social History/Participation
Pt. works part-time in retail home-building store; lives with wife in a retirement community; elevator in building and no stairs.

Prior Level of Function
Prior to this cardiac event, patient was independent with all ADLs and IADLS without an assistive device. He was driving independently and walked 2 miles/day for exercise.

ACTIVITIES
Required mod assist ×2 to roll to side and come to sit on edge of bed. Required mod assist ×1 to maintain sitting position on edge of bed (BP: 136/94). Posture in sitting noted excessive kyphosis, moderate sidebending to L $\overline{c}$ R shoulder elevated. Pt. was able to sit for 2 min $\overline{c}$ mod A before reporting fatigue.

IMPAIRMENTS
Systems Review
Pt. alert but pale; appeared to be resting comfortably. Communication was established using eye blinks (yes/no responses).

Stats
Pt. on ventilator (CPAP). RR 18 beats per minute, TV 8 mL/kg, PEEP 7.0 cm H_2O, PSV 10 cm.

Vitals
HR 98 beats per minute (supine), BP 126/90 mm Hg (supine).

Auscultation
Crackles noted right middle and lower lobes. Heart sounds normal.

Palpation
Pt. had normal chest motion, but excessive use of accessory musculature was noted. No pain reported on palpation.

Skin Integrity
Sternal incision site and bilateral femoral graft site with staples and healing well; no signs of infection.

ROM
Pt. demonstrated full AROM ×4 extremities against gravity. Limitation PROM noted in R ankle DF −5°, L ankle DF 0°.

Strength
BLE 4/5 throughout all pivots and planes of motion.

ASSESSMENT
Pt. is a 72 y.o. male referred to PT following CABG ×4 with complicating renal failure and pneumonia requiring intubation. Pt. presents with decreased strength and activity tolerance and bilaterally decreased ankle DF, which is resulting in a decline in functional mobility including bed mobility, transfers, and ambulation. Pt. requires skilled PT intervention to address impairments and functional limitations denoted above and return patient to his prior level of functioning to facilitate a safe return home.

GOALS
Participation Goals (3 Months)
1. Pt. will return to work part-time without limitation.
2. Pt. will resume walking 2 miles/day for exercise.

Activity Goals (14 Days)
1. Pt. will sit on edge of bed for 5 min $\overline{s}$ assistance.
2. Pt. will transfer from supine ↔ sitting $\overline{c}$ min A ×1.

Impairment Goals (7 Days)
1. Maintain clear airways daily.

PLAN OF CARE
Patient will be seen 5×/wk for 2 wk and then reassessed. Pt. will be D/C to home with support of wife and family as required. Pt. will receive Home Care referral upon D/C—including RN, PT, OT, and ST services as required.

Coordinate with nursing staff for positioning schedule, out-of-bed schedule, and suctioning. Coordinate with D/C planner for home services.

Educational Interventions
Pt. to be instructed in AROM exercises within 1 wk.

Procedural Interventions
Focus on maintaining clear airways and moving toward extubation. Respiratory Rx b.i.d. to include positioning, percussion, and vibration. Suctioning prn following Rx to assist with airway clearance. Inspiratory resistance training and use of pressure support ventilation to begin weaning from ventilator. AAROM strengthening to minimize atrophy and deconditioning, including quad sets, gluts sets, ankle pumps, and AAROM for hip flexion (heel slides) and shoulder flexion (to 90°). Mobility training to include positioning in side lying and semisupine, bed mobility training, and transfers to sitting. Ambulation training for increased activity tolerance.

The findings of this evaluation were discussed with the pt. and he consented to the above intervention plan.

_____   _____
Michael Schultz, Therapist   Date: 6/9/22

CASE EXAMPLE 7.5   Physical Therapy Initial Evaluation   Setting: Long-Term Care

Name: Evelyn Mayer   **DOB:** 12/2/38 **Gender**: Female   **Date of Admission:** 12/21/20
Medicare: #2222222   **Onset Date:** 8/22/23   **Start of Care:** 9/18/23

REASON FOR REFERRAL
Current Condition

Pt. is an 84 y.o. female who is a long-term resident of Whispering Winds Rehabilitation Center. She is A&O ×2. Pt. was diagnosed with LLE cellulitis on 8/22/23 and was treated with antibiotics. She was nonambulatory for a few weeks due to LLE pain. A functional decline is now noted with her bed mobility transfers and ambulation. Her safety awareness is decreased.

PMH

Scoliosis, T12 fracture with vertebroplasty, L1 compression fracture, increased cholesterol, Parkinson disease (PD), dementia, mitral valve prolapse, and urinary tract infection.

Medications

Tylenol prn, Sinemet, Metoprolol, Colace.

Social History/Participation

Pt. has been a resident in this LTC facility for 2.5 yr. She transitioned to this facility as her family was unable to care for her adequately at home as her PD and dementia worsened. She shares a room with a roommate and her living facilities are all on one floor. Her building has elevator access. Her bedroom and bathroom areas are accessible to a W/C. She has assistance for all necessary ADLs and IADLs. Her meals are prepared for her and she eats in the community dining room.

Prior Level of Functioning

Pt. required min A for all bed mobility, min A for bed ↔ w/c and w/c ↔ toilet transfers. She required min A to come to stand at rollator walker. She was able to ambulate 250′ with rollator walker on level carpeted surfaces with CS/CG.

ACTIVITIES
Bed Mobility

Rolling, scooting, and supine ↔ sitting on EOB require max A ×1. HOB is elevated to 45°, and skilled instruction with occasional tactile cues are provided for hand placement and use of bed rails.

Transfers

Sit to stand from bed, w/c, or toilet to rollator walker, require max A. Skilled instruction provided for proper hand placement, as well as to encourage pt. to keep weight forward while coming to stand to prevent LOB posteriorly. Manual guidance provided to keep COM forward while transitioning to stand.

Self-Care

Pt. requires max A for dressing and bathing.

Sitting Balance

Pt. is able to maintain static sitting balance without back support on a firm surface with use of BUE with CS/CG ×3 min.

Standing Balance

Pt. required min A to maintain static standing balance with BUE support of walker ×90 sec. Requires max A to maintain dynamic standing balance, using 1 UE or BUE for functional task while standing. Tinetti score 10/28, indicating high risk for falls.

Ambulation

Pt. ambulates with rollator walker on level carpeted surfaces ×50′ with mod A required to balance. Skilled instruction provided for pt. to drop her heels, as she tends to be a toe walker due to years of wearing high heels. Pt. is unable to manage stairs.

IMPAIRMENTS
Systems Review

HR 96 beats per minute, BP 118/54 mm Hg, RR 22. O_2 saturation is 97% on room air. Pt. does not use oxygen. Pt. is AO ×2. Pt. speaks with a very quiet voice, making it difficult to understand her speech at times.

Skin Integrity

Intact throughout.

Sensory Integrity

Intact throughout extremities ×4 to light touch and sharp/dull discrimination.

Pain

Currently 0/10 t/o. Pt. reports occasional transient low back pain.

ROM

B hip flexion 0°-120°; B knee flexion 0°-130°; B ankle DF 0°-10°. Otherwise, ROM WNL throughout all pivots.

Muscle Performance

Unable to formally assess strength due to increase in tone and difficulty following instructions. Gross functional strength assessed at 3(-)/5 throughout BUE and BLE. Motor planning intact but akinesia noted at initiation of walking and with turns.

Coordination/Tone

Pt. presents with lead-pipe rigidity throughout BUE and BLE with tightness in trunk noted as well. Coordination impaired with finger-to-nose testing, heel-to-shin, and toe tapping, with slow incomplete responses throughout and past pointing noted.

ASSESSMENT

Pt. is an 84 y.o. female referred to PT s/p a period of inactivity due to LLE cellulitis. During the past 4-6 wk, her ambulation activities and overall mobility were placed on hold, and pt. has demonstrated a significant functional decline with bed mobility, transfers, and ambulation. PT evaluation further reveals rigidity, decreased functional strength, poor upright balance with LOB posteriorly, as well as decreased activity tolerance. This has resulted in a decline in functional abilities for bed mobility, transfers, and ambulation, with increased falls risk. Pt. requires skilled PT intervention to address the functional limitations and impairments listed above to return pt. to her prior level of functioning.

GOALS
Short-Term Goals (2 Weeks)

1. Resident will maintain static sitting without upper extremity or back support for 5 min.
2. Resident will demonstrate sit to stand from w/c to rollator walker with min A ×1.
3. Resident will roll R and L in bed using ½ bed rails with min A and skilled instruction for had placement.
4. Resident will ambulate with rollator walker on level tile and carpeted surfaces ×100′ CG.

Long-Term Goals (4 Weeks)

1. Resident will demonstrate safe bed mobility with min A using bed rails and with HOB elevated to 45°.
2. Resident will transfer sit to stand from bed, w/c, toilet and chair ↔ rollator with min A.

(Continued)

CASE EXAMPLE 7.5   Physical Therapy Initial Evaluation   Setting: Long-Term Care—cont'd

Name: Evelyn Mayer   **DOB:** 12/2/38 **Gender**: Female   **Date of Admission:** 12/21/20
Medicare: #2222222   **Onset Date:** 8/22/23   **Start of Care:** 9/18/23

3. Resident will ambulate with rollator walker for >200′ on level tile and carpeted surfaces $\bar{c}$ CS.
4. Resident will ambulate with rollator walker ×100′ on outdoor paved surfaces $\bar{c}$ CS.

PLAN OF CARE
Patient requires restorative physical therapy for 30 days, 5 days a week for minimum 30 min treatment session to address the following: Patient referred to neurologist for workup and to speech therapy for improved vocalization.

Educational Interventions
Patient received skilled instruction to keep her weight forward during sit to stand transfers. This improvement in forward posture will lessen her propensity to fall backward when attempting to come to stand. Further education for fall prevention will include techniques for transfer training in other enviornments.

Interventions
- Gait training to decrease level of assistance and improve activity tolerance.
- Task-specific training including bed mobility and sit to stand training.
- Balance training in sitting and standing to reduce fall risk.
- Therapeutic exercise to increase overall muscle strength and improve coordination.
- Moist heat recommended for transient lumbar pain and facilitate participation in therapeutic activities.

Pt. consented to physical therapy treatment.

_____

Sheryl H., Therapist

CASE EXAMPLE 7.6   Physical Therapy Initial Evaluation   Setting: Inpatient Acute Care

Name: Carl Perez   **D.O.B.:** 07/17/1972   **Gender:** Male   **Date of Eval.:** 1/4/21

REASON FOR REFERRAL
Current Condition
Patient tested COVID + around 12/25/21, presented to emergency department with SOB, found to be saturating in 50 sec on room air, placed on non-rebreather mask and O_2 saturations (SpO_2) improved to 98%. PT eval and treat ordered 1/4/21.

PMH
ESRD on HD, HTN, DM

Medications
Inpatient
Azithromycin IV
Ceftriaxone dexamethasone IV, 6 mg = 0.6 mL, IV
Daily dextrose 50% injection, 25 g = 50 mL, IV push, as directed
PRN dextrose 50% injection, 25 g = 50 mL, IV push, Q15 Min-int
PRN famotidine, 20 mg = 2 mL, IV
Q12hr heparin, 5000 unit(s) = 1 mL, subcut
Q8hr-int insulin regular IV additive 100 unit(s) + NS 0.9% (base) 100 mL
Home Medications
Aspirin 81 mg oral tablet, 81 mg = 1 tablets, oral, daily
Clonidine 0.1 mg oral tablet, as directed
Coreg 25 mg oral tablet, 25 mg = 1 tablet, oral, b.i.d.
Dexamethasone, 2 mg, oral, daily, take 3 tablets daily
Dexilant 60 mg oral delayed release capsule, 60 mg = 1 capsule, oral
Glipizide 2.5 mg oral tablet, extended release, 2.5 mg = 1 tablet, oral, daily
Hydralazine, 50 mg, as directed
Lasix 80 mg oral tablet, 80 mg = 1 tablet, oral, b.i.d., nondialysis
Metolazone 10 mg oral tablet, 10 mg = 1 tablet, oral, daily
Nephro-Vite, oral, daily
Nifedipine 60 mg oral tablet, extended release, 60 mg = 1 tablet, oral, daily
Renagel 800 mg oral tablet, 3 tablets w/meals valsartan 320 mg oral tablet, 320 mg = 1 tablet, oral, daily

Social History/Participation
Lives with wife and 21 y.o. son in single storey studio. Was working full-time as a security guard.

Prior Level of Function
Prior to contracting COVID, patient was independent with all ADLs and IADLS without an assistive device. He was driving independently and walked 8,000-10,000 steps per day when at work.

ACTIVITIES
Pt. desaturates with talking on baseline using high-flow nasal cannula (50 L/65% fraction of inspired oxygen [FiO_2]) thus FiO_2 titrated up to 75% for mobility. Supervised to sit EOB, needs cueing for breath control given desat with too much talking/mobility. Sit to stand and stand pivot transfer to bedside chair, supervised.

IMPAIRMENTS
Systems Review
Systems review unremarkable; cognition and speech intact.

Vitals
Supine/Preactivity
  HR 90, BP 145/72 (mean arterial pressure [MAP] 89), oxygen saturation (SpO_2) 94%, RR 14-18
  Oxygen Flow Rate: 50 L/min via high-flow nasal cannula
  FiO_2: 0.65
  Vital Signs Additional Information: Talking supine: desat to 86% mBORG 7/10 rest
Activity
  EOB: HR 90, BP135/67 (MAP 83), SpO_2 94% RR 14-23
  Oxygen Flow Rate: 50 L/min via high-flow nasal cannula
  FiO_2: 0.75
Postactivity sitting in chair
  HR 87 beats per minute, BP 133/75, SpO_2 96% on 50L/65% high-flow nasal cannula

ROM
Pt. demonstrated full AROM ×4 extremities against gravity.

CASE EXAMPLE 7.6 Physical Therapy Initial Evaluation Setting: Inpatient a Cute Care—cont'd

Name: Carl Perez **D.O.B.**: 07/17/1972 **Gender**: Male **Date of Eval.**: 1/4/21

Strength
BLE 4/5 throughout all pivots and planes of motion.

ASSESSMENT
Pt. is a 48 y.o. male referred to PT following admission for COVID with increased oxygen requirements. Pt. presents at high functional capacity but does present with fragile respiratory reserve as evidenced by desaturation just with talking prior to mobility. Will benefit from skilled acute PT services to progress mobility as tolerated and assist in oxygen weaning as appropriate to return patient to home at his prior level of function.

GOALS
Participation Goal (3 Months)
1. Pt. will return to work part-time without limitation.

Activity Goals (14 Days)
1. Pt. will ambulate × 50 ft, independently, no desaturation on least amount of O$_2$.
2. Pt. will transfer to/from bedside chair independently without desaturation.

Impairment Goals (7 Days)
1. Patient to engage in self-proning at least 8 hr per day.

PLAN OF CARE
Patient will be seen for 3×/wk for PT. Coordinate with nursing staff for assistance with patient self-proning and out-of-bed schedule. Coordinate with D/C planner for home services including potential for home oxygen at initial D/C for airway clearance techniques, balance training, bed mobility training, patient education, therapeutic exercises, and transfer training. Pt. will be D/C to home with support of wife and family as required. Patient may require home oxygen depending on recovery course.

Patient-Related Instruction
Patient instructed on self-proning with assist from RN given high-flow nasal cannula and lines, verbalized understanding.

Procedural Interventions
Pt. to include airway clearance techniques, balance training, bed mobility training, patient education, therapeutic exercises, and transfer training.

CASE EXAMPLE 7.7 Physical Therapy Initial Evaluation Setting: Telehealth

Name: Isabella Granger **DOB**: 5/19/81 **Gender**: Female **Date of Eval.**: 12/10/22
Neurologist: Dr. Simon

REASON FOR REFERRAL
Current Condition
Pt. is a 41 y.o. female referred to PT with a diagnosis of PD. Pt. was diagnosed with PD ×6 mo (in 2022). Hohen and Yahr Stage I. Pt. reports mild PD symptoms, including RUE tremor and slow walking speed, and is taking a low dose of Sinemet. She is worried about the Sinemet on-off states and does not want to up her medication. She is referred to PT to develop a comprehensive exercise program. Pt. is being seen via telehealth due to her distance from a movement disorders specialty clinic. Date of onset for symptoms: 1/18/22. Pt.'s first symptom was twitching of her index finger on her R hand (dominant hand) and a generalized feeling of fatigue.

PMH
Hashimoto disease ×4 yr, history of migraine headaches ×10 yr. No surgical history.

Medications
Sinemet 10/100 (1 pill t.i.d.), Topamax (100 mg 1×/day), Ubrelvy (prn).

Social History/Participation
Pt. lives at home with her wife in a three-level condominium. There are three steps to enter with B hand rails. Inside there are two flights of six steps, separated by a small landing to reach the main floor and another two flights of six steps, separated by a small landing to reach the bedrooms on the top level. All stairs have a single rail that is on the right side when ascending. She currently uses no DME for mobility or safety.
Occupation: Pt. is a residential architect, working full-time for an architectural firm.
Driving: Pt. reports that she drives independently for unlimited distances.

Leisure/Exercise: Pt. reports enjoying the outdoors and takes long walks daily (1-2 miles). Pt. enjoys exercise and tends to focus only on aerobic activities. She also enjoys gardening, playing the guitar, and spending time with her dog.

PRIOR LEVEL OF FUNCTION
Mobility
Pt. is a community ambulator, and repots independence in all mobility without need of an assistive device.

ADLS/IADLS
Pt. reports past and current independence with all ADLs and IADLS. Although she reports that the IADLS currently take her longer to complete than they used to.

Falls
Pt. reports no history of falls.

ACTIVITIES
Bed Mobility
I in all activities.

Transfers
I in transfers from all surfaces including floor to stand.

Ambulation
Pt. able to walk on level surfaces, s̄ AD at an initial gait speed of 1.5 m/sec. Once fatigued, gait speed dropped to 1.2 m/sec. No LOB noted. On uneven surfaces (gravel and grass), pt. walked s AD. Pt. demonstrated occasional unsteadiness but no falls; average gait speed 1.0 m/sec.
Pt. able to ↑↓ 12 steps using a reciprocal gait pattern and R ascending/L descending rail.

(Continued)

CASE EXAMPLE 7.7   Physical Therapy Initial Evaluation   Setting: Telehealth—cont'd

Name: Isabella Granger   **DOB:** 5/19/81   **Gender:** Female   **Date of Evaluation:** 12/10/22
Neurologist: Dr. Simon

Outcome Measures
- Timed Up & Go—12.3 sec
- Timed Up & Go cog—10.8 sec
- MiniBESTest—24/28
- Parkinson Fatigue Scale (PFS)—31/80 (indicating mild to moderate levels of fatigue)

IMPAIRMENTS
Systems Review
Pt. owns electronic BP cuff. Resting BP 122/72, HR 68 beats per minute.

Pain
Pt. reports no pain.

Range of Motion
UEs: WNL except shoulder elevation and abduction to approximately 160 limited by kyphotic posturing. LEs: WNL except hip extension to approximately neutral.

Muscle Function
MMT: BUE and BLE strength grossly 5/5 throughout.

Posture/Observation
Mild resting tremor RUE. Mild forward head, slight kyphosis upper thoracic spine, scapulae are protracted, downwardly rotated bilat, mild winging observed. Mild decreased in lumbar lordosis.

Balance
- *Sitting:* both static and dynamic balance I.
- *Standing:* Static balance I on solid and foam surfaces. Increased postural sway noted on foam surface but WNL. Dynamic standing: pt. able to reach comfortably within her BOS without LOB.

ASSESSMENT
Pt. is a 41 y.o. female diagnosed with early-stage PD on 6/5/2022. Pt. presents with mild RUE tremor that may impact ADLs, as her R hand is her dominant hand. Mild symptoms of fatigue impact her daily activities. Slow gait speed when fatigued impacts her leisure activities. Pt. demonstrates excellent rehabilitation potential and will benefit from 3-4 PT sessions to provide PD education, design a comprehensive exercise program and monitor her response to increasing levels of exercise. Pt. will then be followed biannually in PT, to identify changes in functional status related to disease progression.

PT Goals (4 Weeks)
1. Pt. will be independent, and consistently engage in established HEP.

2. Pt. will be able to explain the importance of high-intensity exercise in slowing the PD progression.
3. Pt. will ambulate 1 mile on paved surfaces without AD, maintaining a gait speed of 1.5 m/sec, 2-3 times/wk.

PLAN OF CARE
Pt. requires consultative PT for 1 sessions/wk for 3-4 wk with training sessions. PT will communicate with pt.'s neurologist to discuss findings and future plan of care. PT will coordinate with nutritionist to make pt. referral.

Educational Interventions
Patient education today included discussions regarding the process of rehabilitation, review of resulting scores on specified outcome measures with plans for additional testing at follow-up. PT POC, discussions on pathology and progression of neurodegenerative diseases with appropriate handouts provided (APDA Facts about Parkinson disease, APDA Be Active and Beyond Booklet, Parkinson's Foundation Exercise Recommendations), review of recent advances in rehabilitation literature with neurodegenerative diseases, importance of engaging in safe, high-intensity cardiovascular exercise, spreading exercise out throughout the day to reduce total sedentary time, incorporation of progressive resistance training, flexibility exercise, and balance training, as well as safety considerations in the home and community environment. The pt. demonstrated and verbalized understanding of all educational material.

Procedural Interventions
PT sessions will include:
- HEP development.
- Flexibility training for improved posture and increased hip ROM.
- Resistance training for increased core muscle strength.
- HIIT training to introduce gradually increasing aerobic exercise challenge to slow disease progression and decrease fatigue.
- Neuromuscular reeducation for high-level balance challenge.

Pt. agrees to goals and treatment plan as stated. Pt. consents to therapy program.

_____   _____

Julie Fineman, Physical Therapist   Date: 12/10/2022

EXERCISE 7.1

In the space provided, identify in which of the six sections of the initial evaluation model the following statements belong (R = Reason for Referral; Ac = Activities; I = Impairments; As = Assessment; G = Goals; PC = Plan of Care). The statements are taken from a variety of initial evaluation reports. See Tables 7.1 to 7.3 and Case Examples 7.1 to 7.5 for help completing this exercise.

1. Child will ride an adaptive tricycle independently for 25 ft in the gym in 8 wk. _____

2. ROM R knee flexion 95°. _____

3. BP 150/90 mm Hg, HR 96 beats per minute. _____

4. Pt. has a 2-yr history of seizures occurring approximately 2×/mo. _____

5. Pt. education will include instructions in home program for walking with self-monitoring of HR and perceived exertion. _____

6. Pt. works as a secretary full-time but is currently restricted to part-time (½ day) due to wrist pain. _____

7. Pt. is able to climb 10 stairs with left hand holding railing in 25 sec. _____

8. Pt. presents with poor expiratory ability 2° to pneumonia, resulting in an ineffective cough and lowered endurance for daily care activities. _____

9. Pt. is a 23 y.o. professional dancer who works 7 days/wk. _____

10. Pt. will be able to stand at bathroom sink for 5 min to brush teeth and wash face and comb hair in 2 wk. _____

11. Intervention will include therapeutic exercise: progressive resistive exercises to quadriceps and strengthening in standing position via squatting and lunging exercises. _____

12. Strength R shoulder flexion 3/5. _____

13. The pt.'s ineffective right toe clearance and weak hip musculature are resulting in slow and unsafe ambulation indoors. _____

14. Pt. can lift a 10-lb box (maximum weight) from floor to waist height. _____

15. Therapist will coordinate training for dressing and bathing with pt.'s OT and nursing staff. _____

Documenting Reason for Referral: Health Condition and Participation

After reading this chapter and completing the exercises, the reader will be able to:

1. Identify and classify various aspects of documenting reason for referral, including a patient's background information, health condition, medications, past medical history, social history/participation, and prior functional status.
2. Explain the three key elements of describing a patient's current health condition.
3. Discuss the implications of direct access for documenting medical diagnoses.
4. Describe the process of conducting an interview to obtain information pertaining to gathering history data.
5. Appropriately document elements of the reason for referral based on case scenarios.

The first section of the initial evaluation report sets the stage for the reason why the patient or client was referred for evaluation and provides critical background information pertaining to what is already known about the patient's condition and situation. We have therefore chosen to title this section Reason for Referral, as it encompasses a range of information, typically gathered from the review of past medical records as well as patient interviews that set the stage and context for the evaluation report. Based on the International Classification of Functioning, Disability and Health (ICF) framework, the Reason for Referral section focuses on information pertaining to health condition, restrictions in participation, as well as personal and environmental factors (Fig. 8.1).

Information about a patient's health condition can be organized in the initial evaluation note in many ways. Different institutions frequently mandate a certain organizational structure, and this structure is often formatted in the electronic medical record or is preprinted on customized initial evaluation forms. The degree to which each of these headings is used differs depending on the institution and patient population. For the general initial evaluation, the following categorization of information is recommended:

- Patient information and demographics
- Current condition
- Past medical history
- Medications
- Social history/participation
- Prior level of function

Table 8.1 provides an overview of the key pieces of information that should be included in these sections, and the content of each subsection is explained in more detail later in this chapter.

HISTORY-TAKING FOR HEALTH CONDITIONS AND PARTICIPATION-BASED INFORMATION: THE FIRST STEP IN PHYSICAL THERAPY DIAGNOSIS

Within the scope of their practice, physical therapists (PTs) encounter patients with a variety of health conditions. *Health condition*, as defined by the ICF framework, is an umbrella term for disease (acute or chronic), disorder, injury, or trauma (see Fig. 8.1). It may also include other circumstances, such as pregnancy, aging, stress, fitness level, congenital anomaly, or genetic predisposition. Health conditions can result from infections, acute or chronic injuries, metabolic imbalances, or degenerative disease processes.

Any physical therapy initial evaluation note must provide specific information about the medical diagnosis or known or suspected pathological conditions. In the *Guide to Physical Therapist Practice 4.0* (APTA, 2014), information pertaining to a patient's health condition is categorized under "History" in the Examination section. Fig. 8.2 illustrates the range of information that can be collected by the PT as part of history-taking. The *Guide* defines *history* as follows: "The *history* is a systematic gathering of data—from both the past and the present—related to why the individual is seeking the services of the physical therapist... While taking the history, the physical therapist also identifies health restoration and prevention needs and coexisting health problems that may have implications for intervention" (APTA, 2014). The relevance of history-taking as it relates to the health condition, therefore, is that it provides the foundation for why the patient is referred for physical therapy, thus setting up the reason for referral. What are the specific medical

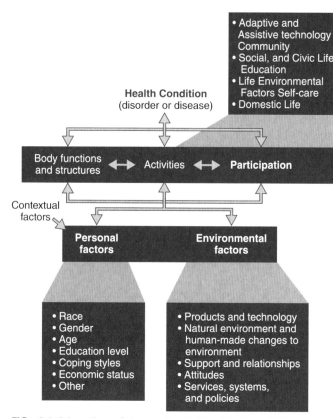

FIG. 8.1 Adaptation of International Classification of Functioning, Disability and Health (ICF) domains and constructs from *The Guide to Physical Therapist Practice 3.0* and *4.0*. Documentation of Reason for Referral encompasses *Health Condition* and *Participation* as well as *Environmental and Personal Factors*.

diagnoses, health problems, or health risk factors that bring the patient to seek the services of a PT?

In general, health condition information is included early in an evaluation report because these data are critical to determining how the PT should proceed with the examination. PTs perform a process known as differential diagnosis (Heick & Lazaro, 2023) in which they gather information to confirm or modify any previously determined diagnoses (from other health care professionals) or develop their own diagnosis (see Chapter 11 for more information on diagnosis by PTs). In addition, therapists will ask health condition-related questions, which help identify possible problems that require consultation with or referral to another provider. Certain conditions raise concerns about whether an underlying condition exists in which physical therapy may be contraindicated or in which referral to another health professional would be warranted.

Detailed information about the health condition is therefore an important part of determining the appropriateness of physical therapy as an intervention. Certain health conditions are appropriate for physical therapy; others are not. However, diagnosis alone does not determine the appropriateness of intervention; instead, the associated or secondary limitations or impairments related to a diagnosis warrant physical therapy intervention.

In some ways, health condition information documented by the PT in this section is somewhat limited. At this point, the therapist simply classifies any facts they have available before

the examination is performed. As the examination proceeds, the PT may uncover information that may help to refine any previously given diagnosis. Any new information obtained during the physical therapy examination that confirms, clarifies, elaborates on, or possibly contradicts the established diagnosis and health condition should be documented in the appropriate section (e.g., Impairments; see Chapter 10) and summarized in the Assessment section (see Chapter 11). Thus information about health conditions and diagnosis does not begin and end in this section.

Another important component of the reason for referral pertains to participation-based information. In contrast to medical or diagnostic information related to health conditions, participation-based information relates to an individual's personal, home, and work life (often referred to as social history), as well as their general level of functioning currently and prior to the onset of this specific medical condition. The focus of documentation of participation and social history varies for different patients and in different settings. Certainly, the primary concern for patients who are very sick in the hospital is working toward the attainment of an independent functional status, such as their ability to dress themselves or take a shower. In fact, in a hospital setting, documentation of a patient's personal and work status often refers to what the patient was doing before being admitted to the hospital. (What was the person's job? What sports and recreational activities did they enjoy participating in?) When the patient is receiving outpatient or home-based services, the focus of documentation should reflect current issues. (Is the patient currently working and, if so, at what functional level? Can they return to recreational sports?)

In the following sections, we outline specific information that may be provided in each of the subsections of Reason for Referral (see Table 8.1 for a detailed outline).

DOCUMENTING REASON FOR REFERRAL

Patient Information and Demographics

General patient information and demographics are the first items included in any medical documentation and typically include the patient's name, date of birth, date evaluation was conducted, gender, and any pertinent demographic information. If the patient's race or ethnic background is relevant, it can be included here. The patient's preferred language can also be included here so that interpretive services can be used as needed to ensure good collaboration and understanding between patient and therapist.

Current Condition

The current condition section includes information pertaining to why the patient was referred for physical therapy and by whom, if it is not evident. This includes information about the current health condition (e.g., diagnosis) for which the patient is being referred for physical therapy, which sets the framework for the reason this evaluation is being performed. In fact, this section is sometimes simply titled "medical diagnosis." In most cases, the PT should go beyond simply restating any previously determined diagnosis and describe a specific precipitating

TABLE 8.1 Components of Documenting Reason for Referral[a]

Component	Information Included
Patient information and demographics	Patient's name
	Date of birth
	Gender
	Other demographic information, such as race or ethnicity, preferred language
Current condition	Reason patient is referred, if not evident
	Concerns that led the patient to seek services of a physical therapist
	Mechanisms of injury or disease, including (see Table 8.2):
	Underlying disease process
	Location
	Time course
	Previous occurrence of current condition
	Results of laboratory or diagnostic tests
	Current and prior therapeutic interventions (if any)
Past medical history	Any prior surgeries, hospitalizations, other diagnoses, or preexisting conditions
	Date or the time course of these surgeries, hospitalizations, or conditions
Medications	Name of medications
	Dosage (if known)
	What the medication is prescribed for
Social history/participation	Living environment (including aids for locomotion, orthotic and prosthetic equipment, seating, and positioning); community characteristics; projected destination at conclusion of care
	Family and caregiver resources
	Cultural beliefs and behaviors
	Work and community integration
	Self-care and domestic life
	Adaptive and Assistive technology (including aids for locomotion, orthotic and prosthetic equipment, seating and positioning)
	Community, Social and Civic life (including social interactions, social activities and support systemts)
	Education Life
	Personal and Environmental Factors
Prior level of function	Patient's level of functioning (work, personal, school, social life) prior to onset of current condition.
Other (as appropriate)	General health status—Can include level of physical fitness, behavioral health risks (tobacco, drug use), general health perceptions; mental functions (e.g., memory, reasoning ability, depression, anxiety); physical function (e.g., mobility, sleep patterns, restricted bed days)
	Developmental history
	Family history

[a]This table incorporates terminology found in the APTA *Guide to Physical Therapist Practice, 4.0*, 2023.

incident, if any, or mechanism of injury. The PT should also report what other treatments have been performed (e.g., consultation with other medical professionals). If a diagnosis is not provided by a referring health care professional, the PT should document any information provided by the patient identifying the primary problem or chief complaint—what is the reason the patient is seeking physical therapy?

Information about the patient's health condition sets the foundation for the physical therapy examination. The PT must gather all relevant information to develop an accurate picture of the patient's medical condition that warrants referral to physical therapy. Whenever possible, three key elements of the patient's current health condition should be specified: the underlying disease process, its location, and the time course (Table 8.2).

If a physician or other health care professional referred the patient to physical therapy, this information should be documented in this section. If applicable, the name of the referring professional should also be listed here in addition to any specific information, orders, or contraindications that they communicated.

PTs who practice in direct-access states face additional issues regarding diagnoses. In many situations under direct access, no medical diagnosis is available. PTs must then determine the diagnosis and health condition through their own evaluation. In some cases, this is not possible within the scope of tests and measures available to PTs and referral to a physician or other health care personnel is warranted. Reports from diagnostic tests such as magnetic resonance imaging scans and x-ray films may be necessary to clarify the patient's health condition.

Activities and Participation

- Current and prior role functions – such as self-care and domestic, education, work, community, social, and civic life – within family, community, and society

Current Condition(s)

- Concerns that led the individual to seek the services of a physical therapist
- Concerns or needs of an individual who requires the services of a physical therapist
- Current and prior therapeutic interventions, including physical therapist services, and surgical or drug management of the condition
- Mechanisms of injury or disease, including date of onset
- Onset, timing, and pattern of symptoms
- Individual, family, significant other, and caregiver expectations and goals for the t herapeutic intervention
- Individual, family, significant other, and caregiver perceptions of individual's psychosocial response to the current clinical situation
- Previous occurrence of current condition(s)

Family History

- Familial health risks

General Demographics

- Age
  Education
- Primary language and preferred method of communication, such as sign language or an interpreter
- Race and ethnicity (belonging to a social group that has a common national or cultural tradition)
- Gender, sex
- Religion, spirituality

General Health Status
(Self-report, family report, caregiver report)

- Behavioral health
- Cognitive function
- General health perceptions
- Physical function

Growth and Development

- Developemental history and milestones
- Birth history
- Hand dominance
- Vulnerability to or history of trauma or violence

Living Environment/Arrangements

- Assistive technology, such as aids for locomotion, orthotic devices, prosthetic requirements, and seating and positioning technology
- Living environment and community characteristics
- Projected destination at conclusion of care
- Accessibility, such as architectural barriers or facilitators
- Level of assistance available at home

Medical (Illnesses)/surgical History

- Cardiovascular
- Endocrine/metabolic
- Eyes, ears, nose, and throat
- Gastrointestinal
- Genitourinary
- Gynecological
- Immune
- Integumentary
- Musculoskeletal
- Neuromuscular
- Obstetrical
- Psychological
- Pulmonary
- Prior hospitalizations (ICU stays, surgeries, and preexisting medical and other health related conditions)

Medications

- Medications for current condition
- Mode of delivery, dosage
- Medications previously taken for current condition
- Medications for other conditions
- Supplements

Other Diagnostic and Clinical Tests

- Laboratory and diagnostic tests, such as bone density and imaging
- Review of available records, such as medical, education, and surgical
- Review of other clinical findings, such as nutrition and hydration

Review of Systems

- Cardiovascular system
- Pulmonary system
- Endocrine system
- Eyes, ears, nose, or throat
- Gastrointestinal system
- Genitourinary/reproductive systems.
- Hematologic/lymphatic systems
- Immune system
- Integumentary system
- Musculoskeletal system
- Neurologic system

Health Habits (past and current)

- Behavioral health risks, such as physical activity; participation in hobbies and sports; exercise; nutritions; sleep quality, hygiene, patterns, and behaviors; stress management; tobacco use; substance use or misuse; and readiness for change

Social History

- Adverse experiences
- Access to care
- Cultural/religious beliefs and behaviors
- Family and caregiver resources, relationships, and interactions, such as codependency and enabling behavior
- Living alone versus with others
- Social interactions, social activities, and support systems
- Neighborhood safety
- Transportation to care

FIG. 8.2 Types of data that may be generated from a patient/client history. (Reprinted with permission from American Physical Therapy Association. *The Guide to Physical Therapist Practice.* <https://guide.apta.org/>; 2023.)

TABLE 8.2   Elements of Documenting Health Condition

Element	Description
Underlying disease process	Type of pathology, such as infection, tumor, or trauma
	• Results of any diagnostic tests (e.g., laboratory tests, magnetic resonance imaging scans, or x-ray films)
	• Any information provided directly from the referring physician that identifies the specific pathology
Location	Specific origin of pathology
	• Includes specific area of the brain, spinal cord, muscles, nerves, joints, or tissues that are affected
Time course	How long the problem has existed
	• Include date of injury or surgery, or date a diagnosis was made

PTs must clearly document all known aspects of a patient's health status relevant to their referral and must be able to make a reasonable differential diagnosis. An important question that each therapist must ask is: "Is the health condition one that is within the scope of practice for a physical therapist, and is it amenable to physical therapy intervention?" Clear, concise, and accurate documentation of the health condition (including disease process, location, and time course) is of utmost importance. In cases where patients are not referred by a physician, aspects of the medical condition obtained from a patient/family interview and chart review should be documented in this first section of the note. However, the PT's final diagnosis should not be documented until the Assessment section because it may depend on physical findings not yet presented.

Past Medical History

Information documented in this category should include any medical history that may be relevant (even indirectly) to the current condition. Past medical history (PMH) can include the following:

- Any prior surgeries, other diagnoses, or preexisting conditions.
- The date or the time course of the medical condition or surgery (e.g., *ACL repair 12/2/21, IDDM ×10 yr, h/o coronary artery disease ×8 yr*).

When physical therapy documentation is included as part of a medical chart in a hospital, nursing home, or rehabilitation setting, PMH may be found in another part of the chart to which all medical professionals can refer. In this case, the PT should document that the PMH was noted and confirmed by the patient and include a reference to where this information can be found.

Medications

PTs should document medications the patient is taking for the current condition, as well as any medications taken for other medical conditions. It is important to document (1) the name of the medication, (2) the dosage (if known), and (3) the reason the medication is being prescribed (e.g., Zoloft 50 mg q.i.d. for depression). Vitamins and over-the-counter medications may also be included, especially if they have known side effects that would be important to consider. Documentation of medications by the PT should occur even in situations when the medications are listed in a medical record. This is because medication information is critical to the understanding of possible patient responses to intervention, and the timing of medication may have a significant impact on a patient's symptoms and functional abilities (e.g., dopamine agonists in patients with Parkinson disease). Furthermore, third-party payers frequently mandate documentation of medications as standard practice in initial evaluation reports.

Social History/Participation

As discussed earlier, social history and participation relate to an individual's personal, home, and work life, as well as the person's general level of functioning. This addresses both environmental and personal factors and describes the ability of a patient or client to perform the specific functions pertinent to their everyday life.

An important concept in conveying participation and social history information is to document how the current condition is affecting an individual's life. What are the patient's current life roles, and is the patient able to perform their roles as a partner or parent? What is the person's home and/or work environment, and how does it affect their ability to function independently? Can the person work in either a paid or volunteer position? Are they able to engage in social and recreational activities?

The first step in obtaining this information is to review the patient's medical record. This minimizes repetitive interviewing of the patient and helps prepare the PT to better organize the examination. The second step is to spend time interviewing patients. Although time is often limited in rehabilitation settings, PTs can prevent many missed diagnoses and develop an appropriate plan of care from the onset if they spend an adequate amount of time gathering pertinent information through history-taking. Simply asking some basic questions can provide the PT with valuable information about the problems affecting a patient's life. Indeed, asking these questions early often saves time because it enables the PT to be more selective in their examination.

Table 8.3 lists various questions that could be asked to ascertain social history and participation information. The type of questions asked during an interview should vary depending on the age and medical diagnosis of the patient. Specifically, the therapist needs to determine the patient's premorbid lifestyle and current goals for regaining that lifestyle. The interview can be conducted with the patient, a caregiver, or both. For young children, interviews are often conducted with the parent or guardian.

TABLE 8.3	**Sample Interview Questions to Ascertain Participation-Based Information**	
	Young Child	**Older Man**
Patient	5 y.o. boy with cerebral palsy; lives at home with parents (interview directed at parent)	64 y.o. semiretired carpenter, with rotator cuff tear; divorced, lives alone, has 2 grandchildren
Social history	• Describe your child's home and living situation. • Do you have any stairs? How many? • Does your child have any siblings? • Who else provides care for your child? • Do you have any cultural or religious beliefs that may affect this evaluation or any future treatment?	• Describe your home and living situation. • Do you have any stairs? How many? • Do your children live close by? • Are they able to assist you in any way with household tasks?
Participation	• Is your child able to participate fully in all school activities, including sitting at his desk during lesson plans and participating in gym class? • What types of play or recreational activities does your child engage in? • Does he have any difficulties or limitations in activities he would like to engage in but is unable? • Does your child participate in age-appropriate chores in the house, such as helping to clean his room? • What types of social interactions does your child engage in? Does your child have any difficulty engaging in play with his peers? • How would you describe your child's overall health?	• To what extent have you recently been involved in your work as a carpenter? • To what degree are you limited in your ability to work? • Are you able to maintain the basic upkeep of your apartment, for example, doing the cleaning or the laundry? • What social and physical activity (e.g., sports, leisure activities) did you engage in before this recent injury? Are you having any difficulty or limitations performing those activities now? • How would you describe your overall health? • Do you smoke?

Assessment of participation clearly sets the rehabilitation professional apart from many other medical professionals. Medical doctors, for example, spend much of their time determining an accurate health condition and relating the patient's impairments to that condition. Conversely, PTs should (and often do) spend a significant amount of their time at the other end of the disability spectrum—focusing on the interrelationship between participation and activities and between activities and impairments. Obtaining this information that encompasses a patient's specific life roles provides the foundation for shaping the rehabilitation process. As noted in Chapter 1, it is the starting point for the process of rehabilitation.

Measurement of participation encompasses a person's involvement in community, social and civic life, which are essential to an individual's quality of life. Providing accurate and reasonable documentation about a person's ability to participate in these activities is critical, particularly to justify services for many patients who may appear "high functioning."

If a patient is working or has recently stopped working because of an injury or illness, the nature of the work should be documented in sufficient detail. Such notations typically include a listing or description of the tasks or activities the patient performs in a typical day (e.g., typing, writing, lifting) and any unique requirements to the patient's job.

Example: *"lifting >50 lb," "standing for >1 hr at a time."*

The therapist should also document here any volunteer work in which the patient is or was participating (e.g., *"volunteers at hospital transporting patients 1×/wk"*) and any of the patient's social activities if this information is pertinent to rehabilitation.

The PT documents a wide range of information pertaining to the patient's home and living situation, often including details about the type of home, the number of floors, and the number and type of stairs (this is typically what is referred to as *social history*). If a patient uses certain medical equipment, such as a wheelchair or a raised toilet seat, this is reported here. The PT should describe the equipment and how it is used in sufficient detail.

Example: *Pt. uses a lightweight wheelchair, with gel cushion and swing-away leg rests, for mobility within the home.*

Descriptions of the patient's family and caregiver resources are also components of the home environment. Cultural beliefs and behaviors, as they are relevant to the rehabilitation process, should also be included here. However, specific details about a patient's personal life that are not pertinent to their current medical condition or reason for referral should not be included in patient documentation. For example, it would rarely be necessary to refer to a patient as "divorced" or to identify a person's specific religious affiliation unless it affected their evaluation or treatment in some way.

Prior Level of Function

It is frequently important to contrast *current* level of functioning and participation with *prior* level of functioning and participation, and therefore therapists commonly document *prior level of function* as a distinct component in the Reason for Referral section. Documenting prior level of function is often a required component of documentation for third-party payers. Prior level of function refers to the degree of functional skill of a patient in self-care, community, civic, and social activities before the onset of the current medical diagnosis or health condition. Determination of prior functional status is particularly relevant for older patients and those with previous medical conditions. Such patients may not have been independent in all activities before the onset of their current condition; they may have had some limitations as a result of other medical conditions or problems related to their current medical condition. For example, a patient who has had a stroke may have had a preexisting condition of chronic obstructive pulmonary disease (COPD). The patient's pulmonary limitations may have reduced the patient's walking distance even before the stroke.

The goal of therapy is often to restore the patient to at least the level of prior functioning. Sometimes the goal is to restore the patient to a higher level of functioning, as in the case of a patient with arthritis who elects to have a total knee replacement. Because that patient's activities may have been significantly limited by the arthritis, the knee replacement may enable the patient to improve to a significantly higher functional level. Importantly, the known prior level of function provides a minimal benchmark for the level of functioning that the patient might be expected to achieve.

Other Information

Several other types of information can be included in this section of a report. These include general health status, developmental history and family history. *General health status* includes information pertaining to the patient's overall health and wellness. This information could include physical and psychological functioning, level of fitness, and behavioral health risks (e.g., history of smoking) or growth and development (in pediatric cases, e.g., date at which child began sitting or walking). A *developmental history* can be used in certain pediatric settings and involves information related to a child's growth and overall development (e.g., the age at which a child first sat up or walked alone). This information would not be pertinent, however, for most adolescent or adult evaluations. A *family history* may be helpful for understanding the patient's medical diagnosis (e.g., a strong family history of heart disease or a history of certain musculoskeletal abnormalities).

SPECIFICITY OF DOCUMENTATION

Information in the Reason for Referral section should be sufficiently detailed so that it is useful to the PT or other personnel reading the report. The information presented in this section helps to shape both the patient's prognosis and the plan of care. Furthermore, it provides the foundation for developing appropriate and realistic goals that will be based on the patient's current level of participation and lifestyle.

An example could be a patient who has had a recent heart attack (myocardial infarction [MI]) and is undergoing cardiac rehabilitation. Consider the specificity of these examples:

Poor Example: *Pt. worked full time prior to MI.*
Better Example: *Pt. worked 50+ hr/wk as a bank VP; pt. reports job was "stressful" and required frequent traveling (3-4×/mo).*
Poor Example: *Pt. led an active lifestyle prior to MI.*
Better Example: *Before heart attack, pt. ran 4 miles 4×/wk and enjoyed sailing his sailboat 1-2×/wk in summer.*

If a goal of this patient is to return to their active lifestyle and level of occupation, documentation of the details of these activities is important.

OUTCOME MEASURES

Table 8.4 provides a list of some commonly used standardized outcome measures that are primarily designed to assess participation (see Chapter 4 for more information on outcome measures). Some of these measures were designed before the implementation of the ICIDH-2 (The International Classification of Functioning, Disability and Health) and thus use the term *disability* rather than *participation*.

It is important to note that most of these measures, indeed probably all, measure not only participation but also some aspects of activity and body structures and function (Perenboom & Chorus, 2003). Those instruments that most closely measure only participation are the Perceived Handicap Questionnaire and the London Handicap Scale (Perenboom & Chorus, 2003). In fact, participation and activities may not be able to be truly differentiated into distinct domains (Jette et al., 2007). Until these constructs can be more clearly defined through research, the authors recommend the two should be documented independently to the extent possible.

Self-Report Measures

The tools listed in Table 8.4 measure life participation obtained by patient self-report. Self-report is a very important piece of an examination, particularly in assessment of outcomes. Patients sometimes have little or no improvement in impairments or even in particular functional abilities, but they may have significantly improved their quality of life or ability to engage in life roles. For example, a patient may have developed strategies for coping with pain or effective compensatory strategies to accomplish tasks. Alternatively, they may show improvement in impairments, such as weakness or limited range of motion, with no corresponding improvement of participation.

Self-report measures are often thought to be less valuable than performance-based measures, which rely on direct observation of abilities, because they are not considered objective. Self-report measures are indeed inherently subjective, which increases the chance that the patient will provide inaccurate or exaggerated information. Nevertheless, a patient's perception of their limitations or problems is just as important as other components of the assessment process, albeit not the only measure. For example, the Oswestry Disability Questionnaire (Roland & Jenner, 1989) was designed for use in patients with back pain and evaluates a person's perceived limitations in various life activities. Such limitations often are difficult to ascertain by physical examination, in part because they measure activities that are not readily evaluated in a clinic setting (e.g., sleeping and traveling).

Quality of Life Measures

Several measures listed in Table 8.4 attempt to measure a construct known as *quality of life*. Quality of life is the degree of well-being felt by an individual or group of people. Although quality of life itself cannot be directly measured, a patient's

TABLE 8.4   Some Commonly Used Standardized Measures of Participation (Listed Alphabetically)[a]

Outcome Measure	Description	Population/Setting
Craig Handicap Assessment and Reporting Technique (CHART) (Whiteneck et al., 1992)	Consists of 32 items across the six WHO domains of handicap, including physical independence, cognitive independence, mobility, occupation, social integration, and economic self-sufficiency	General rehabilitation (e.g., spinal cord injury and traumatic brain injury)
European Quality of Life (EuroQOL)—EQ5D (Brooks et al., 2003)	European quality of life measure; provides a simple descriptive profile and a single index value for health status and is applicable to a wide range of health conditions and treatments	General
Activity Measure for Post Acute Care (AM-PAC)	Generic measure of a patient's function that can be used across an entire episode of care, from acute and postacute care settings and across patient or proxy report	Different patient conditions (e.g., musculoskeletal, neurological, major medical)
Oswestry Disability Index (Fairbank et al., 2000)	Used for evaluation of disability in people with low back pain; assesses disability/participation in 10 functional areas with 6-item responses each	Low back pain
Participation Measure for Post-Acute Care (PM-PAC) (Gandek et al., 2007)	Evaluates participation with 51 items covering nine domains: mobility; role functioning; community, social, and civic life; domestic life/self-care; economic life; interpersonal relationships; communication; work; and education	Acute care
Quebec Back Pain Disability Scale (QBPDS) (Kopec et al., 1995)	20-item self-administered test designed to assess the level of functional disability in individuals with back pain; patients rate level of difficulty in performing various functional tasks	Back pain
Rehabilitation Activities Profile (Jelles et al., 1995)	Consists of 21 items divided into a total of 71 subitems; covers the domains of communication, mobility, personal care, occupation, and relationships; severity of problem as perceived by the patient is rated on a 4-point Likert scale	General rehabilitation
Roland Morris Questionnaire (RDQ) (Roland & Morris, 1983)	A self-report, self-completed questionnaire designed to assess the degree of functional limitation in patients with low back pain in primary care; 24 items selected from Sickness Impact Profile with the term "because of my back" added to each to make it specific to lower back pain	Low back pain
SF-36 (Stewart et al., 1988)	Measure that includes 36 items pertaining to general well-being and quality of life, as well as frequency and degree of participation in daily living, social, and recreational activities	General
Sickness Impact Profile (Bergner et al., 1981; van Straten et al., 1997)	A 136-item questionnaire; includes everyday activities in 12 subscales (sleep and rest; emotional behavior; body care and movement; home management; mobility; social interaction; ambulation; alertness behavior; communication; work; recreation and pastimes; and eating). An adapted version for use in people post stroke contains 30 items.	Back pain
WHO Disability Assessment Schedule 2 (WHODAS II) (www.who.int/icidh/whodas/generalinfo.html)	Assesses day-to-day functioning in six activity domains: understanding and communicating, getting around, self-care, getting along with people, life activities, and participation in society; provides a profile of functioning across the domains and an overall disability score.	General
WHO Quality of Life (WHOQOL) (WHOQOL Group, 1998)	Consists of 26 items in four domains: physical health, psychological health, social relationships, and environment; designed to measure the level of satisfaction in carrying out activities or tasks or in participating in these activities; abbreviated version of the WHOQOL.	General

[a]All participation measures listed here are measured by patient self-report.

perception of their quality of life can. Quality of life and participation are distinct entities, but they are clearly related, and for purposes of documentation, information pertaining to quality of life—and outcome measures related to quality of life—should be included in this section.

Documenting the Results of Outcome Measures

For documentation purposes, we generally recommend that only the scores from standardized tests should be reported in the body of an evaluation report. The PT may choose to summarize components from the tests that are pertinent or

provide a brief interpretation of the test results (see Case Examples 8.1 and 8.3). This applies to all forms of standardized testing, including tests used for activity limitations and impairments (see Chapters 9 and 10, respectively). The completed standardized test form should be included in the patient's record.

PREVENTING PARTICIPATION RESTRICTIONS

Many PTs are currently involved with prevention: primary, secondary, and tertiary. This raises specific issues regarding documentation. For *primary prevention*, there is no present-ing diagnosis or illness. For example, if a therapist performs an evaluation or intervention for a patient who is *at risk* for devel-oping osteoporosis, documentation of pathological information should include why the client is at risk for developing this prob-lem and a discussion of the potential consequences.

Secondary and tertiary prevention are related to current disease processes. *Secondary prevention* consists of decreas-ing the duration of illness, severity of disease, and sequelae through early diagnosis. This would apply, for example, to individuals with certain types of cardiac disease. *Tertiary pre-vention* consists of limiting the degree of disability and pro-moting rehabilitation and restoration of function in patients with chronic and irreversible diseases, such as multiple sclero-sis. Documentation in such cases needs to focus not only on the specific referring health condition (e.g., multiple sclerosis) but also on the subsequent health conditions and/or impair-ments that can be prevented (e.g., muscle contractures). This can be a tricky situation because documentation of prevention is not always well accepted by third-party payers. However, the more frequently PTs document the need for and purpose of preventive intervention, the more likely it will become stan-dard practice.

For some patients, the therapist may be unable to identify a clear restriction in participation. The most obvious example is primary prevention, in which the patient is a healthy indi-vidual with only the risk of developing a disabling illness. In addition, PTs often see patients in the acute stages of an illness or immediately after an injury when a participation restriction is not yet fully understood. Indeed, in such instances the PT actively intervenes to prevent these restrictions from occur-ring (secondary prevention) or limit their severity (tertiary prevention) (Goldston, 1987). For example, a patient who sees a PT for acute low back pain is at risk for developing chronic low back syndrome, which might lead to loss of employment or inability to fulfill other roles. An athlete with a tendon injury might need carefully controlled rest and stabilization to prevent long-term loss of the ability to participate in com-petitive sports. A newborn with *spina bifida* may exhibit few current restrictions in life skills but is clearly at risk for future restrictions; early intervention is designed to minimize these future restrictions.

Identifying potential participation restrictions is therefore an important component of physical therapy practice and affects the plan of care. As an example, consider again the patient with acute low back pain. If the potential restriction in participa-tion is occupational in nature, intervention might be focused on teaching the patient how to perform certain work-related skills safely and alternative ways to accomplish certain tasks. If, however, the potential restriction involves competitive athlet-ics, a very different approach would be used—one with greater emphasis on strengthening muscles and fine-tuning movement strategies so that the patient could continue to perform at a high level without causing further injury.

Clinicians can use a considerable database of evidence to support this concept. Numerous studies have reported that the natural history of certain diseases (and risk factors) lead to predictable participation restrictions (e.g., predictors of low back pain disability: Feuerstein et al., 1999; predictors of func-tional decline in community living elderly: Stuck et al., 1999; risk factors for disability associated with chronic obstructive pulmonary disease: Rodriguez-Rodriguez, 2013; factors associ-ated with mobility limitations in older women with knee pain: Lamb et al., 2000). Clinicians can use this evidence to deter-mine whether a significant risk of future participation restric-tion exists and justify intervention on that basis.

SUMMARY

- Health condition and Participation information form the foundation for the Reason for Referral.
- Medical information and any previously determined diag-noses are included early in an evaluation report because of their importance in shaping the PT's examination.
- Information in this section can typically be organized into the following categories: patient information and demo-graphics, current condition, PMH, medications, social history/participation, prior level of function, and other (including general health status, and family and develop-ment history).
- Documentation of specific health condition information includes providing information about the underlying dis-ease process, the location of the pathological condition, and its time course.
- Documentation of participation and social history ascer-tains information about a patient's life, including their home situation and work.

- Participation is specific to an individual and their environ-ment. In a pediatric setting, participation is often related to a child's ability to play or attend school. For an adult patient, participation encompasses the ability to perform specific functions related to self-care and domestic life; work and education life; and community, social, and civic life.
- Participation information is most commonly obtained through patient and family interviews and from the medi-cal record. Through the interview process the PT ascertains the patient's premorbid lifestyle and determines the patient's current goals for regaining that lifestyle.
- Standardized questionnaires use self-reporting to deter-mine a patient's health perception and participation in recreational, social, occupational, and self-care activities. Such tools provide a patient's perspective on their health status and their level of participation restrictions and are an important adjunct to performance-based measures.

CASE EXAMPLE 8.1   Documenting Reason for Referral   Setting: Outpatient

Name: Rick Quincy   **D.O.B.:** 12/29/70   **Gender**: Male   **Date of Eval.:** 6/14/22

REASON FOR REFERRAL
Current Condition
Patient is a 51 y.o.male referred to PT with dx of L4-5 disc herniation, onset of current symptoms 5/20/22 following heavy lifting at work.

PMH
R rotator cuff tear with surgical repair 2011.

Medications
Etodolac 500 mg 1×/day (for inflammation and pain), low dose aspirin 81 mg 1×/day (cardiac health), multivitamin daily.

Social History/Participation
Lives with wife and two children in two-storey home. Patient has 1 step to enter with no railings. Thirteen steps to the second floor c̄ R ascending rail. His wife has taken responsibility for all household duties and has hired some outside help to assist with gardening and other chores. Pt is currently unable to perform daily household duties (e.g., gardening, taking out trash)

2° to pain. Pt. works as an independent building contractor. He is currently on "light-duty," doing paperwork at his desk and making phone calls but has not yet returned to any physical labor. Job entails 60% moderate-heavy lifting (up to 100 lb) and 40% desk work, requiring sitting at desk and phone for 1-2 hr at a time.

Prior Level of Function
Patient was independent in all ADLs, IADLs, and mobility. Patient was driving independently. Patient worked full time in his own construction business. He managed and participated in all aspects of construction from planning to all physical aspects of carpentry. Pt. enjoyed watching sports (currently able to sit for only 30 min) and attending daughter's softball games (has not attended a game for 2 wk due to inability to sit on bleacher-style seats).

General Health Status
Before onset of LBP, pt. led relatively sedentary lifestyle. Hx of smoking 1 pack/day for past 20 yr. Oswestry Disability Questionnaire Score 28/50 (indicating severe disability).

CASE EXAMPLE 8.2   Documenting Reason for Referral   Setting: Inpatient Acute Care

Name: Lisa Jeter   **D.O.B.:** 5/20/74   **Gender:** Female   **Date of Eval.:** 12/10/22

REASON FOR REFERRAL
Current Condition
Patient is a 48-year-old female referred to PT s/p aortic aneurysm with surgical repair on 12/5/22. Patient is A & O ×4 and is able to communicate without difficulty. She is reporting some double vision and she is having difficulty with her balance.

PMH
Hypothyroidism, cesarean section, kidney stones.

Medications
L-Thyroxine 112 µg.

Social History/Participation
Pt. lives c̄– husband and two teenage children in two-storey home; 5 steps to enter c̄– 2 railings and 12 steps to second floor with one railing (on R to ↑).

Bedrooms and bathroom are on second floor. Pt.'s husband works full time and states that he would need additional support to assist in pt.'s daily care skills if she is not independent when she returns home.

Prior Level of Function
Pt. employed as data analyst; works out of her home 4 days/wk using computer and telephone. Before hospitalization, pt. and her husband split daily household duties. Pt. was responsible for the family's money management, laundry, cooking, and shopping. Pt. led active lifestyle—enjoyed jogging every morning with her daughter; actively coached daughter's soccer team, and her husband reports her health as being excellent. Previous recreational activities include camping trips, skiing, and going to the theater.

CASE EXAMPLE 8.3   Documenting Reason for Referral   Setting: Outpatient

Name: Lucy Quick   **D.O.B.:** 9/24/74   **Gender:** Female   **Date:** 9/29/22

REASON FOR REFERRAL
Current Condition
Pt. is self-referred to PT. RA diagnosed 7/2010, primarily affecting hands, wrists, and knees B. Pt. reports recent flare-up approx. 4 wk ago which resulted in pain, stiffness and residual ↓ in wrist ROM B and required course of prednisone (20 mg ×1 wk and then tapered to 5 mg). Current DAS-28 score: 4.52 indicating moderate disease activity

PMH
Pt. reports L knee arthroscopic surgery 2° to meniscal tear in 2006.

Medications
Embrel IM for Rx of RA, 50 mg 1×/wk; prednisone 5 mg daily.

Social History/Participation
Patient lives with husband and two children on the sixth floor of an apartment building with elevator access. No stairs to enter the building. Home is on one level.

Family History
Pt. has family history of autoimmune diseases, including thyroid disease and pernicious anemia.

Prior Level of Function
Patient is a PT and works full time in a children's hospital. She has full responsibility for the care of her household including shopping, cooking, and cleaning activities. She is a very active and engages in some type of physical activity daily including strength training, Pilates, and cycling. She has given up jogging and yoga due to her RA.

CASE EXAMPLE 8.4 Documenting Reason for Referral Setting: Outpatient—cont'd

Name: Stephen Archer   **D.O.B.:** 5/31/67   **Gender:** Male   **Date of Eval.:** 7/21/22

REASON FOR REFERRAL

Current Condition

Pt. states he has been experiencing increased anal pain over the last 2 weeks. He states the pain started after a more anxiety producing period, insomnia and repeated coughing. This pain increases with sitting and is relieved by patient lying down. Pt. reports he had some pain the first time he experienced a colonoscopy. He did develop an abscess following this which was removed and improved his symptoms initially. He reports that he then felt like he was experiencing hemorrhoids and received multiple injections for management but had no long-term improvement in symptoms. He states that he was diagnosed with anal spasms in January 2022.

Sexual Intercourse:
Reports pain with ejaculation but not erection.

Bowel:
Frequency: daily
Bristol Stool Type: 4-5
Straining: slightly, due to pain
Empty: yes

Bladder: denies changes in urination, reports mild discomfort, no hesitancy, empty bladder

Pain: Description: pain in the L posterior perineum region that radiates up into the lumbar region, constant symptoms currently described as achy, 1-7/10

Aggravating Factors: sitting, hiking, LE lifting (mountain climbers, lunges)

PMH
Aortic root dilatation
Aortic valve sclerosis
Cerebral atherosclerosis
Chest pain
Essential hypertension

Fatigue
Gastroesophageal reflux disease
Headache disorder
Hyperlipidemia
Hypothyroidism
Male hypogonadism
Mycoplasma infection
Palpitations
Prostatitis
Right bundle branch block AND left anterior fascicular block
Colonoscopy
Incision and drainage, perianal abscess, superficial

Medications
Lorazepam 0.5 mg oral tablet
Magnesium oxide 400 mg (241.3 mg elemental magnesium) oral tablet, 800 mg = 2 tablets, oral, daily, 3 refills
Prednisone 20 mg oral tablet
Riboflavin 100 mg oral tablet, 300 mg = 3 tablets, oral, daily, 5 refills
Trazodone 50 mg oral tablet

Social History/Participation
Pt. lives with his roommate in a two-bedroom apartment, fifth floor of building with elevators.

Prior Level of Function
Pt. employed as a composer which he primarily does from home but does spend time in studio 3-5 days/mo. Patient led active lifestyle—working out at gym 5 days/week and hiking ~5 miles on weekends.

EXERCISE 8.1

The following statements are from various sections of an initial evaluation report at a pediatric rehabilitation center. Extract the information that would be appropriate to include in the Reason for Referral section of the report. Indicate to which section each statement belongs according to the following codes:

D = Demographic Information, CC = Current Condition, PMH = Past Medical History, MED = Medications, SOC = Social History/Participation, PLF = Prior Level of Function, OTHER = Other (e.g., general health status, family history, developmental history), or N/A = Not Appropriate to include in this section.

1. Chelsea had a fall 4 years ago resulting in R humerus fracture, requiring casting; healed with residual problems.   _____

2. Chelsea has 3/5 strength (MMT) in B quadriceps.   _____

3. Chelsea has a diagnosis of myotonic dystrophy, a form of muscular dystrophy resulting in muscle weakness and accompanied by myotonia (delayed relaxation of muscles after contraction).   _____

4. She is not currently taking any medications.   _____

5. Chelsea enjoys math and art classes at school.   _____

6. There is a history of myotonic dystrophy in Chelsea's family, so Mrs. Green (mother) and Chelsea were very familiar with related symptoms and problems.

_____

7. Chelsea first began showing symptoms of myotonic dystrophy when she was in third grade.

_____

8. Chelsea was referred by the Smithtown School District for this independent PT evaluation to assist in educational planning.

_____

9. Prior to recent fall, Chelsea was able to ascend and descend 2 flights of stairs with use of railing.

_____

10. Chelsea has not had any surgeries or hospitalizations.

_____

11. She lives in a single-family home, with 4 steps to enter, and one set of 12 stairs to reach bedroom.

_____

12. Chelsea will be able to ascend and descend a full flight of stairs.

_____

13. Chelsea is a 12 y.o. girl.

_____

14. Chelsea attends Jonesbridge Middle School and is in sixth grade.

_____

15. Chelsea's primary concern is that she gets fatigued when walking between classes.

_____

EXERCISE 8.2

Each of the following statements could be found in the current condition section of an initial evaluation. First, identify what is wrong with each statement, using the following key to indicate which components are not specified in enough detail: DP = Disease Process, L = Location, or TC = Time Course. Any one or all three components may be problematic. Rewrite a more appropriate and plausible statement in the space provided.

NOTE: A certain amount of clinical knowledge is necessary to provide a clinically plausible statement. It may be necessary to consult textbooks or other resources based on your current knowledge base in a particular area; however, the purpose of these exercises is not to test your clinical knowledge but to obtain practice in appropriate documentation.

Statement	**What Is Wrong?**	**Rewrite Statement**
EXAMPLE: Patient has a strained muscle.	L, TC; also more detail regarding nature of strain could be provided, if known.	Pt. has grade II strain of R quadriceps, sustained 10/1/23.
1. Pt. had heart surgery yesterday.	_____ _____	_____ _____
2. Pt. reports pain starting 5/10/23.	_____ _____	_____ _____

Statement	What Is Wrong?	Rewrite Statement
3. Pt. had a right-sided stroke.		
4. Pt. is an amputee.		
5. Pt. has typical problems related to aging.		
6. Pt. complains of fatigue.		
7. Pt. has a broken leg.		
8. Pt. diagnosed with cancer Nov. 2020.		

EXERCISE 8.3

Each of the following statements could be found in either the past medical history or medication sections of an initial evaluation. None of the statements provide enough detail. Rewrite a more appropriate and plausible statement in the space provided.

Past Medical History — **Rewrite Statement**

1. Pt. has h/o cardiac problems.

3. Pt. has h/o several surgeries.

Past Medical History

5. Pt. is a diabetic.

Medications

6. Pt. is taking multiple medications for various medical conditions.

8. Pt. is taking antispasticity meds.

10. Pt. takes Flexeril once a day.

Rewrite Statement

_____

_____

_____

_____

_____

_____

_____

_____

EXERCISE 8.4

Identify the errors in the following statements documenting social history/participation. Rewrite a more appropriate statement in the space provided.

Statement	What Is Wrong?	Rewrite Statement
EXAMPLE: Pt. cannot return home.	Not enough detail; provide information about home and why patient cannot return to home.	Pt. cannot return home at this time; there are 2 flights of stairs leading to her apartment, and no modifications can be made.
1. Pt. is confined to a wheelchair.		
2. Has poor motivation to return to work.		
3. Works on a loading dock.		

Statement	What Is Wrong?	Rewrite Statement
4. Client enjoys sports.	_____ _____ _____	_____ _____ _____
5. Pt. cannot return to work 2° to architectural barriers.	_____ _____ _____	_____ _____ _____
6. Pt. was very active before her injury.	_____ _____ _____	_____ _____ _____
7. Pt. is in poor shape.	_____ _____ _____	_____ _____ _____
8. Pt. lives in an apartment.	_____ _____ _____	_____ _____ _____
9. Pt. has a history of bad health habits.	_____ _____ _____	_____ _____ _____
10. Pt. uses adaptive equipment.	_____ _____ _____	_____ _____ _____

EXERCISE 8.5

This exercise is designed to practice patient interview techniques for obtaining participation and social history information and to document the findings in the Reason for Referral section of an initial evaluation. Students should form groups of pairs. Two case reports (A and B) can be found in Appendix C for this exercise. One student (acting as patient) should carefully read Case Report A in Appendix C. The second student (acting as therapist) will ask the patient questions aimed at obtaining a comprehensive assessment of social history and participation. The patient should be careful to answer directly only those questions asked by the therapist, based on information provided in the Case Report, but can improvise as needed. Then students should switch roles for Case Report B. The therapist may choose to record answers on a separate sheet of paper and write the final documentation in the space provided.

CASE REPORT A: Setting: Outpatient

Name: Terry O'Connor   **D.O.B.:** 3/23/49   **Date of Eval.:** 7/2/15

Pt. is a 66-year-old female with diagnosis of right hip bursitis.

REASON FOR REFERRAL
Current Condition:

Medications:

PMH:

Social History/Participation:

Prior Level of Function:

CASE REPORT B: Setting: Inpatient Rehabilitation[1]

Name: Tommy Jones   **D.O.B.:** 5/12/95   **Date of Eval.:** 7/2/15   **Admission Date:** 7/2/15

Pt. is a 20-year-old male s/p C7 incomplete SCI secondary to MVA.

REASON FOR REFERRAL
Current Condition:

Medications:

PMH:

Social History/Participation:

Prior Level of Function:

[1]Note: Patient is in a hospital setting, so participation/social history information will be based mainly on patient's abilities and activities before admission to hospital.

Documenting Activities

LEARNING OBJECTIVES

After reading this chapter and completing the exercises, the reader will be able to:

1. Define activities and function.
2. Discuss the factors involved in deciding which activities should be included in physical therapy documentation, including consideration of benchmark activities.
3. Identify and classify various aspects of documenting activities.
4. Appropriately categorize activities of daily living and instrumental activities of daily living.
5. Document activities using a skill-based framework.

DEFINING AND CATEGORIZING ACTIVITIES

This chapter discusses documentation and categorization of Activities. *Activity* as defined by the International Classification of Functioning, Disability and Health (ICF) is the execution of a task or action by an individual. Physical therapists (PTs) often refer to activities as *function, functional ability, functional status, functional activities,* or *functional limitations.* As discussed in Chapter 1, the ICF has an inherently positive approach toward disablement; thus therapists should be encouraged to document those activities a person is *able* to perform. In most cases, documentation should include abilities *and* limitations as they relate to function. However, the primary purpose of the ICF is to shed a positive light on disablement. In this book, we use the term *Activities,* in accordance with ICF terminology, as a global category for documenting skills, abilities, and limitations related to function.

The term *function* is typically used by rehabilitation professionals to describe a person's performance of skills or tasks that are pertinent to their daily life. If an action is to be considered functional, it must (1) be meaningful to an individual and (2) help an individual fulfill their roles (e.g., spouse, parent, volunteer, worker, student, and pet owner).

The *Guide to Physical Therapist Practice 4.0* (the *Guide*) includes five areas that can distinctly be categorized as measuring activities, as shown in Fig. 9.1:

- Community, Social, and Civic Life
- Education Life
- Mobility
- Self-Care and Domestic Life
- Work and Community Integration

These encompass general areas of participation under which activities can be further evaluated.

The *Guide* further distinguishes tests and measures related to body structures and functions, which are primarily related to measurement at the impairment level (see Chapter 10). The differentiation between body structures and functions and activities is often difficult, as in the case of gait and balance, which are classified as body structures and functions. The task of walking is certainly an activity, but describing the details of the gait pattern or the balance needed to maintain walking is more closely related to impairment of body functions. In fact, the differentiation between impairments and activities may be considered a continuum rather than a strict separation. Fig. 9.2 and Box 9.1 illustrate this concept. This continuum is discussed in more detail below.

Activities are arguably the most important component of physical therapy documentation, particularly when they pertain to function. Performance in functional activities is used to justify the need for physical therapy services as well as to show a patient's improvement over time. From a PT's perspective, health conditions and the resulting impairments are important insofar as they affect a patient's daily functioning. *Functional activities* are those that are meaningful to patients: Can they walk, run, get dressed, reach, and grasp for objects? Improvements in these activities should be a primary outcome of physical therapy intervention.

DOCUMENTING TASK PERFORMANCE

The Task Space

Physical therapy intervention often entails practice of specific actions, such as stepping, squatting, lifting, reaching, and grasping. In effect, these actions can be considered *tasks* that are used in a wide range of activities (walking outside, doing laundry, drinking, and eating). PTs often quantify and qualify performance on tasks as a measure of a patient's functional

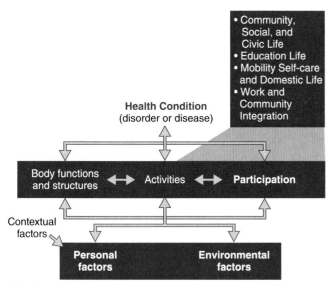

FIG. 9.1 Adaptation of International Classification of Functioning, Disability and Health domains and constructs from *The Guide to Physical Therapist Practice 3.0 and 4.0.* Documentation of Activities encompasses *community, social, and civic life; education life; mobility; self-care and domestic life; work and community integration.*

ability. Stepping, squatting, reaching, and many other types of movement patterns are *elements* of functional activities; they are not functional activities per se. They are not considered activities because they do not have a clearly definable and meaningful goal or purpose. For instance, gait evaluation describes the *movement patterns* used for walking. Gait deviations (e.g., Trendelenburg, excessive circumduction, foot drop) are therefore impairments. Walking to the bathroom and walking outside on the grass to move through a yard describe *activities* because they have a meaningful goal. As stated earlier, functions are actions that are meaningful to an individual and help an individual to fulfill their roles in life. In certain situations, documentation of a patient's performance of tasks outside the context of specific functional activities may be useful.

> **Example:** *A therapist could document a person's ability to reach forward into space or to take steps in the parallel bars. For documentation purposes, such elemental tasks are most logically reported in the Activities section of the report.*

Tasks represent the interface between activities and body structures and functions (see Fig. 9.2). Evaluation of the movement patterns and strategies used to perform such tasks provides important insight into the underlying impairments that affect activities. Task evaluation may bridge many functional skills.

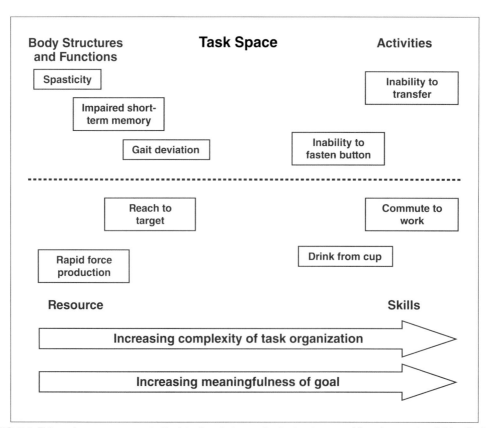

FIG. 9.2 This task space represents the interface between body structures and functions and activities. Tasks can have stronger components of either activities or body functions depending on the nature and goal of the task.

As mentioned in Chapter 1, the ICF model affords different perspectives to describe physical therapy patients and their conditions. A patient's condition can be described in terms of the health condition, body structures and functions, activities, or participation. These are not separate and distinct characteristics of the patient; they are all aspects of the same disabling condition, described in different measurement systems. Furthermore, some overlap occurs between levels of the ICF model.

The classification of an evaluation finding as an impairment versus an activity limitation, and between an activity limitation and participation, is often a slightly gray area.

The crucial distinction between impairments and activity limitations is between means and ends. Activities are described in terms of goals or ends. The impairment level describes means to an end: by what mechanisms the goal is accomplished. This important distinction can be illustrated by comparing assessments of balance and walking.

BALANCE

Balance is a perfect example of a characteristic that is difficult to categorize. In its purest sense, balance is described at the impairment level, reflecting the ability of an individual to maintain an upright position against gravity. However, balance is often evaluated through a set of tasks that might be considered "functional."

> Example: *The ability to stand in one place for more than 30 sec is certainly an activity, as is the ability to reach the floor to pick up an object. Thus if balance is described in terms of the goal, it is an activity. If it is analyzed in terms of the component mechanisms (e.g., increased sway, role of vision), then it is at the impairment level.*

WALKING

Walking is another example of a task that combines both impairments and activity limitations. Therapists often describe walking in functional terms—how long a patient can walk, how quickly, with how much assistance. However, another important component of walking is evaluation of how a person walks—their gait pattern. Gait analysis can be considered a measure at the impairment level.

> Example: *Therapists often describe gait deviations (e.g., a Trendelenburg gait) that reflect the presence of an underlying impairment (gluteus medius weakness). Again, if the walking is measured in terms of goal attainment (e.g., distance, speed), then it is an activity. If gait is analyzed in terms of why the goal is not being achieved (e.g., insufficient knee flexion during swing or inadequate stance phase control of knee extensors), then walking is being described in terms of impairments.*

CLASSIFICATION

Even more problems arise in classification of standardized tests and measures. Standardized tests sometimes measure across different levels of the ICF framework (e.g., measuring some components of activities and some of impairments). This, in fact, may be desirable when a global standardized test is needed.

These difficulties with classification and distinction may seem academic, but documentation can be frustrating if therapists are searching for clear-cut answers (e.g., Is balance an activity or an impairment?). The following strategy is suggested.

All information about a topic (e.g., standing ability, balance control) should be included under one subheading (e.g., standing balance). Even if a particular topic mixes function and impairments, cohesive presentation of that information in the written report is of primary importance (see Case Example 9.1, where standing and sitting ability include components of a balance assessment). Reading a report with information about a single component scattered throughout the report is difficult. Whether the information is categorized under Activities or Impairments can depend on the focus of information being written.

Example: *The ability to squat is an important task for functional activities ranging from using the bathroom to picking up an object. Importantly, therapists may use task analysis to derive a deeper understanding of the contribution of various impairments to activity performance. Documentation of tasks therefore often includes information about how the movement was performed and the effect of any impairments on functional performance.*

Although evaluation of task performance is an important aspect of the physical therapy evaluation process, PTs should give priority to context-based activity assessment.

Example: *Tasks such as reaching and grasping often can be assessed within the context of a functional activity, such as eating or brushing teeth. A person's ability to perform reaching and grasping behaviors is affected by the context in which they are performed (e.g., in a sitting or standing position). Similarly, assessment of gait abnormalities may differ depending on the context in which walking occurs (e.g., walking on tile vs. carpeting).*

Movement Analysis of Tasks

Movement is the process by which an individual acts to achieve goals that are determined by needs, desires, and interactions with the environment. Movements are highly variable, even when an individual is attempting to achieve the same goal (Bernstein, 1967). This variability is a problem when a person is trying to be more consistent in task performance, but it is also necessary during skill acquisition; without variability, an individual may never discover potentially more effective movement patterns. Variability is also important because it is essential for the concept of motor equivalence—that there are usually many ways to achieve a goal.

Analysis of movement during performance of tasks is a core function of physical therapy practice. In 2013 the American Physical Therapy Association (APTA) set forth a vision statement for the physical therapy profession identifying the movement system as central to the identity of physical therapy practice. In 2021 the Academy of Neurologic Physical Therapy's Movement System Task Force proposed a framework for the systematic analysis of movement during tasks (Quinn et al., 2021). This framework supports including core tasks (e.g., sitting, standing, sit to stand, walking, step-ups, and reaching) that should be components of most physical therapy evaluations. In conducting a movement analysis, PTs should observe specific aspects of movement that provide insights into potential motor control impairments (e.g., speed, amplitude, stability, smoothness). Case Example 9.4 provides an example of documentation incorporating movement analysis of tasks.

DOCUMENTING FUNCTIONAL ACTIVITIES

One of the important roles of a PT is to determine *which* activities are meaningful to a specific individual and help that person achieve independence and skill in these activities. Many possible activities could be important for an individual. Pertinent functional activities are those that are related to a person's specific life roles and relevant to the patient's therapy goals. Some activities are common to almost everyone. Other activities are more specific to a person's life roles, such as those required for work or recreational sports.

Box 9.2 presents examples of common activities related to personal, occupational, and leisure roles. Personal activities are further divided into activities of daily living (ADLs) and instrumental activities of daily living (IADLs). ADLs are the basic tasks of everyday life—eating, dressing, bathing, and so on. IADLs are not necessarily critical for everyday functioning but are important for independent functioning within a community—answering the telephone, managing finances, and so on. This list can be used as a guide to documentation of activities. PTs can create subheadings within this section of the report to better organize the information and improve readability (see Case Examples 9.1 to 9.4). It is often useful to group activities or tasks together (e.g., ambulation or transfers) and include all related tasks under their appropriate headings.

BOX 9.2   Documenting Activities: A Suggested List of Activities Related to Personal, Occupational, and Leisure Roles (adapted from the *Guide to Physical Therapist Practice 4.0*). Therapists can use this list as a guideline when determining which activities to document for a patient.

CORE TASKS
- Sitting
- Standing
- Sit to stand
- Walking
- Step-ups/stairs
- Reach, grasp, manipulate

SELF-CARE AND DOMESTIC LIFE
Activities of Daily Living
- Bed mobility
- Transfers
- Dressing
- Toileting
- Grooming
- Oral care
- Bathing
- Self-care
- Eating
- Ambulation and mobility within the home (including wheelchair mobility)
- Climbing stairs

Instrumental Activities of Daily Living
- Ability to use telephone
- Shopping
- Food preparation
- Housekeeping
- Laundry
- Transportation
- Management of medications
- Management of finances

WORK LIFE
- Traveling to work
- Sitting at desk
- Moving around office
- Writing, using computer
- Lifting objects
- Other specific work-related tasks

EDUCATION LIFE
- Traveling to school
- Sitting at desk
- Moving around school
- Writing, using computer
  For young children, this can include play-related activities, such as:
- Ball playing
- Jumping
- Running
- Doing puzzles
- Stacking blocks
- Stringing beads

COMMUNITY, SOCIAL, AND CIVIC LIFE
- Volunteer work, involvement in community organizations
- Going to the movies
- Socializing with friends
- Hobbies (e.g., sewing, stamp collecting)
- Exercising/physical activities
- Playing recreational sports

Documentation of activities should be customized to the particular setting. The focus of activity documentation for a patient who resides in a nursing home would likely be on ADLs. In contrast, a therapist may perform a specific worksite evaluation for a 50-year-old patient with low back pain; in this case, the activity documentation would be limited to occupational activities.

For most patients who reside at home or will be returning home, the PT is responsible for evaluating those activities that are pertinent to different environmental situations. Therapists must consider the type of environment in which the patient will be required to function. Most activities can be performed in many different environments. For instance, the task of "walking" can occur in a controlled, closed environment, such as the physical therapy gym in a hospital. Walking also can occur in a more variable and open environment, such as walking across a busy street. Thus simply documenting the task of "walking" is not particularly meaningful if it is devoid of environmental context. Therapists must take care to assess a range of environmental contexts as they are *meaningful* to a specific patient. (See Gentile's "Taxonomy of Tasks" for more information on environmental and task classification [Gentile, 2000].)

Functional skills for children assume a slightly different meaning. Throughout the course of childhood, the activities and environments that children encounter can change greatly. In early childhood, children need to access various environments—for example, playgrounds, playgroups, cars, or public transportation—and they can perform a wide variety of tasks within those environments, such as climbing, getting up and down from the floor, and walking. As a child gets older, the school environment becomes important, and they would perform activities such as retrieving books from a library shelf, carrying a lunch tray, or navigating hallways.

In addition, although children generally perform many of the same personal roles as adults (e.g., bathing, dressing, eating, and general mobility), their work and leisure activities clearly differ. "Play skills" encompass a child's work and leisure activities, particularly for younger children. In physical therapy, such skills are often categorized as gross motor skills. Documentation of pediatric evaluations often includes a section on gross motor skills and a separate section on self-care or self-help skills (see Chapter 16).

Choosing Which Activities to Document

PTs can document many possible activity limitations. How does a therapist choose which activities to document? In some situations, occupational therapists (OTs) will be involved in functional assessment, particularly for ADLs and IADLs. In such cases, PTs and OTs should collaborate and coordinate their documentation of functional abilities to avoid overlap.

When a PT is the only rehabilitation professional working with a patient, many functions may be relevant to the patient's care. Evaluation and documentation of all functions would be impractical and unnecessarily time-consuming. In those cases, therapists must **prioritize** the functions that are most critical to the patient at the present time.

BOX 9.3   Choosing Which Activities to Measure

The following guidelines should be used in deciding which activities should be measured and documented:
- Consider the practice setting—for example, hospital, outpatient, and home care. It will most significantly influence the PT's choice of functional skill documentation. Some agencies/hospitals mandate evaluation of specific functional skills. Collaboration with other health professionals, such as OTs, will eliminate unnecessary redundancy.
- Choose activities that are meaningful to the patient, family members/caregivers, or both.
- Prioritize activities that are most critical to the patient at this time in their rehabilitation.
- Choose **benchmark** activities—those that are amenable to showing improvement as a result of physical therapy intervention. This will differ depending on the patient and their stage of learning. Simple tasks like transfers may be most useful early in rehabilitation, whereas more complex tasks like shopping or preparing meals are usually more appropriate later.

Example: *An individual who has had a severe brain injury and is just learning to sit and stand without assistance will likely be unable to perform most or all of the personal, occupational, and leisure activities that they were able to perform before the injury. Documentation at an early point in the patient's recovery would likely focus on their ability to perform basic daily care skills. As the patient begins to recover from the head injury, the therapist may begin to evaluate and document different types of skills, such as those related to IADLs or occupational activities. Conversely, a patient with rotator cuff tendonitis may have minimal limitations in functional abilities. The patient may be able to perform all daily living, work, and most leisure activities, and they may be limited only in the ability to participate in a specific recreational sport activity.*

Often the purpose of documenting activities is to demonstrate, at some later point, improvement in these activities over time. In many situations in which a large number of possible functional activities can be measured, therapists can choose to measure and document performance on a few activities that can be used as *benchmarks* (Box 9.3). These activities serve as measures of progress. Therapists should carefully choose as benchmarks those activities that are most meaningful to the patient and sensitive to showing improvement as a result of intervention.

Documentation in the Absence of Activity Limitations

Sometimes therapists report that patients have no specific activity limitations, only impairments that could lead to a potential limitation at some later point if intervention is not provided. For patients who are seen for a current medical condition, third-party payers typically argue that there should be one or more activity limitations to justify *skilled intervention* by a PT.[1] If no activity limitation is present, then the therapist may need to further justify why skilled services are needed.

---

[1]Documentation of skilled intervention is currently a requirement for reimbursement of physical therapy services for Medicare. The key issue is whether the skills of a therapist are needed to treat the illness or injury.

Example: *An elderly client with lack of range of motion of the shoulder joint may be referred for physical therapy. The client has no limitation in performing functional activities but lacks several degrees of joint range of motion in shoulder flexion and abduction (an impairment). The therapist would be prudent to instruct the patient in range of motion and other therapeutic exercises to prevent further loss of range of motion and maintain shoulder strength. However, if this impairment in range of motion does not result in activity limitations or participation restrictions, justifying the need for extended skilled services to third-party payers may be difficult.*

Many therapists provide intervention aimed at *preventing* or *maintaining* participation restrictions and activity limitations. Although it may be difficult to justify the medical necessity for such services, PT intervention may nonetheless be appropriate. Preventive intervention is an important part of PT practice; however, reimbursement by third-party payers may require specific justification and additional documentation. Therapists are encouraged to document *potential* participation restrictions and/or activity limitations that may occur if the underlying pathological condition or impairments are not addressed. In fact, such documentation may be helpful in justifying the role of preventive physical therapy services as standard of care.

MEASUREMENT OF ACTIVITIES

Levels of Assistance

One of the most common ways in which performance of activities, and in particular functional activities, are measured is through level of assistance. Level of assistance refers to how much assistance an individual typically requires to successfully complete a task. Level of assistance is frequently measured by determining an estimated percentage of assistance provided by the therapist or caregiver for performing ADLs (Full & Chui, 2024).

Skill-Based Measurement

Level of assistance provides a relatively small component in the evaluation of a person's functional abilities. In almost all cases, documentation of activities—ADLs, IADLs, or other activities—should exceed simple level of assistance and assess some components of skilled performance. *Skill* can be defined as the ability to achieve a desired outcome with *consistency, flexibility,* and *efficiency* (Gentile, 2000). Table 9.1 outlines a skill-based model for the evaluation of functional activities and provides examples of objective ways in which functional abilities can be documented.

The particular aspects of a skill that a therapist chooses to measure depend on the task and the patient's level of skill. If a patient requires a high level of assistance to accomplish a task, a skill-based assessment may be limited (see Case Example 9.1). Furthermore, documentation of skill can involve any *one* or *all* of these three components: consistency, flexibility, and efficiency.

> **Example:** *In early skill learning the level of assistance and consistency of performance may be more valuable measures than efficiency and flexibility. Such measures may not be meaningful until a higher level of skill is achieved.*

STANDARDIZED TESTS AND MEASURES

Functional and Mobility Assessments

Many different standardized tests and measures are useful in assessing functional skills. Table 9.2 lists some commonly used tests of functional performance and general mobility. Several books and resources provide detailed information on the many functional assessment tools in current use, including their intended purpose (APTA Evidence-Based Practice Resources: www.apta.org/patient-care/evidence-based-practice-resources; Rehabilitation Measures Database-Shirley Ryan Ability Lab: www.sralab.org/rehabilitation-measures; see also Chapter 4 on Standardized Outcome Measures).

TABLE 9.1	A Skill-Based Model of Documenting Functional Performance		
Skill Component	**Definition**	**Examples**	**Documentation Example**
Consistency	Ability to successfully perform a skill repeatedly over multiple trials or days	• Rate of goal achievement (number of successes/number of attempts) • Number of days/week able to perform • Accuracy (spatial measures of errors; number of errors)	*Patient is able to transfer from bed to wheelchair using sliding board 3 out of 5 mornings with assistance of husband only for setup.*
Flexibility	Ability to perform a skill under a variety of environmental conditions	• Height, surface, position of equipment/objects • Environment (e.g., open vs. closed) • Ability to do two tasks at once	*Patient walks up 6 steps in home (8″ high) with railing; unable to carry objects in hands. Requires verbal reminders for foot placement to walk up 4 steps outside (10″ high) with railing.*
Efficiency	Ability to perform a skill within a certain level of energy expenditure (cardiovascular and musculoskeletal)	• Time to complete task • Distance completed • Speed of movement • Heart rate, respiratory rate, or blood pressure changes	*Patient can walk from bed into bathroom (10 ft) in 14.2 sec (average time/3 trials), with increase in heart rate (HR) to 100 bpm.*

TABLE 9.2 Some Commonly Used Standardized Measures of Activities (Listed Alphabetically)[a]

Measure	Purpose	Population/Setting
Activities of Balance Confidence Scale (ABC) (Powell & Meyers, 1995)	Subjective measure of confidence in performing various ambulatory activities without falling or experiencing a sense of unsteadiness	Elderly; general rehabilitation
Acute Care Index of Function (ACIF) (Van Dillen & Roach, 1988)	20-Item scale designed to measure functional status at levels appropriate to acute care setting; items divided into four categories: mental status, bed mobility, transfers, and mobility (wheelchair and ambulation)	Acute care
Barthel Index (Mahoney & Barthel, 1965)	Consists of 10 items that measure a person's daily functioning, specifically activities of daily living (ADLs) and mobility	Elderly; general rehabilitation
Cincinnati Knee Rating Scale Function Assessment (CKRS) (Barber-Westin et al., 1984)	Includes a functional assessment based on six abilities important for participation in sports: walking, using stairs, squatting and kneeling, straight running, jumping and landing, and making hard twist, cuts, and pivots	Patients with knee pain or dysfunction
Disability of the Arm, Shoulder and Hand Questionnaire (DASH) and Quick DASH (Hudak et al., 1996)	30-Item, 5-level ordinal scale (0–4), measuring functional difficulty and symptoms resulting from upper extremity dysfunction; Quick DASH is a shortened version using 11 items	General; for assessment of upper extremity problems
Emory Functional Ambulation Profile (EFAP) (Wolf et al., 1999)	Assesses performance of walking ability based on varying environmental contexts	General rehabilitation
Instrumental Activities of Daily Living (Lawton & Brody, 1969)	Rates ability to perform eight different instrumental ADLs on a 0–2 scale	General rehabilitation
Jebsen test of hand function (Jebsen et al., 1969)	Timed pegboard test with norms established; primarily manipulation and reaching	Hand and upper extremity impairments
Lower Extremity Functional Scale (LEFS) (Binkley et al., 1999)	20-Item, 5-level ordinal scale (0–4); used to evaluate the functional impairment of a patient with a disorder of one or both lower extremities	Orthopedic lower extremity impairments
Motor Assessment Scale (MAS) (Carr & Shepherd, 1998)	Evaluates performance of seven functionally based tasks; rating based on movement patterns used to accomplish the task	Stroke
Outpatient Physical Therapy Improvement in Movement Assessment Log (OPTIMAL) (Guccione et al., 2005)	Measures difficulty and self-confidence in performing 21 movements that are necessary components of various functional activities	Outpatient
Patient-Specific Functional Scale (PSFS) (Stratford et al., 1995)	Individualized measure that asks a patient to list three activities that they are unable to do or have difficulty with and to rate the level of difficulty on a 0–10 scale	General
Six-Minute Walk Test (6MWT) (Guyatt et al., 1985)	Measures the distance a patient can quickly walk on a flat, hard surface in 6 min	Cardiac, adult neurological
Timed Up and Go Test (TUG) (Podsiadlo & Richardson, 1991)	Measures time to stand up from a chair, walk 10 ft, turn around, walk back, and sit down	Geriatric, rehabilitation, falls risk assessment
Tuft's Assessment of Motor Performance (TAMP) (Gans et al., 1988)	Motor assessment for use with adults, with 32 mobility, ADL, and communication test items rated on a 6-point proficiency scale and time recorded for task completion	General rehabilitation

[a]Refer to references listed to determine each measure's proper use and measurement properties.

As discussed in Chapter 4, many standardized assessments measure across more than one level of the ICF model.

Example: *Some tests measure both impairment and activities. An example of such a test is the Berg Balance Scale (Berg et al., 1992). This scale measures standing balance at the impairment level, as in standing with eyes closed or with a narrowed base of support, and at the functional activity level, as in picking up an object from the floor.*

The tests and measures presented in Table 9.2 *primarily* measure performance in functional activities but may have components of participation or impairment assessments or both.

Physical Activity Measures

Measures of physical activity are being used more frequently in rehabilitation, both as an outcome measure as well as a measure of overall health status (see Table 9.3). Direct measures of physical activity use technologies such as pedometers,

TABLE 9.3 List of Commonly Used Standardized Measures of Physical Activity (Indirect Measurement)

Measure	Description/Purpose
7-Day Physical Activity Recall (PAR) (Sallis et al., 1985)	Estimates both work-related and nonwork-related physical activity. For each day of the past week, participants report the approximate number of hours they slept and spent in moderate, hard, and very hard activity.
Community Healthy Activities Model Program for Seniors: Activities Questionnaire for Older Adults (CHAMPS) (Stewart et al., 2001)	Assesses weekly frequency and duration of various physical activities typically undertaken by older adults.
International Physical Activity Questionnaire (IPAQ) (Craig et al., 2003)	The IPAQ includes a short-form and long-form of physical activity questions. The IPAQ has been translated into many different languages and therefore can be used to obtain internationally comparable data on health-related physical activity.
Physical Activity Scale for the Elderly (PASE) (Washburn et al., 1993)	Measures the level of physical activity in individuals aged 65 years and older. It contains measures of self-reported occupational, household, and leisure activities during a 1-week period.
Rapid Assessment of Physical Activity (RAPA) (Topolski et al., 2006)	Designed to provide clinicians with a tool for quickly assessing the level of physical activity of older adult patients. It has been found to be reliable and valid compared with the longer, validated CHAMPS.

accelerometers, indirect calorimetry, and heart rate monitoring to measure such aspects as step counts, energy expenditure, or actual movement. With the rapid development of wearable technologies such as FitBit, Garmin and Apple Watch, to name a few, such assessment of physical activity and general health status may quickly become the norm in standardized rehabilitation assessments.

Such direct measures of physical activity are generally considered more accurate and are not prone to recall biases compared to questionnaires (Kowalski et al., 2012). Physical activity questionnaires depend on the ability of an individual to accurately recall their level of activity, typically over a 1-week period. These are often categorized according to the degree of intensity of the activity, such as light, moderate, or intense, and can include specific activities such as number of steps or time spent walking. Use of quantitative measures of physical activity can be used to evaluate activity levels and to facilitate goal setting (e.g., increasing steps per week).

SUMMARY

- Documenting activities, and in particular functional activities, is likely the most important component of physical therapy documentation and is used to justify the need for physical therapy services.
- For an activity to be considered functional, it must (1) be meaningful to an individual and (2) help an individual to fulfill their life roles.
- A specific function cannot be separated from the context in which it was performed. Thus context-specific documentation is a critical feature of reporting a patient or client's functional status.
- Rather than document all possible activities, the PT should prioritize the activities that are most meaningful to the patient and are amenable to change and should consider benchmark activities: those that are amenable to showing improvement as a result of physical therapy intervention.
- Therapists must document specific activity limitations that are related to certain impairments or a health condition. In preventive care, this may include documenting *potential* participation restrictions, activity limitations, or both.
- Skill can be defined as the ability to achieve a desired outcome with *consistency*, *flexibility*, and *efficiency*. These components can be used to provide reliable and measurable documentation of activities beyond level of assistance.

CASE EXAMPLE 9.1 Documenting Activities Setting: Home Care

Name: Maureen Smith **D.O.B.:** 5/12/61 **Gender:** Female **Date of Eval.:** 7/3/23

Current Condition
A 61 y.o. female c̄ L-sided cerebral hemorrhage 5/14/23 with resulting R-sided hemiparesis; discharged on 7/1/23 from Rehab Center, where she spent 4 wk after acute care stay at Community Hospital.

ACTIVITIES
Standardized Tests
Barthel Index: 25/100 indicating moderate functional impairment requiring assistance for most activities. *Motor Assessment Scale:* 16/48 indicating moderate functional impairment.

Bed Mobility
Pt. is using a hospital bed with trapeze at home. Pt. rolls to R I using side rails; rolls to L c̄ min A to bring R leg over. Needs mod A to position self in bed c̄ use of trapeze.

Sitting Ability
On bed: Bed needs to be positioned so pt.'s feet are flat on floor. Able to sit for 10 min independently (limited due to reported fatigue). Unable to reach >1″ outside arm's length in all directions without LOB in the direction of the reach. **In wheelchair:** Pt. can sit in W/C for up to 30 min; begins to lean to R side after 15 min and cannot straighten self s A.

Sit-to-Stand/Standing Ability
Pt. requires mod A to come to stand with RUE supported on kitchen counter. Once up and positioned, pt. can maintain static standing with RUE support for 20 sec c̄ R AFO and c̄ min A.

Transfer W/C ↔ Bed
Uses SB to transfer from bed →W/C (toward the L side only) and W/C → bed (toward the L side only) with min A to set up SB and begin initial movement on board. Completes task in approx. 1 min.

Mobility
Pt. uses W/C as primary means of mobility in home. Can propel W/C with one-arm drive in home except into bathroom (too narrow). Outside mobility limited to propulsion on level surfaces for 5 min, HR ↑ to 110 beats per minute. Requires A to negotiate curbs, ramps, and uneven terrain.

Feeding
Pt. needs max A to set up for plate, utensils, and cup but can then eat I with spoon or fork with L hand. Uses modified scoop-plate to get food onto utensil. Needs max A to cut foods. Can drink using a light cup or with a straw. Self-care, grooming, and bathroom transfers: Refer to OT eval.

CASE EXAMPLE 9.2 Documenting Activities Setting: Outpatient

Name: Rich Green **D.O.B.:** 8/2/58 **Gender:** Non-Binary **Sex:** Male **Date of Eval.:** 6/15/23

Current Condition
Pt. is a 63 y.o. carpenter s/p R rotator cuff repair on 4/2/23 2° fall from ladder (8-wk postop).

ACTIVITIES
Transportation
Pt. able to drive up to 45 min at a time. Pt. reports pain ↑ from 2/10 at rest to 5/10 while driving >15 min. Reports needing to frequently rest R arm.

Ambulation
No limitations in amb when not carrying items. Pt. is able to carry up to 3-lb item in R hand while walking for up to 1 min before reports of fatigue. Able to ascend/descend full flight of stairs (12 stairs) carrying only up to 5 lb (e.g., tray, laundry basket) with both hands s ↑ in pain.

Household Activities
Pt. is able to reach 2nd shelf (26″ above waist) in cupboard with only minimal elevation of shoulder, with pain rating of 2/10.

Dressing
Able to don a button-down shirt or pullover shirt I within 30 sec.

Outcome Measures
DASH Patient Questionnaire: 49.2% impairment.

CASE EXAMPLE 9.3 Documenting Activities Setting: Inpatient Acute Rehabilitation

Name: Kareem Patel **D.O.B.:** 3/23/48 **Gender:** Male **Date of Eval.:** 6/21/22

Current Condition
Pt. is s/p AAA repair, 10 days postop.

ACTIVITIES
Ambulation
Pt. walks within room unassisted. Requires supervision for ambulation outside room for fatigue monitoring.

6-Minute Walk Test
Distance Walked: 50-foot circuit × 3 for total of 150 ft; *Surface:* Indoor/level/tile; *Device:* Rolling walker; *Bracing:* None; *Assistance:* CG; *Supplemental Oxygen Used:* 2 L/m NC.

Borg Rating of Perceived Fatigue/Exertion
11.

Posttest
HR 70 beats per minute; BP 142/70 mm Hg; RR 24 breaths/min; O_2 saturation 91%.

Stairs
Able to ascend/descend six steps CG, step to step with one hand on railing. HR post: 96 beats per minute; BP: 140/82 mm Hg.

ADLs
Pt. is I in all ADLs. Able to stand for up to 2 min at a time for daily care routine (brushing teeth, combing hair, shaving); takes two breaks in a 5-min period. IADLs assessed by OT.

(Continued)

CASE EXAMPLE 9.3   Documenting Activities   Setting: Inpatient Acute Rehabilitation—cont'd

Name: Kareem Patel   **D.O.B.:** 3/23/48   **Gender:** Male   **Date of Eval.:** 6/21/22

SECTION: GG MOBILITY

	Independent—06	Setup/Cleanup Assist—05	Supervision/Touch Assist—04	Partial/Mod Assist—03	Substantial/Max Assist—02	Dependent—01	Refused—07	NA—Not Performed Prior—09	NA—Envir. Limits—10	NAMedical/Safety—88
Roll left and right										
Lying to sitting on side of bed										
Sit to lying										
Sit to stand										
Chair, bed to chair transfer										
Car transfer										
Picking up object										
Walk 10 ft	X									
Walk 50 ft with 2 turns			X							
Walk 150 ft			X							
Walking 10 ft on uneven surfaces										
1 Step (curb)			X							
4 Steps			X							
12 Steps										X

GG Mobility refers to Section GG is part of a standardized assessment through the Centers for Medicare and Medicaid Services (CMS).

CASE EXAMPLE 9.4   Documenting Activities   Setting: Telerehabilitation

Name: Carter Cornell   **DOB:** 8/30/1969   **Gender:** Male   **Date of Eval.:** 7/27/23

Current Condition

Pt is a 54-year-old male who racially identifies as white, with a past medical history (PMHx) of high cholesterol controlled with atorvastatin. He was diagnosed with Spinocerebellar Ataxia (SCA) Type 2 in 2020 based on clinical presentation and extensive family history of SCA2 with family members having genetic confirmation. Symptoms of ataxia and imbalance began in 2019. The mSARA score for pt denotes early disease, however, progressive symptoms of imbalance and ataxia have led to decreased physical activity. Despite continued home exercise for 30-minutes, 2x/week, they noted disease progression, making them fearful to engage in activities that challenged balance. Pts primary goal was to improve exercise tolerance and balance confidence to continue working.

ACTIVITIES

Patient-reported Measures

Activities Specific Balance Confidence Scale: 72.5%
Exercise Self Efficacy Scale: 46/90 (primary barriers to exercise mood, friends/family, equipment)

Performance-based Measures

30 Second Sit to Stand Test: 10 repetitions (*leaning to R side t/o)
Rise to Toes: 3 seconds without support
Timed Up and Go Test (Single Task): 9.45 seconds
Timed Up and Go Test (Single Task): 12.02 seconds

Gait Speed (over 20 ft): 1.025 m/s
mCTSIB:
FT e/o firm 30 sec
- Quality: Minimal sway, multi-directional, Pt with ankle response.
FT e/o firm 30 sec
- Quality: Mild-moderate multidirectional sway, however predominant retropulsion observed. Clear muscle contraction throughout legs to stabilize.
FT e/o compliant 30 sec
- Quality: Mild sway multi-directional sway but predominant lean to the L
FT e/o compliant 30 sec
- Quality: Mild-moderate directional sway predominant lean to the L
  - Tandem e/o, firm: 16.71 sec
- Quality: Large M/L sway, arms flailing, reaching for support for added balance. Falling towards the R, with LLE back.
  - Tandem e/c, firm: unable
  - Single Leg Stance:
- Left: 1.75 seconds
- Quality: Hip strategy, arms flailing out for added balance. Multi-directional sway.
- Right: 5.45 seconds
- Quality: Hip strategy, arms flailing out for added balance. Multi-directional sway.

CASE EXAMPLE 9.4   Documenting Activities   Setting: Telerehabilitation — cont'd

Movement Analysis of Tasks

Sitting	Participant was able to maintain upright position, very mild intermittent sway ws observed without back support, position maintained without UE stabilization, pt has appropriate BOS. Weight was symmetrical, no symptom provocation.
Sit to Stand	Pt demonstrated appropriate amplitude forward with adequate hip/knee/ankle flexion during early lift phase, a few instances of instability at termination of movement into stance, however pt able to independently recover. Also during movement pt demonstrated listing to the right throughout the entire sit to stand and appropriate extension to hip/knee/ankle during extension however there was a rebound moment at termination which affected stability. Pt was able to independently stabilize. Cautious speed throughout the motion, although speed within normal limits. The task was smooth with the exception of termination rebound, and timing was appropriate.
Standing	Body segments were aligned in all three planes and body oriented with gravity. No UE stabilization required for task, and pt has appropriate BOS, although feet were ER possibly for added stability. No symptom provocation.
Walking	BOS was widened, steps were shortened B with some variability in length. LLE achieved inconsistent foot clearance and frequently did not pass standing limb during swing phase. UE swing was limited bilat with limited trunk rotation although sequencing was appropriate. The body progressed to achieve an adequate trailing limb position B. Turns were segmented, and not fluid (5 steps required). Speed of gait is slow for his age, but appropriate for this setting. When the task was repeated, the pt was consistent with performance. No provocation of symptoms.
Step Up	Placement of the leading limb onto the step was completed with a smooth, continuous and efficient trajectory with RLE lead, but when LLE lead (RLE stance) lack of weight transfer to the right was notable necessitating holding on to external support. Whole body ascent/descent was smooth and fluid B. Appropriate amplitude was demonstrated by the trailing limb B. When repeated, the pt is able to demonstrate learning response and improvement of form with decreased UE support required.

▮ EXERCISE 9.1

Identify the errors in the following statements documenting Activities. Rewrite a more appropriate statement in the space provided.

Statement	Rewrite Statement
EXAMPLE: Demonstrates poor sitting balance.	Pt. is able to sit for 10 sec on side of bed, feet flat on floor, before losing balance to the right side. Needs assistance to return to an upright sitting position.
1. Able to walk 50 ft.	
2. Able to eat with a spoon with occasional assistance.	
3. Pt. is confined to using a wheelchair for long-distance mobility.	
4. Able to climb a few stairs.	

Statement   **Rewrite Statement**

5. Can throw a ball but cannot catch one.

6. Can walk on uneven surfaces.

7. Pt. is not motivated to walk.

8. Dresses upper body with difficulty.

9. Walks slowly.

10. Pt. does not drive.

11. C/o pain during standing.

12. Transfers with assistance.

13. Pt. can lift various sized boxes.

Statement	Rewrite Statement
14. Pt. cannot get up from a low chair.	_____ _____ _____ _____
15. Pt. is having trouble sitting for extended periods at work.	_____ _____ _____

EXERCISE 9.2

The following statements are from an initial evaluation report written in a hospital setting. For statements that do not belong in the Activities section, write NA (not appropriate) on the line provided. For statements that do belong in the Activities section, use Box 9.2 to determine a probable subheading (e.g., transfers, ambulation) under which this information could be listed.
Example: Pt. is able to use commode in her bedroom with min A to transfer. <u>toileting</u>

1. Pt. walks 100 ft in hospital hallway $\bar{c}$ supervision, $\bar{c}$ ↑ in HR to 120 beats per minute. _____

2. Pt. performs daily morning routine of brushing teeth and shaving within 5 min $\bar{s}$ SOB while sitting 2/3 days. _____

3. Pt. can ↑↓ 10 stairs with 1 railing, step over step, in 22 sec. _____

4. Strength B knee extension 4/5. _____

5. Pt. has 20-yr history of Type 1 DM. _____

6. Pt. transfers from bed to W/C $\bar{c}$ supervision. _____

7. Able to stand with min A in hospital room for up to 2 min; limited due to fatigue (HR increase to 102 beats per minute). _____

8. PROM R knee flexion 110°. _____

9. Pt. can ↑↓ 6″ and 8″ curbs $\bar{c}$ CG. _____

10. Pt. performed ADLs I before surgery. _____

11. Able to dress upper body independently; requires mod A to reach down to put on pants and don shoes and socks from a seated position. _____

12. Able to come from supine to sitting on edge of bed with contact guarding. _____

13. Pt. is able to prepare simple meals not requiring stove-top cooking or carrying pots/pans >2 lb. _____

EXERCISE 9.3

For each of the occupations listed, write a list of functional activities that would be most appropriate to document in the Activities section for a theoretical patient. They should be activities specific to the patient's particular occupation.

Bus driver

_____

_____

Homemaker

_____

_____

College student

_____

_____

Administrative assistant

_____

_____

Professional basketball player

_____

_____

Documenting Impairments in Body Structure and Function

LEARNING OBJECTIVES

After reading this chapter and completing the exercises, the reader will be able to:

1. Define impairments in body structure and function.
2. Appropriately classify impairments into categories for documentation purposes.
3. Document impairments concisely using appropriate terminology and abbreviations.
4. Describe the documentation of a systems review.
5. Describe the five characteristics of documenting pain.

DEFINING AND CATEGORIZING IMPAIRMENTS

According to the International Classification of Functioning, Disability and Health (ICF) model, body structures are defined as anatomic parts of the body such as organs, limbs, and their components. Body functions are physiological functions of the body (including psychological functions) (Fig. 10.1). Thus *impairments* are identified problems in body function or structure such as a significant deviation or loss.

Physical therapists (PTs) evaluate the functioning of a wide range of body structures, including those related to the musculoskeletal, neurological, cardiopulmonary, and integumentary systems. In evaluating these systems, PTs attempt to ascertain the nature and extent of any impairments that may be contributing to a patient's activity limitations or participation restrictions. The body structures and functions that a therapist chooses to evaluate for a particular patient are based on the patient's activity limitations and their underlying health condition. A comprehensive consideration of all possible impairments is beyond the scope of this chapter, but the key aspects of documenting commonly assessed impairments are discussed.

The *Guide to Physical Therapist Practice* (the *Guide*) provides a list of the tests and measures typically used by PTs. Fig. 10.1 provides a listing of the tests and measures described in the *Guide* that evaluate the level of body structures and function. As emphasized in Chapter 7, the *Guide* does not organize tests and measures according to impairment and activity. This differentiation is often difficult and may be perceived as a continuum rather than a strict separation (see Fig. 10.2).

When categorizing impairments, it can be useful to create headings that organize impairment documentation in an evaluation report or progress note. The *Guide* presents a categorization of the tests and measures used in physical therapy. These headings can be used for documentation purposes and provide a reasonable approach to organizing this section of an evaluation. However, impairments may be categorized in many ways depending on the patient's medical condition, the facility, and the personal preferences of the therapist (see Case Examples at the end of this chapter).

SYSTEMS REVIEW

Part of the decision-making process in physical therapy involves choosing which impairments to measure based on the patient's activity limitations and their underlying health condition. However, all PTs must perform certain basic assessment procedures and document them accordingly. One such set of measures includes a **systems review**. A systems review includes: (1) a brief or limited hands-on examination of cardiovascular and pulmonary, integumentary, musculoskeletal, and neuromuscular systems; (2) the communication ability, affect, cognition, language, ability to read, and learning style; and (3) movement assessment (*Guide to Physical Therapist Practice 4.0*). Importantly, information included in a systems review is screening, and depending on the nature of the patient's condition and the results of this screening, a more detailed assessment of these areas may be necessary.

For example, if an elderly patient is referred with shoulder pain, the following information would be important to include in a systems review: blood pressure/heart rate (cardiovascular), communication, and cognition. In addition, skin assessment (integumentary), range of motion (ROM), and strength in the lower extremities in addition to the upper extremities (musculoskeletal), and any neurological signs

- Aerobic capacity/
  endurance
- Anthropometric
  characteristics
- Balance
- Circulation
- Cranial and peripheral
  nerve integrity
- Gait
- Integumentary integrity
- Joint integrity and
  mobility
- Motor function
- Muscle performance
- Neuromotor
  development and
  sensory processing
- Pain
- Posture
- Range of motion
- Reflex integrity
- Sensory integrity
- Skeletal integrity
- Ventilation and
  Respiration

Health Condition
(disorder or disease)

Body functions
and structures ◄► Activities ◄► **Participation**

Contextual
factors

**Personal
factors**   **Environmental
factors**

FIG. 10.1 Adaptation of International Classification of Functioning, Disability and Health (ICF) domains and constructs from *Guide to Physical Therapist Practice 4.0.* Documentation of Impairments in Body Structure and Function includes 20 tests and measures listed in the *Guide* (listed alphabetically).

such as sensory changes or reflexes (neuromuscular) should also be assessed as part of general screening.

The cases at the end of this chapter and in Chapter 7 provide examples of systems review documentation for different patient populations.

STRATEGIES FOR DOCUMENTING IMPAIRMENTS

Choosing Which Impairments to Document

The general approach of this text is to evaluate and report those results that are relevant to the patient's current condition and that are necessary to develop an adequate rationale for the diagnosis, goals, and plan of care. Good clinical practice for any PT evaluation typically includes documentation of some specific body functions, including ROM, strength and posture, and a general systems review. Measurement of additional impairments

are then guided by the medical condition and the presentation of activity limitations.

> **Example:** *Assessment of balance and muscle tone would be important in a patient with Parkinson disease who has walking difficulty and has a history of falls.*

If a patient is *at risk* for developing an impairment because of a particular medical condition, the absence of impairment should be documented.

> **Example:** *In a patient with severe diabetes and associated peripheral vascular disease, the skin condition of the feet should be checked regularly and documented because tissue necrosis is a risk in these patients.*

Specificity of Documenting Impairments

Quantifiable and objective data should be provided for impairment measures to be useful for diagnostic or evaluative purposes. Therapists should take care to document impairments with clarity and precision, avoiding vague and ambiguous terminology. Terms such as *minimal*, *moderate*, and *maximal* or *good*, *fair*, and *poor* are not particularly useful in descriptions of impairments and should be used sparingly in favor of more measurable, quantifiable assessments. Case Examples 10.1 to 10.5 give examples of documenting commonly assessed impairments in a concise but specific manner.

Documenting Normal or Typical Findings

An assessment of body structures and functions must include documentation of the results of every test or measure that the therapist has performed, even if the findings were negative (i.e., normal). Documentation of normal findings can occur when the findings are directly relevant to confirming, refuting, or reshaping the movement-based or medical diagnosis.

> **Example:** *If a patient has pain in their shoulder, and strength and ROM of the neck and shoulder are normal, these specific findings would be important to document.*

Therapists sometimes use two general terms, **WNL** (within normal limits) or **WFL** (within functional limits), to indicate "normal" or "typical" findings. The authors strongly discourage the use of WFL, as there is no accepted definition for this term and different professionals reading a note may interpret it in different ways. WNL can be used to describe the results of a quick screening examination, when findings are judged to be within a typically acceptable range, but have not explicitly been measured.

STANDARDIZED TESTS AND MEASURES

Many impairment-based measures used in physical therapy are quantitative, with measurements such as degrees (e.g., ROM), circumference (e.g., limb girth), or force (e.g., muscle strength).

In addition to such measures, therapists can use standardized outcome measures that evaluate a specific impairment-related construct in a structured manner. An example of this is the Berg Balance Scale, which measures the construct of balance using a range of different tasks. Table 10.1 provides a listing of commonly used standardized tests and measures at the impairment level.

Therapists should carefully choose impairment-based measures that have established reliability and validity. As discussed in Chapter 9, several of the standardized outcome measures evaluate at more than one level of the ICF.

Example: *The Short Physical Performance Battery measures impairments (strength and balance) through the performance of specific tasks (standing with feet together, repeated sit-to-stand).*

Chapter 4 provides further details about choosing standardized outcome measures and the importance of evaluation of psychometric properties.

DOCUMENTING STRENGTH AND RANGE OF MOTION

Muscle strength testing and ROM are two of the most common impairment measures for PTs. Both provide numeric data, in strength grade and number of degrees, respectively. Although ROM measurements generally have been found reliable (Reese & Bandy, 2002), manual muscle testing (MMT) has more limited reliability (Escolar et al., 2001; Frese et al., 1987), and its utility as a screening tool for muscle weakness has been questioned (Bohannon, 2005).

TABLE 10.1   Some Commonly Used Standardized Measures of Impairments (Listed Alphabetically)

Measure	Purpose	Population
Berg Balance Scale (Berg et al., 1992)	Measures balance ability on 14 balance items, such as standing with eyes closed, turning in place, and standing on one leg	Any neurological condition, the elderly, individuals with balance problems
Cincinnati Knee Rating System (symptoms) (Barber-Westin et al., 1999)	Measures symptoms related to knee pain, including pain, swelling, and giving way, on a 6-point scale	Patients with knee dysfunction
Constant-Murley Score (Constant & Murley, 1987)	100-point scoring system: 35 points derived from patient's reported pain and function; 65 points from assessment of range of motion (ROM) and strength	Patients with shoulder dysfunction
Fatigue Impact Scale (FIS) and Modified Fatigue Impact Scale (MFIS) (Fisk et al., 1994)	Assesses the effects of fatigue in terms of physical, cognitive, and psychosocial functioning; the FIS has 21 items; the MFIS has 5 items	Multiple sclerosis; traumatic brain injury
Fugl-Meyer (Fugl-Meyer et al., 1975)	Based to a large extent on Brunnstrom's (Smith, 1996) description of the stages of stroke recovery; most items scored on a 3-point scale (0, 1, 2); includes motor function, sensation, ROM, and pain	Stroke
Glasgow Coma Scale (Jennett & Teasdale, 1977)	Rates alertness and cognitive awareness in three categories (eyes, verbal, and motor)	Brain injury
Mini-Mental State Examination (Folstein et al., 1975)	Assesses several categories related to cognition, including memory, recall, and language	Any individual with cognitive deficits or dementia
Motor Assessment Scale (Carr & Shepherd, 1985)	Assesses everyday motor function in individuals after stroke; includes 8-item assessment on a 0-6 point scale	Stroke
National Institutes of Health (NIH) Stroke Scale (Goldstein et al., 1989)	11-Item clinical evaluation tool used to assess neurological outcome and degree of recovery; includes evaluation of level of consciousness, motor function, and language, among others	Stroke
Numeric Pain Rating Scale (McCaffery & Beebe, 1989)	Measures the intensity of pain experienced by a patient in the past 24 hr on a 0 (no pain) to 10 (worst imaginable) scale	All patient populations
Rate of Perceived Exertion (Borg & Linderholm, 1970)	Patients rate their perceived exertion level on a 15-point scale	Cardiopulmonary
Short Physical Performance Battery (Guralnik et al., 1994)	Evaluates balance, gait, strength, and endurance by examining a patient's ability to stand with the feet together in the side-by-side, semitandem, and tandem positions; time to walk 8 ft; and 5 repetition chair stands	General population; elderly patients
Stroke Rehabilitation Assessment of Movement (STREAM) (Daley & Mayo, 1999)	Provides a quantitative assessment of motor functioning in patients after stroke, including upper limb, lower limb, and basic mobility items	Stroke
Tinetti Gait and Balance (Tinetti, 1986)	Developed as a screening tool to identify older adults at risk for falls; balance component measures balance on eight specific tasks; gait component measures specific gait parameters during ambulation; all are scored on a 0-2 scale	Any neurological condition, the elderly, individuals with balance problems

Documenting Strength

Despite its inherent limitations, MMT continues to be the most commonly used method by PTs to measure strength. A typical grading system for MMT uses a numerical rating from 0 to 5, for example:

Right shoulder flexion 4/5
Left knee extension 2/5

These measures, although numerical in nature, are inherently subjective, as they depend on a judgment by the PT about the amount of force production produced by the patient. Other measures, such as handheld dynamometers or isokinetic measurements (e.g., peak torque or torque curves), can provide more reliable and quantitative data to evaluate muscle strength and measure its change over time.

Functional strength tests, such as the Sit-to-Stand test (Csuka & McCarty, 1985) and functional hop test (Booher et al., 1993) can also provide useful information related to muscle strength (Davies et al., 1996). (See Malone et al., 1996, for more information on strength measures and documentation.) In certain cases, a description of functional strength or motor control is most appropriate (see Case Example 10.2).

Documenting Range of Motion

The most common method for recording ROM results is using the 0° to 180° system (Reese & Bandy, 2016). This system defines 0° as the anatomic position for all joints (except supination of the forearm). Despite this relatively simple numerical scoring system, reporting joint ROM can be susceptible to certain ambiguities. For example, consider the following statement:

Knee extension-flexion ROM is 10°-150°

The end of flexion range in this statement is clear (150°), but the end of extension range is ambiguous. Does this statement mean that the individual cannot fully extend the knee (10° knee flexion contracture), or does it mean that the individual has 10° of extension beyond the neutral?

The ambiguity arises in trying to report flexion-extension as a single range of values. Although there are accepted ways to do this (see Reese & Bandy, 2016, for an excellent discussion of the different methods of recording ROM values), the best way to avoid ambiguity is to separate the range into two separate components, one for each direction of movement. For example:

Knee flex: 0°-150°
Knee ext: 0°-10°

This unambiguously states that the individual has 150° of flexion range and 10° of extension beyond neutral. If, instead, the individual has a 10° knee flexion contracture, it would be reported in this way:

Knee flex: 10°-150°
Knee ext: −10°

Note that ROM is always stated as a range of values (e.g., 0°-150°), except when the individual cannot reach the neutral value, in which case the range is stated as a single negative value (see Case Examples 10.1 and 10.2).

A second problem that sometimes arises with reporting of ROM is confusion between active and passive. When *ROM* is used without a modifier, it implies *passive* ROM (PROM). If the writer of the note means active ROM (AROM), then the word "active" must be stated. However, in all cases use of PROM and AROM is preferable so that is it clear whether passive or active ROM was measured.

Using Tables and Checklists

Tables or checklists can be useful to manage a large amount of data. Such forms can be appended to an initial evaluation to simplify it and not clutter the text. This strategy is useful for measures such as ROM or manual muscle tests, which can be cumbersome to document (see Appendix E for examples of forms used to document ROM and muscle testing). In such cases, pertinent findings could be highlighted in the initial evaluation note while referring the reader to additional documentation.

If such forms are used, no line should be left blank; this prevents another party from being able to alter the evaluation without the therapist's knowledge. Also, if a line is left blank, the reason it was left blank is unknown to the reader. The PT must write one of the following on the line:

1. The results of the test, examination findings, or clinical opinion.
2. *N/T* (not tested), which indicates that this item was not tested. This entry in the note should be followed by a reason the item was not tested or a plan for testing in the future (e.g., *N/T 2° to time constraints—to be evaluated 11/1/23*).
3. *N/A* (not applicable), which indicates that this test was not applicable for this particular patient, given their diagnosis or condition. The therapist should state why the test/measure is not applicable (e.g., *N/A—Pt. is currently on ventilator and unconscious; unable to get out of bed*).

DOCUMENTING PAIN

Pain is probably the single most common reported problem that a PT encounters, particularly in clinical practice. Pain, in and of itself, is not considered an impairment, but rather a symptom or reflection of a probable underlying impairment in body structure (e.g., bone fracture) or body function (e.g., muscle imbalance).

Pain symptoms can provide important information to the therapist to aid in developing an accurate clinical diagnosis. Thus pain should be documented precisely and completely.

> **Example:** *It is not enough to write merely that "Pt. c/o pain in L shoulder" or some similar statement. Use of the PQRST mnemonic is helpful in remembering all aspects of pain documentation (Box 10.1).*

The PQRST identifies five key areas to be included in documentation of pain: **p**rovokes (*What provokes the pain?*), **q**uality (*What does it feel like?*), **r**egion/radiation (*Where is it located and does it radiate?*), **s**everity (*How intense is the pain?*), and **t**ime (*When did it start and when does it occur?*). The use of a

BOX 10.1 PQRST for Documentation of Pain

PQRST is a mnemonic commonly used by nurses in the evaluation of pain. It provides a guideline for those aspects to be included in a physical therapist's documentation.

P = Provokes
- What causes pain?
- What makes it better? What makes it worse?

Q = Quality
- What does it feel like?
- Is it sharp? Dull? Stabbing? Burning?

R = Region/Radiation
- Where is the pain located?
- Does the pain radiate, or is it in one place?
- Did it start elsewhere and now localized to one spot?

S = Severity
- How severe is the pain on a scale of 0-10?
- Does it interfere with activities? How bad is it at its worst?

T = Time
- When did the pain start?
- How long did it last?
- How often does it occur: hourly? daily? weekly? monthly? Is it sudden or gradual?

From Budassi-Sheehy S. *Emergency Nursing: Principles and Practice.* 3rd ed. Mosby; 1992.

drawing to indicate the precise location and extent of pain is useful, as shown in Fig. 10.2. Such a pain diagram can also be used to describe the quality of the pain (e.g., stabbing, burning, pins and needles, numbness, or aching).

The intensity of the pain sensation is often assessed verbally by using a numeric pain rating scale (McCaffery & Beebe, 1989). A numeric rating scale, shown at the bottom of Fig. 10.2, requires the patient to rate their pain on a scale of 0-10, where 0 is no pain and 10 is the "worst possible pain." A visual analog

scale, which uses a nonnumerical scale for patients to estimate their degree of pain, can also be used. This type of scale is typically reported as a percentage of maximal pain.

In addition to documenting these key features, it may be important to further document the *setting* in which the pain occurs. Are there environments, personal activities, emotional situations, or other circumstances that bring about the pain? In addition, it may be relevant to document associated manifestations of the pain. Are there other symptoms that occur in conjunction with the pain? Answers to these questions may provide important insights about the underlying pathological conditions contributing to a patient's pain symptoms.

Using the PQRST guideline, the following is an example of documentation of pain in an initial evaluation:

Example: *Pt. reports sharp, stabbing pain (**quality**) in right knee, localized to discrete point in center of patella (**region**), during stance phase of walking. Pt. rates pain 3/10 at comfortable walking speed (**severity**). Pain increases as walking speed increases, is most intense (8/10 during running), and is absent at rest (**provokes**). Onset of pain "about 3 months ago" (**time**). Pain is gradually worsening and is now preventing her from exercising or engaging in recreational sports (e.g., tennis), (**severity**).*

For documentation of an initial evaluation, it is necessary to document these five characteristics of pain. When documenting a progress report or session note, it would be redundant for the PT to document each of these characteristics, particularly if they had not changed. In a session note, a PT may choose to document only the patient's pain rating on a 0-10 scale if all other aspects remain the same.

For children, ascertaining the type and degree of pain can be difficult. In such situations, facial expressions are frequently used and should be included in an evaluation report. The Wong-Baker FACES Pain Rating Scale is a useful tool that has demonstrated validity and reliability (Wong & Baker, 1988). This may also be an option if an interpreter is temporarily unavailable with individuals for whom English is not their primary language.

SUMMARY

- Impairment-based documentation should be categorized into test and measure headings to provide a concise and organized written report.
- Therapists should document a systems review, which is a screening of key body systems that may or may not be related to the patient's current condition.
- Impairment-based documentation should include all tests and measures that were performed but should highlight impairments that contribute to the observed activity limitations or participation restrictions.
- Whenever possible, impairment documentation should be quantitative. Standardized tests and measures can provide a reliable means for reporting impairments quantitatively.

- *WNL* can be used to describe the results of a quick screening examination (e.g., for ROM or strength), when findings are judged to be within a typically acceptable range, but have not explicitly been measured. *WFL* is an ambiguous term and should generally be avoided.
- Pain is one of the most commonly documented types of impairments. Although it is not an impairment in and of itself, it is a reflection of an underlying impairment. Documentation of pain should be detailed, including the following characteristics: What provokes the pain, the quality of the pain, the region the pain is located or where it radiates to, the severity, and the timing of the pain (PQRST).

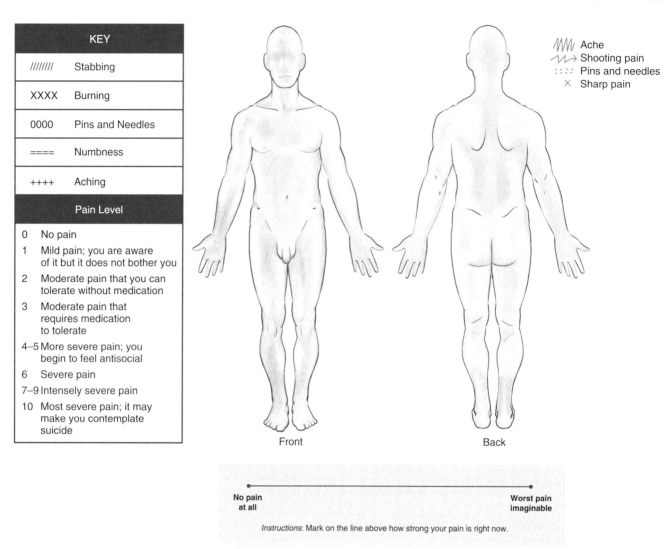

KEY	
////////	Stabbing
XXXX	Burning
0000	Pins and Needles
====	Numbness
++++	Aching
Pain Level	

0   No pain

1   Mild pain; you are aware of it but it does not bother you

2   Moderate pain that you can tolerate without medication

3   Moderate pain that requires medication to tolerate

4–5 More severe pain; you begin to feel antisocial

6   Severe pain

7–9 Intensely severe pain

10 Most severe pain; it may make you contemplate suicide

∿∿∿ Ache
∿∿→ Shooting pain
: : : : Pins and needles
× Sharp pain

Front   Back

No pain at all ●————————————————● Worst pain imaginable

Instructions: Mark on the line above how strong your pain is right now.

FIG. 10.2 Body diagrams for marking the location and nature of pain. (Modified from Cameron MH, Monroe, LG. *Physical Rehabilitation: Evidence-Based Examination, Evaluation, and Intervention.* Saunders; 2007.)

CASE EXAMPLE 10.1   Documenting Impairments   Setting: Outpatient

Name: Jose Rodriguez   **D.O.B.:** 12/29/2000   **Gender:** Male   **Date of Eval.:** 2/25/23

Current Condition

22 y.o. college student with medical diagnosis of R grade 2, ACL sprain on 2/22/23.

IMPAIRMENTS

Systems Review

Skin intact. No evidence of cardiovascular problems; HR 60 beats per minute; BP 120/78 mm Hg. Cognition and communication intact.

ROM: Hip and ankle AROM assessed in all planes with no limitations noted.

AROM	Left	Right
Knee ext	0°-5°	10°-8° with empty end-feel
Knee flex	0°-135°	10°-115° with empty end-feel
PROM		
Knee ext	0°-10°	10°-5° with empty end-feel
Knee flex	0°-145°	5°-120° with empty end-feel

CASE EXAMPLE 10.1   Documenting Impairments   Setting: Outpatient—cont'd

Name: Jose Rodriguez   **D.O.B.:** 12/29/2000   **Gender:** Male   **Date of Eval.:** 2/25/23

Strength (Manual Muscle Tests): Hip and ankle strength assessed in all planes and 5/5.

Strength	Left	Right
Knee ext	5/5	3+/5 with pain
Knee flex	5/5	4/5

	Left	Right
Reflex Integrity		
Patellar tendon	2+	Not tested due to pain in region
Achilles tendon	2+	2+
Special Tests		
	−Lachman test	+ Lachman test (grade 2; firm end-feel)
	−Pivot shift test	+ Pivot shift test (grade 1)
Anthropometric Characteristics		
Inferior pole of patella	34.0 cm	35.0 cm
Superior pole of patella	35.0 cm	36.0 cm
3 cm proximal to superior pole of patella	36.5 cm	37.5 cm
15 cm proximal to superior pole of patella	43.0 cm	42.5 cm

Integumentary Integrity

Moderate erythema and tenderness to palpation along the anteromedial joint line, as well as the MCL insertion.

Pain

Average pain over last 3 days 3/10 at rest; throbbing, aching pain at anteromedial aspect of tibiofemoral joint.

7/10 while ↑↓ stairs and doing any twisting motion; described as "sharp" pain in anteromedial aspect of tibiofemoral joint with sensation of knee "buckling."

Outcome Measures

IKDC Subjective Knee Evaluation Form; 39/87 (44.8%).

CASE EXAMPLE 10.2 Documenting Impairments   Setting: Nursing Home

Name: Marjorie Jones   **D.O.B.:** 5/12/41   **Gender:** Female   **Date of Eval.:** 7/3/23

Current Condition

Pt. is an 82 y.o. female dx PD with a history of multiple falls.

IMPAIRMENTS

Systems Review

HR 68 beats per minute; RR 15 breaths/min; BP 120/78 mm Hg.

Integumentary

+2 pitting edema noted in both lower legs and feet.

Posture

Forward head, thoracic kyphosis, posterior pelvic tilt, and flexion at B hips and knees in standing.

ROM

Limited PROM as follows: B hip extension −10°; B hip flexion 10°-100°; B knee extension −10°; **R shoulder** flexion 0°-160°, ER 0°-45°, abduction 0°-140°; **L shoulder** flexion 0°-140°, ER 0°-40°, abduction 0°-120°. All other joints and directions WNL.

Muscle Tone

Modified Ashworth Scale 3/4 indicating moderate rigidity (cogwheel) evident in PROM ×4 extremities, all directions.

Motor Control

Able to move all 4 extremities against minimal resistance. Rapid alternating movements of UEs are slowed. Resting tremor B hands; does not interfere c̄ hand fx.

Sensation

Intact to light touch B UEs and LEs.

Balance and Gait

Tinetti Gait and Balance[1]: scored 14/28, indicating high risk for falls.

Pt. exhibits a shuffling gait with foot flat initial contact; takes small steps, and has a fast cadence (140 steps/min). She also has a narrow step width c̄ R foot occasionally crossing midline. Pt. demonstrates occasional freezing episodes while ambulating in narrow/small areas, crossing thresholds and when walking through doorways. Hips and knees are flexed throughout gait cycle, and there is no visible trunk rotation and decreased arm swing.

[1]The complete scoring sheet for the Tinetti Gait and Balance tests could be included as part of the documentation, typically attached to the evaluation report.

CASE EXAMPLE 10.3   Documenting Impairments   Setting: Hospital Inpatient[2]

Name: Gareth Jones   **D.O.B.:** 6/12/51   **Gender:** Male

Date of Eval.: 8/2/22

Current Condition
Pt. is a 71 y.o. male c̄ dx of COPD h/o frequent acute exacerbations.

IMPAIRMENTS
Systems Review
Pt. is communicative and A&O ×4. Vitals: HR 130 beats per minute; RR 20 breaths/min; BP 148/88 mm Hg. No limitations noted. B UE and LE ROM.

Ventilation/Respiration
Dyspnea, wheeze, productive cough (mucopurulent sputum); chest pain left side. Use of accessory muscles of inspiration, hyperinflated chest, Hoover's sign, peripheral cyanosis, raised jugular venous pressure, and pursed-lip breathing.

Palpation
Limited thoracic expansion, decreased movement noted at the left lower zone, vocal fremitus on left.

Percussion
Hyper resonant ++ all zones although ↓ resonance (dull) left base.

Auscultation
Fine crackles and wheeze all zones, c/o plural rub left base.

Integumentary Integrity
Peripheral pitting edema noted in B LEs BK.

Aerobic Capacity/Endurance
Unable to stand due to breathlessness.

[2]Note that in this example some different headings than those recommended by the *Guide to Physical Therapist Practice* are used. PTs should choose headings that best fit the clinical setting in which they are working.

CASE EXAMPLE 10.4   Documenting Impairments   Setting: Outpatient

Name: Kate Davis   **D.O.B.:** 5/7/1969   **Gender:** Female

Date of Eval.: 5/19/2022

Current Condition
Pt. is a 53-year-old right hand dominant woman with family history of breast cancer who is status post right nipple-sparing mastectomy with SNLB with immediate DIEP flap reconstruction on 10/26/2021. Final pathology revealed: pTisN0, DCIS, 2.6 cm size, all margins negative, 0/4 sentinel nodes negative, ER/PR +. No radiation or chemotherapy treatment is advised. She was pre-scribed letrozole starting the end of November 2021 and is tolerating it well. She reports some knee weakness and hand joint swelling. She reports that her R shoulder range has been very limited since her surgery even after 10-12 sessions of physical therapy from February to March 2022. She reports that her shoulder is limited by pain.

IMPAIRMENTS
Systems Review
Pt. is communicative and A&O ×4. Vitals: HR 95 beats per minute; RR 14 breaths/min; BP 125/78 mm Hg.

Integumentary Integrity
Palpation—No areas of increased skin temperature or pitting edema throughout B UE. No visible or palpable trunkal edema in bilateral upper anterior and lateral quadrants.
Observation—No significant redness or rash. No visible difference in limb girth in B UE.

Posture
Mild forward head posture. B forward rounded shoulder with mild upper thoracic excessive kyphosis.

ROM
Shoulder:

AROM	Right	Left	Comments
Flexion	105	140	Early upward rotation and excessive elevation of R scapula
Abduction	80	150	Early upward rotation and excessive elevation of R scapula
Functional external rotation reach	T1	T2	
Functional internal rotation reach	R side of trunk	T8	Most painful movement on R

Muscle Performance
MMT-Shoulder:

	Strength Right	Strength Left
Anterior deltoid	4 (Good)	4 (Good)
Supraspinatus	4 (Good)	4 (Good)
Infraspinatus	4 (Good)	4 (Good)
Subscapularis	4 (Good)	4 (Good)

MMT-Upper Arm

	Strength Right	Strength Left
Biceps, long head	4 (Good)	4 (Good)
Triceps	4 (Good)	4 (Good)

Joint Integrity
R glenohumeral joint hypomobile in inferior and posterior directions.

CASE EXAMPLE 10.5 Documenting Impairments   Setting: SNF

Name: Gladys Winter   **D.O.B.:** 8/6/1952   **Gender:** Female   **Date of Eval.:** 8/20/2022

Current Condition

Pt. is a 70 y.o. female with dx of BLE venous wounds. These have been recurrent over the last 5 years. Patient reports that she does not consistently wear her compression garments in the summer months because they are "too hot." She has been primarily functioning from a wheelchair level for the past 3 weeks due to increased difficulty with walking.

IMPAIRMENTS
Systems Review

Pt. is communicative and A&O ×4. Vitals: HR 90 beats per minute; RR 13 breaths/min; BP 130/72 mm Hg. No limitations noted in B UE ROM. Pt. reports her legs feeling "heavy," which increases as the day goes on. States that elevating her legs helps them feel better.

Wound Characteristics

R medial LE (proximal to malleolus)—4.2 × 3.4 cm partial thickness wound with 60% dermis and 40% inflammatory by-product in wound bed. Moderate serosanguineous drainage present. Immediate periwound is macerated with hemosiderin staining noted to extended periwound.

L medial LE (proximal to malleolus)—3.7 × 2.2 cm partial thickness wound with 80% dermis and 20% inflammatory by-product in wound bed. Minimal serosanguineous drainage present. Hemosiderin staining noted to extended periwound.

Integumentary Integrity

2+ edema present to bilateral lower legs and feet. No induration, no temperature change.

ROM

B ankle DF AROM is limited by 10°, PROM limited by 5° due to soft tissue approximation from significant B LE edema.

EXERCISE 10.1

The following statements could be written in an Impairment section of an evaluation report. In the space provided, classify each of the following statements into the appropriate Impairment category from Fig. 10.1. This exercise should be completed with reference to the specific tests and measures listed and defined in the *Guide to Physical Therapist Practice*.

Impairment Statement	Impairment Category
1. R elbow flexion PROM 0°-60°.	_____
2. Walks with uneven step lengths and ↑ weight-bearing time on the R side.	_____
3. Sensation intact B LEs below knee, 10/10 correct responses.	_____
4. Mini-Mental State Examination score 19/30 (cognitive assessment).	_____
5. AROM B UEs—no limitations noted.	_____
6. Right facial nerve intact.	_____
7. Circumference midpatella L knee: 10″; R knee: 9.25″.	_____
8. Rates pain in low back 5/10 sitting for 10 min, pain described as aching/throbbing.	_____
9. Skin intact B LE and trunk.	_____
10. Berg Balance Scale score = 31/56, indicating high risk for falls.	_____
11. Demonstrates antalgic gait pattern.	_____
12. B patellar tendon reflexes 2+.	_____

Impairment Statement	**Impairment Category**
13. B lung fields clear to auscultation.	_____
14. Incentive spirometry in sitting $\bar{c}$ maximal volume = 1750 mL.	_____
15. Pt. has forward head and flattened lumbar lordosis.	_____
16. Pt. is alert and oriented to ×2 (person and place).	_____
17. HR ↑'d to 110 beats/min $\bar{p}$ 5 min walking at 1.0 m/sec.	_____
18. Proprioception sensation impaired L ankle 2/8 correct responses.	_____
19. R hand grip strength 15 kg as measured by handheld dynamometer, avg. 3 trials.	_____
20. Eye movements, smooth pursuit, and visual fields intact (cranial nerves II, III, IV, and VI).	_____

EXERCISE 10.2

Identify the errors in the following statements documenting impairments. Write a more appropriate statement in the space provided. Use the Case Examples at the end of this chapter for guidance.

Statement	**Rewrite Statement**
EXAMPLE: Demonstrates poor standing balance.	Pt. unable to stand in place >10 sec $\bar{s}$ LOB.
1. Sensation is impaired.	_____ _____
2. ROM is moderately limited.	_____ _____
3. Pt. c/o excruciating pain.	_____ _____
4. Pt. has L leg edema.	_____ _____
5. Pt. demonstrates a significant ↑ in HR $\bar{c}$ stair climbing.	_____ _____
6. Pt.'s reflexes are hyperactive.	_____ _____
7. Pt. does not know what is going on.	_____ _____

Statement

Rewrite Statement

8. Pt. has abnormal gait pattern.

_____

_____

9. Pt. has poor endurance.

_____

_____

10. Pt. walks c̄ L knee pain.

_____

_____

Documenting the Assessment: Summary and Diagnosis

LEARNING OBJECTIVES

After reading this chapter and completing the exercises, the reader will be able to:

1. Explain the role of physical therapists in establishing and documenting a diagnosis.

2. Describe the elements of the Assessment section of an evaluation report.

3. Appropriately document an Assessment for different case scenarios.

This chapter presents the Assessment section of the initial evaluation documentation by the physical therapist (PT). The assessment is a pivotal section of the initial evaluation. In it, the PT draws on information presented in the previous sections to arrive at a decision regarding the main problems to be addressed in therapy and the probable causes of those problems. The sections of the initial evaluation that follow the Assessment are used to propose goals and a plan for achieving those goals.

The Assessment section has three purposes:

1. To provide a summary of the evaluation and the PT's clinical judgments about the case
2. To confirm, extend, or, if necessary, question the referral diagnosis
3. To justify the necessity of physical therapy intervention

The notion that PTs make a diagnosis is an important one and has become more readily accepted within the physical therapy and medical communities. Therefore this chapter begins with an explanation of diagnosis and a consideration of the rationale for diagnosis by PTs. The case examples at the end of this chapter provide sample documentation of the Assessment section in various clinical settings.

DIAGNOSIS BY PHYSICAL THERAPISTS

Definition of Diagnosis

The term *diagnosis* refers to both a process and the product of that process. In a general sense, diagnosis as a process is an investigation or analysis of the cause or nature of a condition, situation, or problem. Diagnosis as a product is a statement or conclusion from such an analysis, typically a recognizable label that identifies the nature or the cause of the problem. Thus an auto mechanic can diagnose what is wrong with a car, or an electronics technician can arrive at a diagnosis as to what is wrong with a computer. In medicine, diagnosis has traditionally referred to the act of identifying a disease from its signs

and symptoms as well as the decision reached by that process. In medicine, the diagnostic label often identifies the pathology or disease process presumed to be the underlying cause of the patient's signs and symptoms.

Diagnosis in physical therapy has been considered controversial, although recently has become more widely accepted across the profession. (Jiandani & Mhatre 2018; Sahrmann 2020). Some people have argued that PTs neither have the training to make a correct diagnosis of a patient's condition nor are they able to order and interpret the myriad of tests available to the modern physician. However, this perspective is based on a narrow definition of diagnosis—that it is the act of determining the nature and location of a pathological condition. If a broader view is used—that diagnosis is the process by which any professional, not just a physician, determines the cause of a problem—then the term can be used to describe the process that PTs use to determine the causes of the problems faced by their patients.

Diagnostic Process

The term *diagnosis* refers to a process that all PTs engage in: the act of evaluating the physical and subjective findings to make a decision about whether physical therapy will be helpful to a patient and, if so, what kind of therapy the patient should receive. The diagnostic process involves making a clinical judgment based on information obtained from history, signs, symptoms, examination, and tests that the therapist performs or requests. According to the *Guide to Physical Therapist Practice 4.0*, the diagnostic process "leads to a diagnostic label and directs the therapist's priorities toward alleviating symptoms, remediating impairments in body structures and function, and restoring the individual to the highest levels of activity and participation" (Chapter 4).

Over time, the American Physical Therapy Association's (APTA) House of Delegates has shifted its position from one that recognizes the right of a PT to make a diagnosis ("may establish" in 1984; APTA HOD, 1984) to one that requires a diagnosis

BOX 11.1 Resolutions of the American Physical Therapy Association House of Delegates Relevant to Diagnosis

DIAGNOSIS BY PHYSICAL THERAPISTS HOD P06-12-10-09 (Amended HOD P06-08-06-07; HOD P06-97-06-19; HOD 06-95-12-07; HOD 06-94-22-35; Initial HOD 06-84-19-78) (Position)

PTs shall establish a diagnosis for each patient/client. Prior to making a patient/client management decision, PTs shall utilize the diagnostic process in order to establish a diagnosis for the specific conditions in need of the PT's attention.

A diagnosis is a label encompassing a cluster of signs and symptoms commonly associated with a disorder or syndrome or category of impairments in body structures and function, activity limitations, or participation restrictions. It is the decision reached as a result of the diagnostic process, which is the evaluation of information obtained from the patient/client examination. The purpose of the diagnosis is to guide the PT in determining the most appropriate intervention strategy for each patient/client. In the event the diagnostic process does not yield an identifiable cluster, disorder, syndrome, or category, intervention may be directed toward the alleviation of symptoms and remediation of impairments in body structures and function, activity limitations, or participation restrictions. The PT's responsibility in the diagnostic process is to organize and interpret all relevant information collected.

The diagnostic process includes obtaining relevant history, performing systems review, and selecting and administering specific tests and measures. When indicated, PTs order appropriate tests, including but not limited to imaging and other studies, that are performed and interpreted by other health professionals. PTs may also perform or interpret selected imaging or other studies.

In performing the diagnostic process, PTs may need to obtain additional information (including diagnostic labels) from other health professionals. In addition, as the diagnostic process continues, PTs may identify findings that should be shared with other health professionals, including referral sources, to ensure optimal patient/client care. When the patient/client is referred with a previously established diagnosis, the PT should determine that the clinical findings are consistent with that diagnosis. If the diagnostic process reveals findings that are outside the scope of the PT's knowledge, experience, or expertise, the PT should then refer the patient/client to an appropriate practitioner.

for each patient ("shall establish" in 2007; APTA HOD, 2007) (Box 11.1). However, any diagnosis or classification should be within the legal realm of physical therapy, as defined by state practice acts.

Thus the PT has a professional responsibility to engage in the diagnostic process even when the patient has been referred with a diagnostic label previously determined by a physician. First and foremost, the PT must determine whether the patient's condition is appropriate for physical therapy intervention. Going through the process of ruling out medical conditions that would be inappropriate requires, in effect, that the therapist make a *diagnostic decision* regarding the nature of the pathology and its severity. Deciding that the pathology causing a patient's pain is *not* cancer, *not* myocardial infarction, and *not* an infection in the kidney requires a diagnostic process in which the nature of the pathology is investigated. Thus the PT is making a diagnostic decision, even though they may not actually be making the final determination of the diagnostic label.

Although this process may be referred to as screening, the reality is that PTs engage in the process of *differential diagnosis* when they perform a general systems review to rule out serious pathological conditions, such as tumors or heart disease, that are not appropriate for physical therapy intervention (Heick & Lazaro 2023). If evidence of such a pathological condition is found, the PT must refer the patient to an appropriate practitioner for further testing. This requires the therapist to at least consider the possible pathological conditions, even if they will not verify the presence or absence. The specific tests and measures used in the differential diagnosis process should be documented in the evaluation, and any modifications to the diagnostic label should be documented in the Assessment.

In addition, in the course of assessing the patient, and especially when a patient does not respond to treatment, information is often uncovered that may necessitate modification or rethinking of the original diagnostic label. In this case, it is the legal and professional responsibility of the PT to bring this information to the attention of the referring practitioner.

Diagnostic Label

Although there is widespread agreement among PTs about the importance of the diagnostic process, real questions exist regarding the form of the result (the diagnostic label). The APTA House of Delegates' position on the Management of the Movement System (HOD P06-15-25-24) states: "APTA endorses the development of diagnostic labels and/or classification systems that reflect and contribute to the physical therapists' ability to properly and effectively manage disorders of the movement system." The *Guide to Physical Therapist Practice 4.0* defines a diagnosis as "a label encompassing a cluster of signs and symptoms commonly associated with a disorder or syndrome or category of impairments in body structures and function, activity limitations, or participation restrictions" (Chapter 4). Hedman et al. (2018) have outlined several characteristics of developing clinically meaningful movement system diagnoses, which include that they should represent a unique cluster of movement observations and associated examination findings that can impact a variety of tasks and provide unique and nonambiguous labels for each diagnosis. The APTA Board of Directors adopted the following recommendations with regard to developing a diagnostic label:

- Use recognized movement-related terms to describe the condition or syndrome of the movement system.
- Include, if necessary, the name of the pathology, disease, disorder, anatomical or physiological terms, and stage of recovery associated with the diagnosis.
- Be as succinct and direct as possible to improve clinical usefulness.
- Strive for movement system diagnoses that span all populations, health conditions, and life spans. Whenever possible, use similar movement-related terms to describe similar movements, regardless of pathology or other characteristics of the individual.

While there are no currently universally accepted movement system diagnostic labels, there is emerging literature describing a range of diagnoses in neurological conditions (Scheets et al., 2007; Gill-Body et al., 2021), general orthopedic conditions (Sahrmann et al., 2017), low back dysfunction (Delitto et al., 2012), shoulder pain (Kelley et al., 2013), and neck pain (Fritz & Brennan, 2007). We anticipate there will be continued development of diagnostic labels, and their use will become more routinely incorporated into physical therapy documentation.

Further Classification of Medical Diagnosis

Apart from differential diagnosis, which includes identifying the target disorder, which may be a disease or a pathology resulting from injury, therapists may provide further classification of any established medical diagnosis. Documentation of the diagnosis should almost always include some statement about the stage of recovery, which is usually stated as acute, subacute, or chronic (Box 11.2). Another very important role of classification in diagnosis is the determination of etiology (what caused the disorder). In many instances, especially when there is a musculoskeletal disorder, the PT should determine whether the patient's abnormal movement or postural patterns caused the disorder (kinesiopathology) or are the result of the disorder (pathokinesiology) (Sahrmann, 2014). Many current classification systems emphasize this distinction. Other classification schemes are based on what types of treatment approaches the disorder is most likely to respond to (e.g., Airwaily et al., 2017).

Disablement Analysis

Guccione (1991) advocated for diagnosis by PTs to be focused on the relation between impairments and functional limitations, based on the Nagi Model. Indeed, we advocated for a similar definition in the first edition of this textbook in 2000. With the adoption of the *International Classification of Functioning, Disability and Health* (ICF) framework and terminology, a more global classification system for considering diagnosis is warranted. We argue that diagnoses within the ICF framework should not just link two of the levels (impairments and activities) but should include links within all levels of the framework (health condition, body structures and functions, activities and participation as well as personal and societal factors). A framework for disablement analysis is presented in Fig. 11.1.

How to Document the Diagnosis

Given the complex and evolving landscape of diagnosis by PTs, how should the diagnosis be documented? Think of the diagnostic statement as more than merely a label; it is the summary of the diagnostic process by the PT. We therefore recommend a three-part diagnostic statement:

1. Differential diagnosis: This is the health condition or target disorder, if available; it may be elaborated on, extended, or questioned.
2. Further classification: If possible, include further classification regarding the stage of recovery, etiology, movement system impairment, or other evidence-based classification system.
3. Disablement analysis: Elucidate the causal relation of impairments to activity limitations and participation restrictions; explain how the health condition is affecting or will affect the patient's abilities and roles if untreated.

Table 11.1 shows examples of diagnostic statements. In some cases, it includes further specification regarding location or type of tissue involved, beyond what was indicated in the referring diagnosis. Classification is highly recommended, especially regarding stage and etiology. The relation of the impairments in body structure and function to activity and participation should be explicitly stated. Indeed, this is the key component of clinical decision-making by the PT.

ASSESSMENT SECTION

The extended discussion of diagnosis in this chapter is necessary because a primary purpose of the Assessment section of the initial evaluation is to present a diagnosis of the patient's problems. In effect, the Assessment presents the outcome of the clinical decision-making process. If the first three sections of the initial evaluation (Reason for Referral, Chapter 8; Activities, Chapter 9; and Impairments, Chapter 10) have been developed as proposed in the preceding chapters, then the Assessment should be relatively easy to write.

It is useful to structure the Assessment as a summary statement, highlighting the key problems along with the diagnosis and adding a statement of the patient's overall prognosis or potential to benefit from physical therapy. One important reason to do this is that some professionals reading the evaluation will skip directly to the Assessment. In addition, it is often useful to have a succinct summary statement ready to insert directly for letters to referral sources or insurance companies. For this reason, it is important to minimize the use of abbreviations and provide clear, unambiguous statements in this section.

BOX 11.2   Terms to Describe Stages of Recovery

The terms *acute* and *chronic* refer to two ends of the spectrum in describing the time course of recovery:

Acute refers to the initial stages of a disease process or the immediate aftermath of an injury. During this period of time, the effects of the pathology are still evolving, often rapidly. Signs and symptoms are usually most severe during the acute phase, but this is not always the case.

Chronic refers to a condition that has become a long-term problem. Usually, the severity of the condition is relatively stable during the chronic phase, although signs and symptoms may fluctuate.

Two other terms are often used:

Subacute refers to a condition that is still relatively recent in onset, but signs and symptoms are no longer evolving rapidly. A subacute condition may resolve and never progress to chronic, or it may gradually become a long-term chronic condition.

Recurrent refers to a condition that appears to be fully resolved but occurs repeatedly over a long period.

The actual time courses associated with each of these terms depend on the specific nature of the pathology. For many diagnoses, there are generally accepted norms associated with each term. For an example of the time courses typically associated with low back pain, see the clinical practice guidelines authored by Delitto and colleagues (2012).

The Process of Disablement Analysis

1. Participation (or Potential Disability)

- Why has the patient come to, or been referred to, physical therapy?
- What is the referring diagnosis, if any?
- What are the patient's desired or required roles, occupations, life goals?
- Does the current condition interfere with these, or does it have the potential to interfere?

> *Identify disability or potential disability*

2. Activity Limitations

- What is the patient's current and prior functional status?
- What are the critical skills that the patient needs to perform to be able to overcome or prevent disability?

> *Identify functional problems – critical functional activities*

3. Impairments in Body Structures and Functions

- Why can't the patient carry out required functional activities?
- What are the causes of the activity limitation?
- What impairments contribute to the activity limitation?

> *Identify causes of the activity limitations and contributing factors*

4. Health Condition

- Can the referring diagnosis be further specified?
- What is the stage of healing or recovery?
- Is there potential for development of secondary impairments?
- Should the patient be referred to other practitioners?

> *Identify clarifications of medical diagnosis, recovery stage, and requirements for prevention*

Fig. 11.1 The process of developing a physical therapy diagnosis includes the analysis of problems at all levels of International Classification of Functioning, Disability and Health model.

TABLE 11.1 Examples of Diagnostic Statements

Referring Diagnosis	Differential Diagnosis	Further Classification and Disablement Analysis
COPD, acute pneumonia	COPD 2° to emphysema with pneumonia	Acute pneumonia and impaired cough result in inadequate clearance of airway secretions with potential for fluid accumulation in lungs and infection. Long-term COPD leads to poor endurance during upper extremity functional activities, and patient therefore requires assist with ADLs.
s/p R medial meniscus tear	Medial meniscus tear R knee	Acute phase: joint effusion, pain, and limitation in ROM of right knee resulting in potential muscle atrophy and prolongation of healing. Pain prevents patient from walking long distances and up/down stairs and driving a car. Unable to participate in classes at college.
Left hemiplegia 2° to stroke	L anterior cerebral artery stroke	Subacute phase: 1° impairment of force production deficit resulting in impaired mobility and standing balance, which in turn lead to inability to walk independently at home.
R shoulder pain	R shoulder pain with muscle power deficits/rotator cuff syndrome	Acute strain likely the result of repetitive overhead activities while painting at home. Pain and weakness interfere with normal ADLs, especially dressing, and require rest and treatment to prevent progression to chronic pain and weakness.

ADLs, Activities of daily living; *COPD,* chronic obstructive pulmonary disease; *L,* left; *R,* right; *ROM,* range of motion; *s/p,* status post.

When structured as a summary statement, the Assessment section includes three specific components as follows (Box 11-3):

> ### BOX 11.3   Three Components of the Assessment
>
> 1. **Summary statement:** The introductory sentence(s) should briefly describe the patient and summarize the background information.
> 2. **Diagnosis:** Next, state the differential diagnosis or health condition (if applicable) along with further movement system diagnosis. It may be necessary here to present an alternative or extension to the referring diagnosis, along with a rationale. Finally, describe the patient's activity limitations, key impairments contributing to those limitations, and participation restrictions or potential participation restrictions that will result from those limitations.
> 3. **Potential to benefit from physical therapy:** Conclude with a statement summarizing the patient's potential to benefit from physical therapy and the reasons why physical therapy intervention is or is not indicated. This can include a summary of the types of interventions that the patient requires.

The PT must always be alert to the possibility of secondary and tertiary impairments that might develop as a result of the original health condition. These impairments may in turn exacerbate the health condition or produce new disorders. It is appropriate to document these risks in the Assessment section. The Assessment section also serves an important function to summarize the medical necessity for intervention (see Chapter 5). If there is a medical necessity for physical therapy intervention, it is important to state that the patient "requires" physical therapy services rather than "would benefit" from these services. As seen in the case examples at the end of this chapter and in Chapter 7, all Assessments end with a similar statement that addresses medical necessity.

COMMON PITFALLS IN ASSESSMENT DOCUMENTATION

There are several common pitfalls in writing the Assessment section. These usually result from an overly general or vague statement.

Poor Example: *Pt. has decreased strength and ROM, which is leading to limitations in ADLs.*

This statement could apply to many patients seen by a PT and should be more specific.

Better Example: *Weakness in knee and hip extensors and limitation in hip extension PROM prevent pt. from being able to perform bed mobility and transfers independently.*

Another common example of an overly general statement is the following:

Poor Example: *Pt. is a good rehab candidate.*

This does not sound so bad until we imagine the converse statement:

Pt. is a poor rehab candidate.

Neither of these statements is particularly helpful. What is meant by *good* or *poor*? Both statements merely label the patient; the latter in a way that seems unfair and arbitrary. A better approach is to state more objectively what specific functional limitations might be remediated by a course of rehabilitation therapy.

Better Example: *Pt. requires 6-8 sessions of strengthening exercises and functional training to become sufficiently skilled in transfers and self-care to function independently at home.*

This statement merely implies that the patient is a "good" candidate for rehabilitation because they will benefit from it. If the patient will not likely benefit from further rehabilitation, a clear reason should be given.

Better Example: *Pt. has insufficient voluntary movement in the fingers of the right hand to benefit from therapy to increase the usage of the right arm.*

Or

Pt. is no longer showing improvement in walking velocity and will therefore not benefit from further therapy related to this functional goal.

In general, it is probably not a good idea to make blanket statements about the rehabilitation potential of any patient. Instead, limit statements about prognosis to specific functions for which there is clear evidence one way or the other.

▌ SUMMARY

- The Assessment section of the initial evaluation is used to summarize the findings of the evaluation and to present the diagnosis.
- The Assessment section is often structured as follows: (1) a summary statement, (2) diagnosis, and (3) a general statement regarding the patient's medical need for physical therapy.
- Documenting diagnosis is a key component of the assessment, and we advocate use of pathology-based medical terminology as the principal diagnostic label, and when applicable an additional relevant movement-based label can be used.
- The diagnostic process by PTs has three components: (1) differential diagnosis; (2) further classification by stage of recovery, etiology, movement system, or treatment response; and (3) determination of the fundamental relations among health condition, impairments, activity limitations, and participation restrictions as well as contributions of personal and societal factors.

CASE EXAMPLE 11.1   Documenting Assessment   Setting: Inpatient Rehabilitation

Name: Jose Martinez   **D.O.B.:** 8/31/99   **Gender:** Male   **Date of Eval.:** 10/5/23

Current Condition

6 wk s/p TBI 2° to MVA

ASSESSMENT

Pt. is a 24 y.o. patient 6 wk s/p TBI and presents with residual cognitive and motor impairments. Pt. is impulsive, confused, and easily agitated. His memory deficits limit his cognitive abilities, and learning new tasks is difficult. These cognitive impairments, in addition to L-sided weakness and spasticity, have led to limitations in pt.'s ability to safely and independently perform tasks related to bed mobility, self-care, transfers, ambulation, and wheelchair mobility. Pt. also presents with impaired anticipatory and reactive standing balance, which is the primary factor limiting his ambulation ability at this time. Before injury, the patient was a full-time student, living with his family, and he enjoyed active leisure activities. His residual cognitive and motor limitations have led to safety concerns and lack of independence in functional abilities and significant limitations in social, personal, and occupational life roles. Pt. requires intensive 1:1, 6 days/wk b.i.d. physical therapy to address the above-stated impairments and activity limitations in light of his cognitive and behavioral impairments.

CASE EXAMPLE 11.2   Documenting Assessment   Setting: Inpatient Acute Care

Name: Jessie Goldstein   **D.O.B.:** 2/3/61   **Gender:** Female   **Date of Eval.:** 5/31/23

Current Condition

s/p radical hysterectomy 5/29/12 2° to cervical CA

ASSESSMENT

Pt. is a 62 y.o. patient s/p radical hysterectomy 2° to cervical CA. Incision site is healing well, but pt. reports significant pain and discomfort in abdominal area. Pt. has limitations in trunk mobility and abdominal strength 2° to surgery. These impairments are limiting pt.'s independence in bed mobility, transfers, and ambulation as well as overall comfort in a sitting and supine position. Pt. requires skilled physical therapy intervention daily to improve overall strength and endurance, education regarding appropriate mobility and pain management techniques, and instruction in home program to facilitate recovery and safe D/C home. Patient will be referred to home care services for continued intervention after D/C.

CASE EXAMPLE 11.3   Documenting Assessment   Setting: Health/Wellness Center/OPPT

Name: Emily Ko   **D.O.B.:** 9/1/38   **Gender:** Female   **Date of Eval.:** 12/2/23

Current Condition

Pt. is 85 y.o. patient self-referred for Falls Risk Assessment; hx of two falls in the past month

ASSESSMENT

Pt. is an 85 y.o. patient who came to PT for a falls risk assessment. Based on examination today, pt. presents with a primary diagnosis of Deficit in Anticipatory Postural Control related to impairments in motor control. Underlying contributors to impaired postural control are decreased BLE strength, impaired coordination, and decreased ankle DF ROM bilaterally. Pt.'s scores on Berg Balance and Timed Up and Go assessments indicate a high risk for falls. She also reports a decline in her usual activity level over the last 2 months and is deconditioned. Given these findings, she is at risk for declining independence, limitations in functional activities, and is at significant risk for future falls during dynamic activities such as reaching, walking, or turning. Pt. requires skilled PT intervention 2×/wk for 6 wk to address these specific impairments and activity limitations and to reduce fall risk.

CASE EXAMPLE 11.4   Documenting Assessment   Setting: Outpatient

Name: Zachary Brown   **D.O.B.:** 6/17/57   **Gender:** Male   **Date of Eval.:** 3/16/23

Current Condition

s/p R knee arthroscopy on 3/9/23 for menisectomy and arthritic debridement secondary to presentation of signs and symptoms related to Tibiofemoral Hypomobility Syndrome.

ASSESSMENT

Pt. is a 65 y/o patient who is 1-week s/p R knee arthroscopic menisectomy and arthritic debridement with subsequent impairments in lower extremity strength and balance/stability, increased pain, and limitations in functional mobility. The pt.'s post-op pain and weakness have caused difficulty with stair negotiation, community ambulation, and sit ⇔ stand transfers in the home and in/out of the car. Pt. has a prior h/o falls, and their current scores on the Berg Balance and Timed Up and Go indicate a continued risk for future falls and injury. Prior to surgery the pt. was very active and enjoyed biking, hiking, and camping. They are currently unable to participate in these activities due to their post-op status. Pt. requires physical therapy to address their impairments and functional limitations in order to return to their PLOF.

EXERCISE 11.1

In each of the following cases, a therapist's rough notes appear in the left column. Using these as a guide, formulate a plausible Assessment that includes (1) a summary statement, (2) diagnosis, and (3) potential for physical therapy. It may be necessary to refer to other diagnosis-specific resources to create the most clinically accurate assessment. Refer to the Case Examples and guidelines in this chapter and Chapter 7 as needed.

CASE 1: OUTPATIENT

Case Information

59 y.o. man, s/p R THR 2° to osteoarthritis, 3 wk previous. Pt. past acute stage; no significant pain or swelling; incision well healed.

Participation
Sales representative, travels by car, unable to work since surgery.

Activity Limitations
Needs assist for transfers into car, walks slowly with walker, up to 100 ft at a time, needs assist on steps.

Impairments
Weakness in R hip flexors, abductors, and extensors; habitual gait deviations from preop antalgic gait. R hip ✓ and abduction ROM limited.

Assessment

CASE 2: OUTPATIENT

Case Information

43 y.o. female with multiple sclerosis diagnosed 3 yr back; recovering from recent exacerbation.

Participation
Clerical worker in major downtown office building; rides train and bus to work; resists using cane. Pt. is fearful of falling during commute and needs extra time during commute.

Activity Limitations
Requires assist to go up and down steps; walks slowly; walking difficulties exacerbated in crowded places.

Impairments
Only mild weakness; standing balance easily disturbed, esp. when patient is distracted. Pt. has particular difficulty with motor/cognitive simple and complex dual tasks.

Assessment

CASE 3: INPATIENT*

Case Information

48 y.o. woman admitted to an acute care hospital with complaints of severe abdominal pain, diminished appetite with nausea and diarrhea for 4 days. PMH, end-stage liver disease; liver transplant 4 yr ago, end-stage renal disease with hemodialysis 2×/wk, hypertension and sacral pressure injury onset ×4 mo.

Activity Limitations
Mobility limited to wheelchair. Mod. to maximal assistance for all bed mobility and transfers.

Impairments
Muscle strength: 2+/5 gross lower extremity strength, 3−/5 gross upper extremity strength. Wound: 3.7 × 3.4 × 1.4 cm with 2.2 cm of undermining from 12:00 to 4:00; 85% yellow rubbery eschar; 15% red granulation.

Assessment

CASE 4: OUTPATIENT

Case Information

39 y.o. female c̄ diagnosis of cervical strain. Onset of symptoms occurred 6 wk ago.

Participation
CPA at local firm, currently unable to tolerate typical 8- to 10-hr workday 2° to symptoms. Majority of time typically spent on phone and computer.

Activity Limitations
Occasionally requires pain medication to assist with sleeping at night. Unable to talk on phone 2° to pain with phone cradling position. Unable to tolerate computer work >2 hr 2° to increased pain.

Impairments
Static sitting posture presents with a decrease in cervical lordosis and an increase in thoracic kyphosis. Limited AROM with R-side flexion and rotation at C-spine. Flexed, rotated, and side-bent left at C5 and C6. Weakness in bilateral lower trapezius: 3/5, bilateral middle trapezius/rhomboids: 4/5, and cervical extensors: 3+/5. Pain rated as 3/10 at rest and 6/10 after working 2 hr; described as throbbing and occasionally shooting.

Assessment

CASE 5: INPATIENT REHABILITATION—BURN CENTER[†]

Case Information

23 y.o. female college student sustained 11% TBSA full-thickness scald burn to right anterior thigh, anterior lower leg, and dorsal foot. s/p surgery to excise burn eschar followed by split-thickness skin graft 5 days ago.

Participation
Previously active in playing tennis weekly. Full-time graduate student; lives in apartment with two roommates; elevator to enter; all living on one floor.

Activity Limitations
Able to amb. independently 20 ft in 19.5 sec; step to gait; Tinetti Gait assessment 7/12. Stands independently without support; independent and safe with transfers.

Impairments
11% TBSA, full-thickness burns to right anterior thigh, anterior lower leg, dorsal foot; potential for scarring after healing/surgery. Pain in right lower extremity: 4/10 at rest, 6/10 with movement. ROM: R knee ext/flex 0°-90°; right ankle dorsiflexion 5°, plantar flexion 20°. Edema noted right lower extremity.

Assessment

*Adapted from Hamm RL. Tissue healing and pressure ulcers. In: Cameron M, Monroe LG, eds. *Physical Rehabilitation: Evidence-Based Examination, Evaluation, and Intervention.* Philadelphia: Saunders Elsevier; 2007.
[†]Adapted from Ward RS. Burns. In: Cameron M, Monroe LG, eds. *Physical Rehabilitation: Evidence-Based Examination, Evaluation, and Intervention.* Philadelphia: Saunders Elsevier; 2007.

Developing and Documenting Effective Goals

LEARNING OBJECTIVES

After reading this chapter and completing the exercises, the reader will be able to:

1. Differentiate between goals and outcomes.
2. Describe the important aspects of writing goals at the participation, activity, and impairment levels.
3. Distinguish between short-term and long-term goals.
4. Describe the essential components of a well-written functional goal.
5. Identify poorly written goals and make modifications to goals.
6. Appropriately document participation and activity goals for a written report.

The *Guide to Physical Therapist Practice 4.0* defines *goals* as "Goals are the intended impact on functioning (body functions and structures, activities, and participation) as a result of implementing the management plan. Goals are measurable, functionally driven, and time limited, and, when applicable, classified as short term and long term…. The primary criterion for conclusion of physical therapist services is the achievement of the individual's goals" (See Chapter 4).

Therapists work in collaboration with patients to set goals that are designed to measure progress toward specific expected *outcomes*. Outcomes are the actual result of implementing the plan of care. Thus the goals are what the patient and therapist hope to achieve; the outcomes are what are actually achieved. Outcomes can be measured by evaluating the degree to which goals have been achieved, but they can also be measured by utilizing outcome measures (as discussed in Chapter 4 of this textbook).

THE GOAL-SETTING PROCESS

Goal setting is the process by which a rehabilitation professional or team, together with the patient and/or their family, negotiate and formulate goals. Goal setting has several important purposes, as described by Wade (2009), including the following:

1. As motivation for the patient
2. To ensure that all team members (including health care professionals, caregivers, family members, and the patient) are working toward the same goals
3. To allow monitoring of change on an ongoing basis to enable quick changes in intervention strategies, if needed

Collaborative goal setting and shared decision-making has become standard practice in most rehabilitation settings, as it is the process by which the therapist works together with the patient, other health care professionals, caregivers, and family members to develop goals and establish a plan of care (Fig. 12.1).

This ensures that the patient is fully aware of the goals that are being formulated and that they are meaningful to them (Melin et al., 2021). Further to this concept, Randall and McEwen (2000) have described *patient-centered* goals as being central to goal writing; this emphasizes that goals be focused on what is important and meaningful to the patient. As the authors comment, "for goals to be truly patient-centered, they should be relevant to the patient's desired outcomes, not to what the therapist thinks is 'best' for the patient" (Randall & McEwen, 2000).

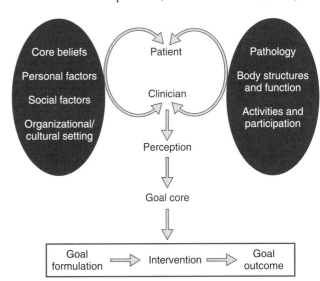

FIG. 12.1 Elements that are considered important in the goal-setting process. Goal setting requires consideration of individual patient factors, including the patient's core beliefs, personal factors, social factors, and organizational/cultural settings. The patient and therapist work together to develop the goal core and to formulate the written goal(s). Following an intervention, goal outcomes are then assessed. (From Playford ED, Siegert R, Levack W, Freeman J. Areas of consensus and controversy about goal-setting in rehabilitation: a conference report. *Clin Rehabil.* 2009;23:334–344.)

Of course, such an approach has some inherent concerns, not the least of which is that this approach may be limited in patients with cognitive abilities who might have difficulty expressing goals that are achievable. Furthermore, such an approach assumes that the patient's needs or wants should prevail, even when a therapist or other health care professional may not believe the goal is realistic or attainable and may require excessive use of resources to achieve. We would argue, therefore, that therapists consider adopting a utilitarian approach to goal planning, which requires that patient-centered goal planning is balanced with an overarching view regarding the best use of health care resources for all patients (see Levack, 2009, for an overview of this approach and its relationship to goal planning).

The therapist's role in the goal-setting process is to provide guidance to facilitate the formulation of goals that are challenging, yet achievable. Therapists use their knowledge of a patient's specific medical diagnosis and related impairments in combination with their knowledge of personal and environmental factors to formulate a prognosis, which provides the foundation for developing an intervention plan specific to the individual patient's needs. In establishing goals, the physical therapist (PT) makes a professional judgment about the patient's prognosis, that is, the likelihood of functional recovery. The prognosis is, in effect, a prediction about the future, and therefore it depends on a certain level of skill, knowledge, and experience. Nevertheless, it should not be assumed that establishing a prognosis requires years of experience. Indeed, one of the most beneficial aspects of evidence-based practice is the increased availability of information about prognosis for a wide range of medical conditions.

If rehabilitation is perceived as a journey, goals are a statement of the destination that the patient and the PT are collaboratively attempting to reach. Goals are central to guiding the therapeutic decision-making process throughout its course. For goals to function effectively as a guide, they should be referred to during every treatment session. Thus goals are not simply documented during the initial evaluation; they should be referred to or addressed in every daily progress note, so the progress toward goals is continually monitored. A method for doing this using the SOAP note format is presented in Chapter 14. The Case Examples at the end of this chapter provide sample documentation of goals written in initial evaluation reports in various clinical settings.

A TRADITIONAL APPROACH: SHORT-TERM AND LONG-TERM GOALS

The traditional approach to documenting goals has been to differentiate between short- and long-term goals. The major distinguishing factor between such goals is the time frame in which they can be achieved. The factor that drives whether a goal is considered long term or short term is frequently the expected time course of rehabilitation. For example, a typical long-term goal in outpatient rehabilitation for a patient post stroke might be:

Patient will walk independently for distances up to 1000 ft outdoors without an assistive device within 1 mo.

A short-term goal related to this long-term goal might be:

Patient will walk 200 ft on level surfaces indoors with a quad cane and require contact guarding within 1 wk.

Thus the concept of a short-term goal is that it is an intermediate step toward achieving the long-term goal. Such a goal can directly relate to a long-term goal, for example, walking 200 ft for the short-term goal versus walking 1000 ft for the long-term goal. Short-term goals can also be distinctly different goals than long-term goals, but they are judged to be achievable in a shorter time frame. An example of this is provided in Case Example 12.1, where the short-term goals (donning a residual limb shrinker, standing ability, transfer ability) need to be achieved before the long-term goals (walking independently at home and in the community) can reasonably be expected to be achieved.

An approach using long-term and short-term goals can be useful, especially in rehabilitation and home care settings where treatment may continue for an extended period. However, with changes in the health care system and especially in payment policy, patients are less likely to be treated over an extended period by a PT. A notable exception is pediatric school-based therapy, where children are often seen over the course of a year. In this situation, long-term goals and short-term objectives are typically written (see Chapter 16).

WRITING GOALS AT THREE DIFFERENT LEVELS

Another approach to writing goals is consideration of the ICF levels: participation goals, activity goals, and impairment goals.

Participation Goals

Participation goals express the expected outcomes in terms of the specific roles in which the patient wishes to be able to participate. These goals provide the "big picture"—what is the overall purpose of the physical therapy intervention? Participation goals relate to specific areas of life participation, as discussed in Chapter 8. Participation encompasses a person's ability to be involved in community, leisure, and social activities. It also relates to a person's life roles—e.g., occupational, volunteer work, and personal. Goals written at the participation level are broadly defined and address general involvement in a range of activities related to one or more life roles.

The type of participation goals written for a patient depends on a number of factors, including the patient's medical condition and the location of therapy services. For example, patients in an acute care hospital or rehabilitation center may simply have immediate goals to become independent in daily personal care or to be able to care for children. However, for patients in outpatient centers who are living at home, a participation goal may be to return to work or to be able to travel to and attend church services.

Activity (or Functional) Goals

Activity goals express the expected outcomes in terms of the skills needed to participate in necessary or desired roles. Activity goals are the key component of any goal section and should always be included. An activity goal may be to walk from the bed to the bathroom, to put on a shirt, or to drink from a cup. Activity goals can also be termed functional goals because they typically focus on specific functions that are pertinent to a person's life.

Because of their importance, writing activity goals is the focus of the remainder of the chapter.

Impairment Goals

Impairment goals express the expected outcomes in terms of the specific impairments in body structures or functions that contribute to the functional limitations. We would argue that although addressing impairments in body structure and function is clearly an important component of almost any physical therapy intervention, it does not necessitate writing a specific goal or goals to address those impairments. In most cases, addressing impairments is actually a reflection of the plan of care and does not need to be explicitly written as a goal per se.

In some situations, however, one or more goals of therapy are to explicitly reduce or eliminate certain impairments. In such cases, setting of impairment goals is reasonable so that outcomes can be monitored. Impairment goals may be viewed as short-term goals used as benchmarks on the way to attain activity goals. These goals are particularly important for patients who may have serious activity limitations, such as immediately after a stroke or spinal cord injury. Changes in impairments, such as strength, may be the only immediate demonstration of improvement in the patient's status, and therefore they may be more sensitive indicators of progress. The goal of therapy is then for the improvements in impairments to ultimately result in improved activities.

FUNDAMENTALS OF WELL-WRITTEN GOALS

SMART Goals

Skillful goal writing is deceptively difficult; one strategy for developing well-written goals uses the acronym *SMART* (Fig. 12.2). The concept of SMART goals was first developed for use in business and setting personal goals (Doran et al., 1981) and has since been adapted almost universally, including in health care settings. Most health care professionals use SMART goals as

Goals Should be SMART

Specific	Target a specific area for improvement
Measurable	Use quantifiable measures as indicators of progress
Assignable	Able to specify who will complete the task
Realistic	Can be achieved with the current resources (e.g., personal, physical, financial)
Time-bound	Time to achieve goal is specified

FIG. 12.2 Elements of writing SMART goals. (Adapted from Doran GT. There's a S.M.A.R.T. way to write management's goals and objectives. *Management Review.* 1981;70(11):35-36.

a means to confirm that goals are specific, measurable, assignable, realistic, and timely. Although writing SMART goals can be a useful formula for clinical goal writing, it should not necessarily be applied rigidly, and some clinicians and researchers believe other characteristics of goals are more meaningful than SMART ones. Following we describe some of these characteristics that we believe are essential to developing well-written goals.

Goals Are Outcomes, Not Processes

The process of learning how to write goals begins by defining the fundamental characteristics of goals and illustrating some of the pitfalls. The single most important characteristic of goals is that they are *outcomes*, not *processes*. This is also the characteristic that is most often forgotten, especially by beginning students. A goal is something that the *patient*, not the PT, will do. The goal defines an end state, not the process that results in that state. The following shows a poorly written goal:

Pt. will be taught proper precautions following hip replacement surgery.

This is not a goal, but rather a plan for achieving a goal. The goal is for the patient to know the precautions, which can be incorporated into a goal, such as follows:

Pt. will be able to state proper hip replacement precautions.

A better, more specific goal would be as follows:

Pt. will be able to demonstrate proper hip replacement precautions during bed mobility, sitting, and transfer tasks.

The use of *able to* in these statements is an excellent way to ensure that the goal is defining an end state—that is, an ability or skill. However, it is not essential in writing the goal. The previous goal could be written without those words, as in the following example:

Pt. will demonstrate proper hip replacement precautions during bed mobility, sitting, and transfer tasks.

If the patient demonstrates the precautions, it can be assumed that they are "able to." Nevertheless, often the PT should at least mentally include the words "able to," especially if the therapist is unsure whether the goal is being properly stated.

Goals Should be Concrete, Not Abstract

One of the most challenging aspects of writing goals is expressing them in concrete terms. The following goal highlights this challenge:

Pt. will demonstrate increased control during reaching movements.

This statement is too general and abstract. What is meant by "control during reaching movements"? Ideally, goals should be stated in terms of an action or functional activity that the individual will perform and must include a concretely stated outcome, such as follows:

Pt. will reach to pick up a cup.

Too often goals are written in such general terms as to be almost useless. For example, the following goals, written in clinical shorthand, are poorly written:

Ind. ambulation
Ind. ADL
Functional strength in UEs

Such goals should be avoided in favor of measuring performance on concrete, specific tasks, or activities.

Well-Written Goals Are Measurable and Testable

A goal should be stated in such a way that the measurement or testing procedure is explicit. The following goal is neither measurable nor testable:

Good sitting balance.

One of the (many) problems with this goal is that it is unclear how sitting balance will be tested. In particular, use of terms such as *good, fair,* and *poor* is not recommended because these terms usually imply something different for each person. A better way to write the goal is as follows:

Pt. will be able to sit unsupported on the edge of a mat table for up to 1 min.

Here, the goal is stated in such a way that the test is embedded in the goal itself. One of the reasons goals are so important is that they provide a way of determining whether progress is being made in therapy. Therefore frequent testing is essential.

Goals Are Predictive

Setting goals requires PTs to generate a prediction. The goal states that the patient will be able to accomplish something in the future that they cannot accomplish now. The prediction must be feasible and at the same time challenging. The PT must also set a specific time within which this goal will be reached. As noted earlier, this aspect is especially challenging for student PTs who have little or no previous experience. Two suggestions may help students to deal with this problem. First, the rehabilitation literature is an excellent starting point for researching typical times required for achieving certain functional outcomes. Second, goals are not written in stone. As a patient progresses in a rehabilitation program, it is appropriate for goals to be revised to reflect the patient's current status and projected capabilities.

The predictions that therapists make in setting goals will therefore not be perfectly accurate because individual patients differ from one another and from the average results in clinical studies. In general, it is better to err on the side of being too optimistic, expecting a bit more from the patients than they may be capable of achieving. If the PT is wrong, then the consequence is that patients do not quite make it, but they are (usually) no worse than if more modest goals had been set. If, on the other hand, the PT errs on the side of being too conservative in setting a patient's goals, the consequence may be that the patient does not accomplish what they are capable of. This approach does not advocate unrealistic optimism in setting goals but instead reflects a preference to challenge patients.

Goals Are Determined in Collaboration With the Patient and the Patient's Family or Caregivers

Collaboration with the patient and their family or caregiver is the most obvious of the fundamental characteristics of goals and yet is the most consistently violated principle. Crawford et al., (2022) highlighted several barriers to implementation of patient-centered goal setting in physical therapy practice including therapist's lack of skill in setting patient-centered goals, and poor integration of goal setting into clinical routines. Even more detrimental to the rehabilitation process is that the patient may not even be told what the goals are, or they are related only in the most general terms. If the goal is for the patient to be able to walk 500 ft in 2 min, this goal should have been determined in collaboration with the patient. When patients are aware of the specific aspects of a goal, they often are more dedicated to achieving that goal.

A FORMULA FOR WRITING GOALS - ABCDE

Goals have a specific structure, and the first step in learning to write goals is to learn to apply this structure in the process. Applying the principles developed in this chapter, a goal has five necessary components (adapted from Mager et al., 1977):

1. The person who will accomplish the goal (Actor).
2. The task or functional activity that the individual will be able to perform (Behavior).
3. The context, circumstances, and support needed to carry out the task (Condition).
4. A quantitative specification of performance (Degree).
5. The time period within which the goal will be achieved (Expected time).

These components of a goal are illustrated in Fig. 12.3, which provides a flowchart for writing goals using this ABCDE format.

The five components shown in Fig. 12.3 are most readily applied for the documentation of activity goals. Some of these components are not pertinent when writing disability or impairment goals (covered later in this chapter). Nevertheless, all properly written activity goals should include all five components. Thus the following formula can be applied to writing an activity goal:

$$Goal = A + B + C + D + E$$

Using this formula, as shown in Fig. 12.3, the following goal might be constructed:

Mr. McCarthy (actor) will walk (behavior) in hospital corridor with rolling walker and supervision (conditions) for 100 ft in less than 2 min (degree) within 1 wk (expected time).

This goal can easily be modified by substituting different components as follows:

Mr. McCarthy will walk in hospital corridor with rolling walker and min A for 500 ft in 4 min (different degree) within 2 wk (different expected time).

Or

Mr. McCarthy will walk outdoors on uneven surfaces with a cane and min A (different conditions) for 100 ft in 2 min within 1 wk.

Flowchart for Writing Goals

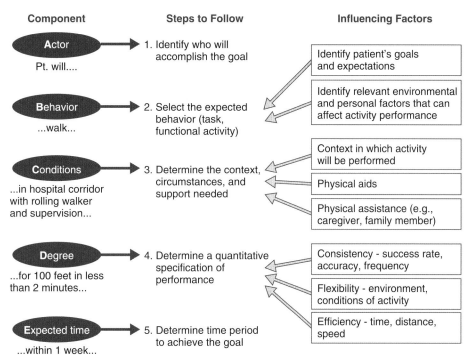

FIG. 12.3 A flowchart for writing goals. The five necessary components of a goal (ABCDE) include the actor (A), behavior (B), conditions (C), degree (D), and expected time frame (E). To ensure a well-written goal, therapists can implement the steps to follow considering influencing factors specific to their patient or client. (Adapted from Kettenbach G. *Writing SOAP Notes*. 3rd ed. FA Davis; 2003; Bovend'Eerdt T, Botell R, Wade D. Writing SMART rehabilitation goals and achieving goal attainment scaling: a practical guide. *Clin Rehabil*. 2009;23:352–361.)

TABLE 12.1   A Table Used in an Outpatient Physical Therapy Clinic to Document Activity Goals for a Patient S/P Spinal Fusion Surgery

Activity	Target Performance	Rationale	Method of Assessment	Due Date
Pain-free sitting	45 min	To allow for community transportation	Patient report	14 days
Pain-free side lying	Up to 8 hr	To allow for restful sleep	Patient report	7 days
Even-terrain ambulation	45 min pain free	To allow for community and household ambulation	Patient report	14 days
Uneven-terrain ambulation	20-25 ft	To maximize safety with community ambulation	Observation	21 days
Stair-climbing	20 stairs, ascend and descend without railing	To allow for independent household ambulation	Observation and patient report	21 days

Thus by mixing and matching the different components, a wide range of goals can be constructed. The benefits of this approach are twofold. First, goals will be properly written, that is, not missing any essential components. Second, this approach is designed to encourage functionally oriented goals because the focus is on the patient and the behavior, or activity, that they will be performing.

Time-Saving Strategies

Writing goals, particularly well-written goals, can be very time-consuming. One strategy that therapists can use to write goals more efficiently is to use a table format. Table 12.1 provides an example of outcome goals listed in such a format. In this table, several shortcuts have been taken. First, the actor is omitted (because it is assumed to be the patient). However, each of the goals lists a behavior, condition, degree, and expected time. In addition, a rationale is provided for each goal, providing further clarification for third-party payers. Second, by eliminating full sentences for the goals, fewer words are written, thus saving a significant amount of time. Note that in this table the goals are still patient-centered and not generalized goals that could be applied to any patient.

THE ART OF WRITING PATIENT-CENTERED GOALS: GOING BEYOND THE FORMULA

While structured formulas are helpful to get started with goal writing, individualized goals created in collaboration with the patient will guide the therapeutic process toward the best possible outcome. Importantly, patient-centered goals are expressed in terms of specific activities that are meaningful to the patient. As an example, let us start with a fairly generic but still acceptable goal:

Pt. will walk on level surfaces with a walker and min A for a distance of 100 ft in 2 min within 1 wk.

The goal can be reformulated so that it is more patient-centered as follows:

Pt. will walk from his bedroom to his kitchen with a walker and his wife's assistance in 2 min within 1 wk.

A simple change makes the goal much more meaningful to the individual. Another example starts with a fairly generic goal:

Pt. will feed herself independently within 1 wk.

Again, the goal can be reformulated in a way that is more patient-centered:

Pt. will eat full bowl of dry cereal and milk c̄ a spoon using R hand in 10 min within 1 wk.

Of course, the assumption here is that Ms. Henry wants to be able to eat cereal in the morning. The patient-centered goal, in addition to being more relevant to the patient, is intrinsically more testable and measurable.

Randall and McEwen (2000) state that the main reason for writing patient-centered functional goals is that "people are likely to make the greatest gains when therapy and the related goals focus on activities that are related to them and that make a difference in their lives." The key to this is taking the time to discuss the goals with the patient so that the goals are formulated in terms that are meaningful to them. Then the goal is stated in as concrete a manner as possible.

DETERMINING EXPECTED TIME FRAMES FOR GOALS

Determining the appropriate expected time frames for a goal can be particularly challenging. Inevitably, the PT makes an educated guess about how the health condition, medical history, and many other factors will affect how quickly a patient will achieve a goal. Although determining expected time frames can be subjective, PTs should use current research and their clinical experience and judgment to determine the most reasonable time frame.

Expected time frames are typically written in weeks. In certain settings where the length of stay is typically short, such as acute care hospital settings, goals can be set in terms of days. Time frames can also be written in terms of number of physical therapy sessions by which they are likely to be achieved (e.g., *Pt. will walk 200 ft in hospital corridor c̄ min A within 6 sessions*).

CHOOSING WHICH GOALS TO MEASURE: PRIORITIZING AND BENCHMARKING

As with documentation of activities, choosing which goals to measure can be tricky. Sometimes it is relatively straightforward—if the patient's primary functional problems are related to pain while walking, the focus of the activity goals will be on walking. However, sometimes there are many different goals that can be chosen. In these situations, two specific strategies can be implemented for choosing appropriate goals: prioritizing and benchmarking.

Prioritizing Goals

Prioritization of goals should take into consideration not only those goals that are most important to the patient but also those that are necessary for the patient to achieve their highest level of functioning. Take, for example, the case of a patient who is acutely ill in the hospital who is currently dependent in all activities of daily living and requires maximal assistance for bed mobility, transfers, and standing. In such a situation, a therapist should probably not choose the task of walking down the hall as the first goal. The therapist should, in coordination with the patient and their family, prioritize the patient's needs. In this situation, establishing a goal of independent bed mobility and transition to sitting may be a more appropriate early goal.

Benchmarking

As discussed in Chapter 9, benchmark activities are those that are amenable to showing improvement as a result of physical therapy intervention. Therapists can thus choose benchmark goals, which will differ depending on the patient and their stage of learning.

> **Example:** *If a patient is referred for hand therapy after a tendon transfer and is unable to perform a wide range of hand-related skills, such as writing, typing, eating, buttoning, and manipulating money, the therapist and patient can work together to determine two or three of these tasks to be used as benchmark tasks; improvement in performance of these tasks would be representative of general progress in hand function.*

GOAL ATTAINMENT SCALING

Goal attainment scaling (GAS) is an individualized, criterion-reference measure of change using goals specific to an individual patient (King et al., 1999). In developing a GAS for a patient, tasks or activities are individually identified using an approach similar to that discussed in this chapter. Goals should be at the activity level, be set in collaboration with the patient, and be meaningful and relevant. Five levels of achievement of that goal are then individually set around a patient's current and expected levels of performance. Fig. 12.4 shows the rating scale used for GAS.

Table 12.2 shows an example of using GAS in a research study in an adult receiving home care services. As shown in this table, GAS incorporates one overall functional goal, which is then

−2	−1	0	+1	+2
Baseline	Less than expected outcome	Expected outcome	Greater than expected outcome	Much greater than expected outcome

FIG. 12.4 Scoring criteria for use with goal attainment scaling.

TABLE 12.2 A Sample Goal Attainment Scaling (Gas) Record for a Patient with Huntington Disease Receiving Home-Based Physical Therapy Services

GAS Score	Goals
Participant Goal: To Be Quicker at Walking From House Around Park	
+2	Participant will be able to walk from house, around park, and back with no rests in 23 min.
+1	Participant will be able to walk from house, around park, and back with no rests in 27 min.
0	Participant will be able to walk from house, around park, and back with no more than 1 rest in 30 min.
−1	Participant will be able to walk from house, around park, and back (1.1 miles) with 2 rests in 35 min.
−2	Participant will be able to walk from house, around park, and back with up to 4 rests in 40 min.

Adapted from Quinn L, Debono K, Dawes H, et al. Task-specific training in Huntington disease: a randomized controlled feasibility trial. *Phys Ther.* 2014;94:1555–1568.

broken down into five possible outcomes. One level, typically −2, reflects the current level (representing no change on outcome assessment). Level −1 represents a less than expected outcome. Levels 0, 1, and 2 reflect outcomes that are expected, greater than expected, or much greater than expected, respectively.

The intervals between levels of the scale should ideally be similar. For example, the jump from +1 to +2 should require the same degree of change as a jump from −2 to −1 (McDougal & King, 2007). Importantly, the amount of change between these levels must also be clinically relevant; for example, a difference of 5 or 10 ft in walking distance is not likely to be relevant for a person who ambulates independently in the community. Finally, improvement in the goal should be measured using only one variable of change, keeping the other variables constant. For example, if a goal is related to decreasing the level of assistance needed to perform a transfer task, then all features of the task should remain constant (e.g., the chair/bed used for the transfer or the equipment used), while the level of assistance is changed.

Although GAS is not necessarily an appropriate tool in all clinical settings, it can be useful particularly in rehabilitation, in home care settings, and in pediatrics as an objective measure of progress toward functional goals. Further information and examples of using the GAS can be found in Chapter 16.

WRITING PARTICIPATION AND IMPAIRMENT GOALS

In this chapter, most of the discussion has focused on techniques that are appropriate for writing activity goals. Factors that should be considered when the PT writes participation goals and impairment goals are now considered.

Participation Goals

Generally, participation goals can and should be written just as activity goals are written. The difference is that the activity that is the subject of the goal is stated in more general terms (overall participation in work, home, recreation, etc.) than it would be in an activity goal, where the focus is on performing specific tasks or skills. The following statements are examples of participation goals.

Example 1: *Mr. Rasheed (A) will return to work (B) as a bus driver (C) able to accomplish all regular duties (D) within 1 month (E).*

Example 2: *Ms. Loring (A) will take care (B) of her two children at home (C) without daytime assistance (D) within 2 months (E).*

Example 3: *Mr. Fox (A) will attend (B) church services (C) daily (D) within 6 wk (E).*

Example 4: *Ms. Samson (A) will return (B) to jogging for fitness and recreation (C) 4×/wk (D) within 2 months (E).*

In participation goals, the condition typically clarifies the nature of the activity or activities. These goals make little sense if they are not followed up by activity goals that detail the specific skills needed to fulfill these roles. It may not always be the case that the activity goals will directly lead to the participation goal. The participation goal may be a goal that is not attainable for several months, which may be beyond the patient's expected duration of treatment in the current setting. In this case, the patient will likely undergo two separate episodes of PT—one immediately after the accident (for which the goals are listed), which may last only a few weeks, and another episode after the fractures have healed. The participation goal, however, is still stated as a long-term outcome for the patient—to return to school in their full capacity.

Impairment Goals

In certain situations, one or more goals of therapy are to explicitly reduce or eliminate certain impairments. Impairment goals are considered optional for most evaluation reports and should be used sparingly. In some clinical settings, these are referred to as *therapy goals*. As mentioned earlier, short-term goals can be focused on impairments and long-term goals on functional activities.

It is very important that the impairment goals are linked in some way to activity goals. The link should be clearly stated in the Assessment section of the initial evaluation, or it could be linked to an activity or function at the end of the goal. Some examples would be:

Example: *PROM of L knee flexion (C) will increase (B) to 110° (D) within 3 wk (E) so that patient can transfer to floor.*

Example: *Shoulder flexion AROM will increase from 100° to 140° so that patient can reach items in high kitchen cabinets.*

Although this is an acceptable strategy that is often recommended, it may be more concise and clearer to simply write a functional goal related to reaching items in high kitchen cabinets. The increase in shoulder flexion may or may not be an important impairment/short-term goal, depending on the factors contributing to the activity limitations.

A primary reason that such goals often are not useful is that typically more than one impairment contributes to an activity limitation. In the previous example, the patient may have a strength deficit in addition to loss of range of motion (ROM) in the shoulder. Thus the patient could attain the goal of improving ROM in the shoulder, but if strength was not improved, the patient would still not be able to reach items in a tall cabinet. The discussion of the often-complex link between any observed limitations and impairments may therefore be more appropriate for the Assessment section. In summary, the focus of therapy should almost always be on achieving meaningful activities, and reaching the impairment goals should be subordinate to attaining the activity goals.

Impairment goals are often not written with the actor specified, as it is assumed that the statement is made with relation to the patient. Furthermore, it would not sound incorrect if a goal read "Pt. will increase ROM in R knee." Thus impairment goals are often stated without the actor explicitly specified, although

the behavior (B), condition (C), degree (D), and expected time (E) should be included. Some more examples include:

Example 1: *Strength R shoulder flexion (C) will increase (B) to 4/5 (D) within 3 wk (E).*

Example 2: *Single limb stance on R leg (C) will improve (B) to 10 sec (D) within 2 wk (E).*

Example 3: *Pain in R shoulder (C) will decrease (B) to 2/10 (D) within 1 wk (E).*

Example 4: *Circumference of R anterior thigh wound (C) will decrease (B) to 2 cm (D) within 4 wk (E).*

A common pitfall when documenting impairment goals is to not specify the degree (D). Some examples include:

↑ *strength R biceps*
↓ *pain in L ankle*

These goals are not well written because they do not include specific measures. In the first example, if a patient's strength increased even a minimal amount, the goal could be met. This might make it difficult to justify the need for continued intervention to achieve even greater strength in the biceps. If, however, the amount of strength (e.g., manual muscle testing grade) was specified as a goal, this would allow all involved parties to be aware of the specific expected outcomes.

SUMMARY

- Therapists work in collaboration with patients to set *goals* that are designed to measure progress toward specific expected *outcomes*.
- Goals can be written based on time frame (short term or long term) or based on levels of the ICF (participation, activity, impairment)..
- Well-written goals have certain fundamental characteristics. They are focused on outcomes, not processes. They are concrete, not abstract. They are measurable and testable. They

are predictive and are based on collaboration between therapist and patient.
- Goals have five essential components: the actor, the behavior, the condition, the degree, and the expected time.
- Although these components can be used to construct a goal in a mechanical way, therapists are expected to go beyond the formula to create goals that are patient-centered, that is, stated in terms of activities and environments that are meaningful to the patient.

CASE EXAMPLE 12.1 **Documenting Goals** **Setting: Home Care**

Name: Martin Jones   **D.O.B.:** 5/7/68   **Gender:** Male   **Date of Eval.:** 5/10/23

Current Condition
55 y.o. patient, hx of diabetes, s/p B transtibial amputation (left: 4 yr ago; right: 4 wk ago)

PARTICIPATION GOAL
Pt. will live in apartment independently and will return to duties as cantor in temple within 3 mo.

LONG-TERM ACTIVITY GOALS
1. Pt. will walk through all rooms inside apartment I c̄ walker and B prostheses within 8 wk.
2. Pt. will walk three blocks home ↔ temple c̄ crutches and B prostheses c̄ supervision of housekeeper or friend in 20 min within 12 wk.

SHORT-TERM ACTIVITY GOALS
1. Pt. will don shrinker to R residual limb c̄ correct technique whenever OOB within 2 days.
2. Pt. will demonstrate proper performance of LE preprosthetic strengthening exercises within 2 days.
3. Pt. will stand at edge of bed c̄ CG of therapist c̄ walker and L prosthesis for up to 5 min within 2 days.
4. Pt. will transfer independently bed ↔ W/C c̄ only L prosthesis within 1 wk.
5. Pt. will walk with walker from bedroom ↔ kitchen (15′) I c̄ walker and L prosthesis in 2 min within 3 wk.

IMPAIRMENT GOAL
1. Circumferential measurement of R distal limb will decrease by 1″ overall within 4 wk for permanent prosthesis fitting.

CASE EXAMPLE 12.2 Documenting Goals — Setting: Acute Care Hospital

Name: Mario Nieto **D.O.B.:** 10/14/47 **Gender:** Male **Date of Eval.:** 11/5/23

Current Condition
76 y.o. patient s/p R THR on 11/4/23 2° degenerative joint disease; PWB R LE.

ACTIVITY GOALS
1. Pt. will demonstrate proper THR precautions during transfers and dressing 3/3 trials within 1 day.
2. Pt. will transfer bed ↔ chair with armrests 3/4 trials with CS within 2 days.
3. Pt. will walk independently with walker for 100 ft in 3 min indoors on level carpeted and tiled surfaces within 3 days.

CASE EXAMPLE 12.3 Documenting Goals — Setting: Outpatient

Name: Keisha Brown **D.O.B.:** 1/9/2007 **Gender:** Female **Date of Eval.:** 2/12/23

Current Condition
16 y.o. patient s/p fx R distal tibia and fx R proximal humerus 1 wk ago 2° to MVA; NWB R LE.

PARTICIPATION GOAL
Pt. will attend regular classroom in high school and participate in all activities, including extracurricular sports, within 4 mo.

ACTIVITY GOALS
1. Pt. will demonstrate proper performance of home exercise program within 3 days.
2. Pt. will transfer wheelchair ↔ car using a stand-pivot transfer c̄ min A of a parent within 2 wk.
3. Pt. will use knee walker/scooter independently in school hallways, elevators, and outside paved areas, while effectively avoiding obstacles within 2 wk.
4. Pt. will tolerate sitting in class with R leg in dependent position for 30 min within 1 wk.

CASE EXAMPLE 12.4 Documenting Goals — Setting: IP Acute Rehabilitation

Name: RJ Jones **D.O.B.:** 2/5/03 **Gender:** Male **Date of Eval.:** 3/17/23

Current Condition
Pt. is a 20 y.o. patient who sustained a TBI 2° to a MVA 4 weeks ago on 2/22/23. Pt. is emerging from coma in a minimally conscious state, trach (for suctioning only) and g-tube and indwelling catheter in place.

SHORT-TERM GOALS (2 WEEKS)
1. Pt. will tolerate the tilt table while maintaining NWB precautions for 15 min at 60° with stable vital signs, to prepare for upright pregait tasks
2. Pt. will reach across midline with LUE on verbal command 3 out of 5 trials, to initiate bed mobility
3. Pt. will turn head to the right of midline with auditory stimulus 3 out of 5 trials, to initiate bed mobility.
4. Pt. will tolerate head of bed at 70° for 25 min while PT performs ROM activities with stable vital signs, to initiate sitting activities.

CASE EXAMPLE 12.5 Documenting Goals — Setting: OP-Maintenance Therapy

Name: Sylvia Bacchus **DOB:** 6/16/1972 **Gender:** Female **Date of Eval.:** 5/5/2023

Current Condition
Pt. is a 55 y.o. patient diagnosed with Parkinson disease 10 years ago in February 2013. Pt. is currently being seen in OP rehabilitation for a PT maintenance program.

PARTICIPATION GOALS (8 WEEKS)
Pt. will maintain their functional mobility level to enable weekly attendance at church on Sundays.

ACTIVITY GOALS (4 WEEKS)
1. Pt. will maintain their ability to ambulate 250' on level indoor surfaces using rollator walker 5/5 times.
2. Pt. will maintain their ability to transition from sit to stand with CS, from recliner chair and toilet, pushing up with BUE 5/5 trials.
3. Pt. will identify potential fall hazards in ambulation path, with 80% accuracy during skilled physical therapy sessions.
4. Pt. will maintain the ability to complete a complex standing task for 5 min to allow for grooming/hygiene tasks without demonstrating SOB or excessive fatigue.

IMPAIRMENT GOALS (4 WEEKS)
1. Pt. will maintain the ability to achieve 0°-5° of hip extension bilaterally to allow for full uptight posture and prevent loss of balance anteriorly.

EXERCISE 12.1

For each goal, indicate what type of goal it is (Participation or Activity). Write one or more letters in the column at the right to indicate the missing or problematic component (A = actor; B = behavior; C = conditions; D = degree; E = expected time). More than one component may be missing or problematic in a single example. Rewrite each goal in the space below, adding or changing the missing or problematic components using plausible details. Identify A, B, C, D, and E in each answer.

EXAMPLE: Patient will walk 300 ft in 4 min c̄ walker and require contact guarding.

Type:
Activity

Answer: **Patient (A) will walk (B) on level hallway surface (C) 300 ft (D) in 4 min (D) using walker (C) and requiring contact guarding (D) within 5 days (E).**

Problem:
C, E

1. Independent in transfers in 2 wk.

Type:

Problem:

2. Patient will be functional in ADLs within 3 wk.

Type:

Problem:

3. Return to work in 3 mo.

Type:

Problem:

4. Pt. will ↑↓1 flight of stairs in 1 min.

Type:

Problem:

5. Pt. will return to school.

Type:

Problem:

_____

_____

_____

6. Pt. will get from his room to therapy.

Type:

Problem:

_____

_____

_____

EXERCISE 12.2

Identify the errors in the following statements documenting Activity goals. Rewrite a more appropriate statement in the space provided.

Statement	**Rewrite Statement**
EXAMPLE: Transfers will improve.	Pt. will transfer from bed ↔ w/c c̄ min A, within 1 wk.
1. Pt. will experience less pain.	_____
	_____
2. Pt. will progress from a walker to a cane within 3 wk.	_____
	_____
3. Educate pt. on hip precautions within two sessions.	_____
	_____
4. Pt. will walk with a normal gait pattern within 4 wk.	_____
	_____
5. ADLs in 2 wk.	_____
	_____
6. Pt. will ascend and descend stairs within 3 days.	_____
	_____

Statement	**Rewrite Statement**
7. Pt. will not have pain when reaching.	_____ _____
8. Pt. will sit for 5 min.	_____ _____
9. Pt. will improve standing balance.	_____ _____
10. Pt. will transfer from sit → stand in 2 wk.	_____ _____

Documenting the Plan of Care

LEARNING OBJECTIVES

After reading this chapter and completing the exercises, the reader will be able to:
1. Identify and describe the components of documentation of the management plan/plan of care.
2. Appropriately document a plan of care as part of an initial evaluation.
3. Discuss the importance of documenting informed consent.

The Plan of Care section details the overall management strategy that will be used by the physical therapist (PT) to accomplish the stated activity goals. The Plan of Care encompasses coordination and communication with other health care professionals and/or caregivers and family members, educational instruction, and physical therapy procedural interventions. The *Guide to Physical Therapist Practice 4.0* defines interventions as "purposeful interaction of the physical therapist and physical therapist assistant (PTA) across numerous practice settings and via electronic platforms used in telehealth." The Guide further states that "through clinical reasoning, based on examination findings, diagnosis, and prognosis, PTs select, prescribe and implement relevant interventions targeted toward established goals."

The Plan of Care includes the framework for the PT services to be provided and should be developed in collaboration with the patient and other providers involved in their care. In documenting the Plan of Care, the PT usually states the proposed frequency and duration of physical therapy visits in addition to a tentative date for reevaluation. The plan can also include coordination/communication with other health care professionals/team members. Categorizing the interventions into two distinct areas (educational and procedural) can help organize this section but is not required. This categorization is useful because PTs often focus exclusively on describing the procedural interventions and minimize or even omit interventions involving coordination of care, communication with individuals involved in the patient's care, and educational instruction.

DOCUMENTING THE PLAN OF CARE

Before documenting the components of the Plan of Care, the PT should first indicate the recommended frequency and duration of this plan.

Example: *Pt. will be seen 2×/wk, 30-min sessions for 6 wk.*

If appropriate, the PT can also document when the patient will be reevaluated.

The PT should also document the coordination of care that occurs directly with a patient, their family members, or any individuals directly involved in the patient's care. Such individuals may include PTAs, other medical personnel, caregivers, or teachers.

Example: *Diagnosis and plan of care were discussed with PTA, who met pt. and pt.'s family at the completion of the evaluation.*

In an initial evaluation report the PT also reports their plan for any anticipated coordination or communication that is relevant to physical therapy.

Example: *Pt.'s HHA will be instructed in appropriate guarding during standing activities and ambulation to maximize pt.'s safety while facilitating active participation by pt.*

Example: *(PT will) coordinate with John's SLP re: strategies to maintain upright positioning in W/C and possible use of adaptive equipment during mealtimes.*

Documenting Educational Interventions

All physical therapy intervention involves some aspect of patient education or instruction. This section should include a general description of the nature of the instruction. For example, the therapist can report as follows:

Pt. will be instructed in care of wound.

Although the specific details of this instruction may not need to be documented in the evaluation report, the inclusion of any educational materials given to the patient to be kept in the medical record or chart is helpful. Another example that could be included in a report is as follows:

Pt. will be educated on proper positioning in bed.

It could be argued that this statement does not provide enough detail about specifically what is meant by "proper positioning" or why positioning is important for this patient. An alternative documentation that provides more detail would be:

Pt. will be educated on positioning self in side-lying position with pillow between knees to maintain back alignment and improve comfort while sleeping.

Documenting Procedural Interventions

The Procedural Intervention section of the Plan of Care can include a wide variety of interventions, ranging from therapeutic exercise to training in self-care skills to airway clearance techniques (Table 13.1). First, documentation of interventions should flow logically and systematically from other aspects of the report. For example, if stair-climbing is identified as an

TABLE 13.1 Categories for Documenting the Plan of Care (with adaptations from the *Guide to Physical Therapist Practice 3.0 and 4.0*)

Section	Description
Plan of Care	Describe the interventions (educational and procedural) that will be administered by the PT
Educational interventions	
	Includes instruction in the following:
	• Cognitive and behavioral techniques to increase functioning and/or modulate pain (including motivational interviewing)
	• Health, wellness, and fitness programs (e.g., mindfulness, meditation)
	• Impairments in body functions and structures, activity limitations, and participation restrictions
	• Lifestyle intervention (e.g., stress management, sleep hygiene, physical activity, nutritional recommendations, addressing environmental factors and exposures)
	• Pathology or health condition
	• Performance enhancement
	• Psychosocial influences on treatment (e.g., fear-avoidance beliefs, behavioral change techniques)
	• Risk factor mitigation
	• Transitions across new settings and to new roles
Procedural interventions	
Adaptive and assistive technology	Includes prescription, application, and, as appropriate, fabrication or modification of splinting, bracing, taping, casting, seating, and positioning technologies; aids for locomotion; orthotic devices; prosthetic devices; robotics; sensors; and other adaptive technologies to improve functioning
Biophysical agents	Includes modalities such as cryotherapy, thermotherapy, compression therapy, biofeedback, sound agents, light agents, hydrotherapy, mechanical devices, hyperbaric oxygen, and electrical stimulation
Functional training in self-care and domestic, work, community, social, and civic life	Includes training in functional tasks related to: • Activities of daily living training • Barrier accommodations or modifications • Developmental activities • Device and equipment use and training • Functional training programs • Instrumental activities of daily living • Injury prevention or reduction
Integumentary repair and protection techniques	Includes biophysical agents, debridement, dressing application, and topical agent application
Manual therapy	Includes manual lymphatic drainage, manual traction, massage, mobilization/manipulation, neural tissue mobilization, passive range of motion, and dry needling
Motor function/movement training	Includes agility training, balance training, dual-task training, environmental stimulus training, gait training, manual guidance, mental rehearsal, pain modulating movement training, observational modeling, perceptual training, proprioception training, sensory integration, sports-specific movement training, task-specific training, virtual reality adaptive training, practice of closed and open skills to enhance motor performance, and environmental manipulation
Respiratory and ventilatory techniques for enhanced respiratory function	Includes the following: *Strategies:* active cycle of breathing or forced expiratory techniques, assisted cough and huff techniques, and autogenic drainage *Manual and mechanical techniques:* assistive devices (e.g., AMBU [artificial manual breathing unit] bag, incentive spirometry); chest percussion, vibration, and shaking; suctioning *Positioning:* to alter work of breathing, to maximize ventilation and perfusion, and pulmonary postural drainage
Therapeutic exercise	Includes aerobic and endurance conditioning and reconditioning; flexibility exercises; neuromotor development training; relaxation; strength, power, and endurance training for head, neck, limb, pelvic floor, trunk, and ventilatory muscles; balance training; gait and locomotion training; posture training; graded motor imagery

Adapted from the *Guide to Physical Therapist Practice*, 4.0.

activity limitation and improved speed and efficiency in stair-climbing is listed as an activity goal, then part of the intervention would logically entail training in stair-climbing skills. Sometimes, however, the justification for physical therapy interventions is not so readily apparent. For example, therapists use electrotherapeutic modalities for many different reasons, including muscle reeducation and reduction of swelling. When the purpose for using a particular intervention is not clear, the therapist must take the time to document in the report a concise rationale for the intervention chosen.

> **Example:** *NMES to R quads for muscle reeducation.*
> *US to proximal extensor carpi radialis to promote tissue healing.*

As with other sections of the physical therapy report, documentation of interventions should be detailed appropriately. For example, simply stating "gait training" is too vague. Specification of more detail about the gait training—such as to improve safety during outdoor ambulation or to improve endurance, speed, or efficiency of gait pattern—is essential. Alternatively, providing too much detail in this section wastes the therapist's time and clouds the report with extraneous information. For example, if progressive resistive strengthening exercise for the right quadriceps and hamstrings is one of the procedural interventions for a particular patient, the PT need not document the specific number of repetitions, sets, positioning, or exact types of exercises that will be performed. Similarly, documentation of modalities in the initial evaluation need not include specific parameters. This information is more appropriately conveyed in each session note documentation, as the parameters are likely to change over the course of the episode of care.

DOCUMENTING SKILLED INTERVENTION

An important component of documenting the Plan of Care is to demonstrate to third-party payers that the intervention proposed for the patient is medically necessary and requires the skilled services of a PT. The interventions listed in the Plan of Care section therefore need to encompass those interventions that are within the PT's scope of practice (based on state law).

PTs may have difficulty justifying the need for their services if the intervention plan includes a statement similar to the following:

> *Practice walking on a variety of surfaces.*

It is unclear from this statement *why* the skilled services of a PT are needed. Instead, terms such as *gait training* are useful. PTs should also consider further justification of the need for a therapist's skilled intervention, such as:

> *Gait training to improve effective foot clearance and maximize safety.*

To depict skilled interventions in your initial evaluation report, it is important to *describe* what *you* (as the PT) will do during the interventions. If a PT or PTA is the only

---

BOX 13.1   Terminology That Indicates Skilled Performance

Some terminology that indicates skilled performance include the following:
- Adjust
- Analyze
- Assess
- Direct
- Downgrade
- Educate
- Establish
- Implement
- Modify
- Progress
- Revise
- Teach
- Upgrade

If a caregiver can perform a task or activity with a client, then that intervention is generally *not* considered skilled. Some terminology that is indicative of *unskilled* interventions include the following:
- Supervise
- Observe
- Monitor
- Maintain
- Practice

Adapted with permission from Preferred Therapy Solutions, Wethersfield, Connecticut.

---

one who can do what you are proposing, then it is skilled. Box 13.1 shows sample terminology that is indicative of skilled interventions.

DOCUMENTING INFORMED CONSENT

The principle of informed consent is integral to health care. Whereas traditionally such consent was taken for granted, the modern approach is to verify informed consent in writing. Documenting informed consent has two benefits: it serves as evidence that informed consent was obtained, if there is a dispute at a later date, and (perhaps more important) it reminds practitioners to take this crucial last step before beginning treatment. It therefore reflects the concept of shared decision-making, where patients are informed of potential benefits and risks of interventions and alternatives, and health care professionals work together with patients to develop goals and a Plan of Care (Hoffman et al., 2022).

Informed consent can be documented either by (1) having the patient (or responsible family member) sign a standard form or (2) reporting that verbal consent was obtained at the end of the written initial evaluation. In the absence of a standard form, an appropriate variant of the following statement should be inserted at the end of the Plan of Care section:

> *The findings of this evaluation were discussed with (insert name of the patient or responsible party) and they consented to the above plan of care.*

If the patient is a minor or not competent to give informed consent, then the evaluation and Plan of Care should be discussed with a responsible person (e.g., parent, guardian, or spouse). If other persons are present during the discussion of informed consent, the PT should indicate who they are.

Finally, the concept of informed consent implies that the patient or responsible party has the right to *not* consent to the recommended plan, either in whole or in part. If that occurs, the PT should indicate in detail those parts of the Plan of Care with which the patient disagrees and briefly summarize the reasons given.

SUMMARY

- The therapist documents the details of the patient's activity limitations and impairments throughout the functional outcome report; these details should logically lead to specific goals and an appropriate Plan of Care designed to achieve those goals.
- The Plan of Care is typically the last section in a physical therapy report. It reflects the compiling of information from all other aspects of the report and can be the most highly scrutinized section.
- Although the Plan of Care of an initial evaluation report can be short and concise, it should provide sufficient detail so that the justifications for the chosen interventions are clear.

- The Plan of Care must document the need for skilled interventions, and it is important to describe what you (as the PT) will do during the interventions. If a PT or PTA is the only one who can do what you are proposing, then the intervention can be considered skilled.
- The Plan of Care should reflect shared decision-making, where patients PTs and patients work collaboratively toward meaningful goals.
- Following the Plan of Care, a statement indicating that informed consent was obtained should be included.

CASE EXAMPLE 13.1   Documenting Plan of Care   Setting: Outpatient Cardiac Rehabilitation

Name: Jason Press   **D.O.B.:** 3/15/66   **Gender**: Male   **Date of Eval.:** 9/10/22

Current Condition
s/p percutaneous transluminal coronary angioplasty 8/27/22.

PLAN OF CARE
Pt. will be seen for skilled PT cardiac rehabilitation 3×/wk with 45-min sessions for 6 wk.

Educational Interventions
1. Review cardiac guidelines with patient and wife; discuss strategies for exercising at home. Review Rate of Perceived Exertion (RPE) scale and warning signs.

2. Pt. will be instructed in HEP to include progressive walking routine and use of heart rate monitor and home blood pressure monitor. Discussed lifestyle modifications (activity level; weight loss).

Procedural Interventions
1. Phase II cardiac rehabilitation including monitored activity (treadmill walking, stationary bike, and UE ergometry), performed at 70% of maximal HR and <11-13 RPE, HR no greater than 30 beats per minute above resting.
2. Warm-up and cool-down prior to aerobic activity, with emphasis on total body flexibility routine.
3. Introduction to UE strength training with handheld weights (2 kg to start).

CASE EXAMPLE 13.2   Documenting Plan of Care   Setting: Acute Care Hospital

Name: Joseph Jacobs   **D.O.B.:** 6/17/53   **Gender**: Male   **Date of Eval.:** 5/1/23

Current Condition
1 day s/p right total hip replacement.

PLAN OF CARE
Pt. will receive PT 2×/day, anticipated D/C 7/4/23. F/u with hospital social worker re: D/C plan: 1. Home care PT/OT services for the evaluation of home safety and furthering community access. 2. Necessary adaptive equipment—raised toilet seat, tub bench, walker.

Educational Interventions
Pt. was instructed in total hip precautions and exercises (hip isometrics, ankle pumps, glut sets, quad sets) preop on 6/20/24 (handout given). Will continue reviewing precautions and exercises each session. Exercises to be performed 3×/day.

Procedural Interventions
1. AROM exercises B LEs—progression from ankle pumps, glut sets, and quad sets to active knee flexion/extension, hip flexion, abduction, and extension following THR precautions.
2. Bed mobility and transfer trng while maintaining hip precautions, maximizing independence.
3. Balance trng in standing to improve standing tolerance during functional activities.
4. Gait trng for short distances (10-20 ft) with standard walker, progressively increasing distance and decreasing skilled instruction for safety and foot placement.
5. Elevation trng: curbs and stairs to promote independence and safety.

CASE EXAMPLE 13.3   Documenting Plan of Care   Setting: Outpatient

Name: Brian Jones   **D.O.B.:** 4/23/06   **Gender:** Male   **Date of Eval.:** 6/15/23

Current Condition

1 wk s/p R ACL reconstruction with hamstring autograft.

PLAN OF CARE

Pt. will be seen for PT 3 days/wk for 12 wk, 45-min sessions. Reassess pt. status in 2 wk to determine the ability to progress interventions in accordance with the MD's postop protocol. Follow-up the phone call with MD prior to pt.'s next appointment to coordinate progression of exercise program. Consult with athletic trainer at school who will be working with Brian within 2 wk.

Educational Interventions

Brian will be instructed in the following:

1. PROM exercises for knee flexion and extension for inclusion in HEP and in the clinic.
2. Patellofemoral self-mobilization to increase joint mobility.

3. Isometric quad sets.
4. Instruction in safe use of crutches in all environments.
5. Use of ice and elevation to reduce swelling and pain.

Procedural Interventions

1. Retrograde massage to improve circulation and decrease LE edema.
2. NMES to R quads for neuromuscular reeducation.
3. AROM and progressive resistive strengthening exercises to increase the strength of R quadriceps, hamstrings, and gastroc/soleus as per MD protocol.
4. Gait trng to improve safety and endurance during ambulation, including uneven surfaces, ramps, and stairs.
5. Balance activities in standing to improve RLE stability.
6. Progressive trng, once appropriate, on stationary bike, NordicTrack, and treadmill to increase cardiovascular and muscular endurance.
7. Plyometric trng in preparation for return to sport as per MD protocol.

CASE EXAMPLE 13.4   Documenting Plan of Care   Setting: Inpatient Subacute Rehabilitation

Name: Alice Hawkins   **D.O.B.:** 2/16/ 64   **Gender:** Female   **Date of Eval.:** 8/12/22

Current Condition

2 weeks s/p L CVA with R hemiplegia.

PLAN OF CARE

Pt. will be seen for skilled PT intervention: 5-6 days/wk for 6 wk. Consult with orthotist regarding possible R AFO for improved gait stability. Coordinate with family regarding home evaluation to assess home environment prior to D/C. Coordinate with social work regarding home PT/OT/ST services at D/C for assessment of home safety, DME ordering, and to further community access.

Educational Interventions

Pt's family will be instructed in the following: safe sequencing, hand placement and guarding techniques for all bed mobility skills, sit-to-stand/stand-pivot transfers from bed←↑w/c, w/c←↑ toilet, and sit←↑stand with rolling walker.

Pt. will be instructed in seated ther-ex HEP for continued mobility and strengthening outside sessions and will be given ADL training videos to watch in evenings. PT will begin self-management education prior to D/C.

Procedural Interventions

1. AAROM/AROM and progressive resistive strengthening exercises to increase strength of RUE and RLE throughout all pivots.
2. Static and dynamic balance activities in standing to improve RLE and core stability.
3. Bed mobility trng with and without the use of side rails to improve mobility in preparation for transfers.
4. Transfer trng to improve forward momentum, facilitating a safer sit-to-stand motion.
5. Gait trng to improve safety and endurance during ambulation, including level and uneven surfaces, ramps, curbs, and stairs with progressively decreasing AD as tolerated.

CASE EXAMPLE: 13.5   Documenting Plan of Care   Setting: OP Pelvic Health/Female

Name: Joanne Lewe   **D.O.B.:** 10/22/82   **Gender:** Female   **Date of Eval.:** 9/1/22

Current Condition

Difficulty with urinating, incomplete defecation, and pelvic pain.

PLAN OF CARE

Pt. will receive PT 1×/wk for 12 weeks. Discuss progress with OBGYN as needed.

Educational Interventions

Pt. instructed in stretching (butterfly stretch, happy baby, and hip flexor stretch in Thomas test position—all with 60-sec hold × 5 repetitions) and diaphragmatic

breathing (10 repetitions in hook-lying position). Will continue to review and advance HEP as able at each session. Exercises to be performed daily.

Procedural Interventions

1. Down-training of pelvic floor muscles to address hypertonicity currently present.
2. Manual therapy to address increased tone of pelvic floor muscles.
3. Trunk stabilization training to limit pelvic floor muscle overuse.

EXERCISE 13.1

Identify the errors in the following statements documenting the Plan of Care. Rewrite a more appropriate statement in the space provided.

Statement	**Rewrite Statement**
EXAMPLE: Gait training.	Gait trng within the home with manual and verbal cues to improve gait symmetry and speed.
1. Practice walking.	
2. Apply hot packs.	
3. Pt. will be able to walk 10 ft to the bathroom.	
4. Pt. will be given strengthening exercises.	
5. Coordinate care with all nursing personnel.	
6. Assess work environment.	
7. Pt. will increase right hamstring strength.	
8. Balance training.	
9. Pt. will receive ultrasound at 1.0 W/cm², 1 MHz to R quadriceps (VMO), in a 10-cm area just proximal and slightly medial to R knee, moving ultrasound head slowly in circular fashion for 10 min, each session.	
10. Pt. will take pain relief medication as needed.	

Statement	**Rewrite Statement**
11. Home evaluation.	_____ _____
12. Reduce R ankle edema.	_____ _____
13. Teach family to care for pt.	_____ _____
14. Practice pressure-relief techniques.	_____ _____
15. E-stim to anterior tibialis.	_____ _____

Session Notes and Progress Notes Using a Modified SOAP Format

LEARNING OBJECTIVES

After reading this chapter and completing the exercises, the reader will be able to:
1. Identify and describe the key components of a session note.
2. Identify and describe the key components of a progress note.

3. Explain the key legal issues pertinent to session note documentation.
4. Appropriately document components of session notes and progress notes using a modified SOAP format.

Session notes and progress notes are key components of physical therapy documentation. In fact, many therapists spend a majority of their documentation time writing these types of notes. Although the focus of this book thus far has been on documenting the initial evaluation, all elements included in session or progress notes are essentially components of the initial evaluation. The concepts discussed in Chapters 7–13 all apply here.

Although there are no formal guidelines from either the American Physical Therapy Association (APTA) or the Centers for Medicare and Medicaid Services regarding the structure of session or progress notes, such documentation can become unwieldy without some organization. The SOAP note is a commonly used format and is one with which most medical personnel are familiar (see Chapter 2 for the history and development of the SOAP note). The SOAP format is relatively easy to master and provides a quick format for writing a session note. This chapter presents a format for writing both session notes and progress notes using a modified SOAP format.

MODIFIED SOAP FORMAT

The acronym SOAP stands for *subjective, objective, assessment,* and *plan* (Weed, 1971). This format was discussed briefly in Chapter 2 and is presented here as a framework for session and progress note documentation. However, the original design for use of the SOAP note is not how it is currently used by most medical professionals. The SOAP note was designed to promote a sequential rather than an integrative approach to clinical decision-making and was linked to the problem-oriented medical record, which is no longer routinely used. However, with some modifications the SOAP note can provide the foundation for efficient, effective functional outcomes documentation in rehabilitation.

The tables in this chapter outline key components of these notes to meet criteria necessary for optimal clinical decision-making, third-party payment, and legal purposes. Because

BOX 14.1 Time-Saving Tips for Writing Session Notes

- Keep a printout of patient's goals readily visible in the front of the patient's chart.
- Use tables and flowcharts whenever possible Case Example 14.5 for documenting both interventions and outcomes.
- When documenting tests and measures, focus on *changes* to patient's status.
- Use electronic documentation whenever possible. Even if your facility has not yet implemented a complete system, use a computer and write your own documentation template.

session notes must serve such diverse purposes, there may be a tendency for therapists to write excessively long notes. Strategies for simplifying documentation are provided in Box 14.1. Furthermore, the case examples at the end of this chapter demonstrate how such notes are modified for different patients in different practice settings.

SESSION NOTES

Session notes are written for each encounter a physical therapist (PT) or physical therapist assistant has with a patient (Case Examples 14.1 to 14.5). Although APTA documentation guidelines and most third-party payers require documentation for each physical therapy encounter, the format of session note documentation is at the discretion of each therapist or institution.

Session notes are written for four distinct reasons:
1. *Legal documentation:* A session note importantly provides a legal record of what was done in a therapy session and why. For this reason, documentation of the specifics of the interventions performed and the patient's reaction to those interventions is critical (see Chapter 13).
2. *Third-party payment:* Third-party payers typically request that session notes be provided as proof of service. Medicare, for example, requires documentation to create a record of all

treatments and skilled interventions to justify the use of billing codes (see Chapter 5).

3. *Facilitation of functional outcomes and clinical decision-making:* Writing a session note that focuses on functional outcomes helps maintain a therapist's attention on patient-specific goals. Each session note allows the therapist the time to reevaluate the patient's progress and goals and to consider changes to the plan of care.

4. *Record for other therapists in case of absence:* In the event that a therapist is absent, it is important for any covering therapist to have a complete record of the specific interventions that were performed with a patient.

For the session note to address these varying aspects, the following information should be included (adapted from APTA's Defensive Documentation[1]):

1. Patient/client or caregiver report.
2. Interventions provided, including frequency, intensity, time, duration, and level of physical and/or cognitive assistance provided as appropriate.
3. Patient/client response to treatments/interventions.
4. Patient or client response to treatments.
5. Communication and collaboration with other providers, patient or client, and family, caregiver, and significant others as applicable or indicated.
6. Verbal communication other than orders, including phone calls or contact with the patient or client, their family or other caregivers, a patient's other health care provider and any other professionals involved in the individual's care also should be documented.
7. Factors that modify frequency or intensity of intervention and progression within the plan of care.
8. Plan for next visit(s) including interventions with objectives, progression parameters, and precautions, if indicated within the PT's plan of care.

Framework for Session Note Documentation— Modified SOAP Note

The recommended framework for session note documentation is based on the modified SOAP note and includes goals, subjective (S), objective (O), assessment (A), and plan (P) (Table 14.1).

Goals

From a functional outcomes perspective, the focus of session notes should be on the specific goals that are being addressed. Thus the goals should be readily visible to the therapist as he or she writes the session note. This can be accomplished by adding a statement at the beginning of the SOAP note that identifies the goals, possibly including only those that were the focus of that treatment (restatement of the goals that were set at the time of the initial evaluation or last progress note). Alternatively, therapists can easily have the patient's goals reproduced at the beginning of the SOAP note. This can be more easily accomplished using computerized documentation.

Common Pitfall. Goals are not included. Restating the goal(s) forces the therapist to maintain a focus on the outcomes toward which therapeutic intervention is directed.

[1]https://www.apta.org/your-practice/documentation.

TABLE 14.1 Framework for Writing Session Notes Using a Modified SOAP Format

Goal	• List goals for patient.
S—Subjective	• Patient's subjective response to interventions (including any adverse reactions). • Patient's report of changes in participation or activity limitations.
O—Objective	• Status update: Indicate any objective, measurable changes in patient's status with regard to activity limitations or impairments. • Intervention (Rx): Outline interventions that were performed, including communication and/or education with health care providers, patient, family, or significant others. Include frequency, duration, and intensity, if appropriate, as well as any equipment provided.
A—Assessment	• Indicate the progress being made toward patient's goals, including adherence to patient-related instructions. • Discuss factors that modify frequency or intensity of intervention and progression toward anticipated goals. • Modify or set new goals if necessary.
P—Plan	• State specific intervention plan for upcoming sessions. • Report what patient will be doing between sessions (e.g., home program, other interventions/tests).

Note: Framework for session note documentation using a modified SOAP format. Recommendations from American Physical Therapy Association and current Centers for Medicare and Medicaid Services requirements for session note documentation are incorporated into this framework.

Subjective (S)

In the Subjective section of the session note, the therapist documents the patient's subjective responses to interventions and any changes in participation or activity limitations. This section could include any relevant statements or reports made by the patient, patient's family members, and/or caregivers. The purpose of this section is to detail the patient's own perception of his or her condition, which can relate to impairments (e.g., pain), activities (e.g., ability to walk), or participation (e.g., ability to work). Box 14.2 provides more information on documenting pain in session notes.

This section of the note does *not* include direct observations made by the therapist. Therapists can report a patient's or caregiver's remarks in quotation marks if the exact phrasing is somehow pertinent. Documentation of subjective information should incorporate information that is relevant to the patient's progress in rehabilitation and specifically related to changes in functional performance or quality of life. It should not include extraneous information that is not directly related to the patient's current condition.

Common Pitfall. Documentation is not specific enough.

Example: *Pt. reports pain is getting better.*

Such a statement needs to be more specific.

Better Example: *Pt. reports pain in left hip during walking has improved from 6/10 to 4/10.*

The therapist could also document nonpertinent information. For example, a therapist might write:

Example: *Pt. reports she did not like her last PT.*

BOX 14.2   Documenting Pain in Session Notes and Progress Notes

In the initial evaluation, a detailed description of pain is recommended, including what provokes the pain, the quality, the region or any radiating pain, the severity and the timing (PQRST) (see Box 10.1). The setting in which pain occurs and any associated manifestations may also be included.

In the session note or progress note documentation, a change in any component of pain is worthy of documentation. Decrease in pain severity (e.g., "Pt. reports pain has decreased to 2/10") or quality (e.g., "Pt. reports pain has gone from a burning, stabbing pain to an aching pain") can be indicators of patient improvement. It is not essential in the session note or progress note to completely redocument the detailed pain assessment provided in an initial note. Rather, *changes* in the patient's report of pain should be specifically documented.

Reports of pain (because they are inherently subjective) should typically be documented in the Subjective section of a session note or a progress note. However, if report of pain is incidental to an Objective statement, then it can be included in the Objective section, for example, "Pt. performed 10 reps ×3 sets SLR with no increase in pain." This statement's focus is on the intervention being performed.

This statement is not pertinent to the therapy program and should not be included in documentation.

Better Example: *Pt. reports she was "unsatisfied with her previous treatment results" and is hoping for more significant improvement in her walking ability.*

This statement is more specific to the patient's concern.

Objective (O)

The focus of the Objective section is twofold: (1) to document the results of any tests and measures performed, specifically those that relate to achievement of the stated goal(s) (Status Update) and (2) to provide details of the interventions performed (Rx) (see Case Examples). The Status Update should include any examination findings that were performed or observed (e.g., range of motion, walking speed). Documentation of the interventions should include the procedural interventions that were performed, including location, frequency, intensity, duration, and/or repetitions, as appropriate. Some of this information can be recorded in table or flowchart form. However, the documentation must clearly show evidence of skilled intervention and the interaction between the patient and therapist (see Chapter 13). For example,[2]

- Did you teach, educate, direct, progress, adjust, modify, revise?
- Did you challenge the client's ability to perform a task or activity?
- Did you facilitate some function during a task to improve it?
- Did you focus on something specific to bring about a change or improvement in function?
- If you provide "cues," they must be skilled, specific, and detailed. Avoid general cues such as *cues for safety and hand placement to push to stand.*

Common Pitfall. Not enough detail is provided regarding specific interventions. Therapists may generalize the interventions performed in a session note.

Example: *"E-stim" or "MH" or "Ther ex."*

---

[2]Adapted with permission from Preferred Therapy Solutions, Wethersfield, Connecticut.

Instead, specific details should be provided for each intervention performed.

Better Example: *Ther ex. seated knee ext through full range, 30 lb, 8 reps ×3; prone knee flex through full range, 20 lb, 10 reps ×3.*

Assessment (A)

In the Assessment section, the therapist indicates the progress being made toward the patient's goals, discusses factors that would modify frequency or intensity of intervention, and reports progress toward anticipated goals. The therapist should summarize the patient's progress and discuss those factors contributing to or hindering progress. Therapists should report modification of goals or document any new goals in this section.

Common Pitfall. The Assessment is too vague and not meaningful.

Example: *"Pt. tol Rx well" or "Pt. is improving."*

Such statements provide little insight into the effectiveness of the intervention. A better example would be:

Example: *Pt. has demonstrated improved tolerance to performing ther ex. regimen and has reported an increase in sitting tolerance time at work.*

Plan (P)

The final section of the session note outlines the Plan. Any specific interventions for upcoming sessions should be documented, including any changes in the intervention strategy.

Common Pitfall. The upcoming plan is not documented.

Example: *"Cont Rx,"; "Cont per plan."*

Although sometimes appropriate, statements such as these provide no information about how the therapist plans to continue to help the patient's progress.

Better Example: *Increase number of repetitions in squatting and wall slide exercises to 20.*

As the therapist reviews the patient's record at the next visit, this statement will serve as a reminder of the intended plan.

Legal Issues for Session Notes

As mentioned earlier, session note documentation is important for legal purposes (see also Chapter 3 for more information on legal aspects of documentation). If issues or conflicts arise as a result of the therapy intervention, the session notes will be highly scrutinized. A note that is poorly documented opens the door in support of a lawsuit or legal proceedings, even if the accusations are not well-founded.

Some important documentation guidelines for session notes follow (Scott, 2011):

1. *Timeliness:* Therapists should write session notes as soon as possible after a session. This helps keep information fresh in their mind and minimizes the chance of errors.
2. *Decision-making rationale:* Each section should flow logically from the next, and the therapist's decisions about assessment, goals, and interventions should be supported by concrete data.
3. *Patient/client behavior:* Missed or canceled appointments must be documented in the patient's medical record.

Example: *Pt. called at 9:00 AM to cancel 1:30 PM appt. Pt. reports his L shoulder was sore from doing too much lifting yesterday. Next appt scheduled in 2 days.*

This provides the time the appointment was canceled, detailed information as to the reason the appointment was canceled, and information about future appointments. A patient's noncompliance with recommendations or instructions given by a therapist must also be carefully and objectively documented.

4. *Prior and concurrent treatment:* Therapists should document any other interventions a patient is currently undergoing or has undergone in the past.

   Example: *Pt. reports he has begun acupuncture 2×/wk to facilitate back pain relief.*

5. *Communications:* Any conversations (oral or written) pertinent to the patient and the rehabilitation program should be documented. Such documentation should include the name, time, issues discussed, and the resolution or action.

   Example: *PT called pt.'s orthopedic surgeon, Dr. Smith, to discuss pt.'s report of increased pain in L ankle at the fracture site. MD stated to D/C PT immediately and refer pt. back to him for evaluation.*

6. *Informed consent and referral:* Documentation of informed consent in an initial evaluation is discussed in Chapter 3. In a session note, informed consent should be documented if changes to the plan of care are being implemented.

   Example: *Pt. was informed of phone conversation and MD's orders and was instructed to call MD immediately for an appt. Pt. agreed to this and stated he would call MD upon returning home.*

7. *Adverse incidents:* Therapists should follow their institutions' guidelines for documentation of an adverse incident. Typically, this is done on an incident report. Therapists should document in the medical record only pertinent clinical findings, and it is not necessary to indicate that an incident report has been filed separately (Scott, 2011) (Case Examples 14.1 to 14.5).

Progress Notes

Progress notes are written to provide an update of a patient's status; these notes often are based on a reexamination (Case Examples 14.6 to 14.10). The progress note typically covers multiple visits and therefore provides a summary of the patient's

TABLE 14.2	Framework for Writing Progress Notes Using a Modified SOAP Format
Goal	• List goals for a patient.
S—Subjective	• Patient's subjective response to interventions (including any adverse reactions).
	• Patient's report of changes in participation or activity limitations.
O—Objective	• Status update: Indicate any objective, measurable changes in patient's status with regard to activity limitations or impairments.
	• Intervention (Rx): Provide summary of interventions that were performed, including communication and/or education with health care providers, patient, family, or significant others. Include frequency, duration, and intensity, if appropriate, as well as any equipment provided. Evidence should be provided that skilled intervention was required to achieve the stated goals (particularly important for Medicare documentation).
A—Assessment	• Indicate the progress being made toward patient's goals, including adherence to patient-related instructions.
	• Discuss factors that modify frequency or intensity of intervention and progression toward anticipated goals.
	• Provide justification for continuation of therapy (state medical necessity).
	• Modify or set new goals if necessary.
P—Plan	• State specific intervention plan for upcoming sessions, with revision of original plan of care if needed.
	• Report what patient will be doing between sessions (e.g., home program, other interventions/tests).

Note: Framework for progress note documentation using a modified SOAP format. Recommendations from American Physical Therapy Association and current Centers for Medicare and Medicaid Services requirements for progress note documentation are incorporated into this framework.

progress to date. A progress note can have a format similar to an initial evaluation, and the functional outcomes framework presented in earlier chapters can be used. However, the SOAP format can also be used.

Table 14.2 outlines the key elements of each section of the progress note based on a SOAP format. Progress notes should be succinct and easy to read because they often are used by third-party payers to justify the need for skilled therapeutic intervention (see Chapter 5). Comparisons of preintervention and postintervention functional performance are especially useful. Therapists should document any interventions that were performed during the reevaluation period and provide justification for the need for continued therapy.

SUMMARY

- Session notes and progress notes can be organized as a functional outcomes report using a modified SOAP format.
- Documentation is required for every physical therapy encounter and should include information about the interventions provided and progress toward stated goals.
- Session notes are important legal records. Therapists should carefully document all aspects directly pertinent to

a patient's current physical therapy intervention and his or her current condition.

- Progress notes provide an update of a patient's status. Progress toward the stated goals is discussed, and justification for continued therapy is provided.

CASE EXAMPLE 14.1 Session Note   Setting: Outpatient

Name: Emily Rodriguez   **D.O.B.:** 2/3/92   **Gender:** Female   **Date of Eval.:** 1/5/23

Current Condition
31 y.o. female 12-wk postpartum c̄ onset of stress incontinence p vaginal delivery of first child.

Goal
Decrease urine losses from 2× daily to 1×/wk.

S: Pt. reports urinary losses of 1 tablespoon have decreased to 1×/day over past 3 days. Occurs primarily when coughing or during physical activities, such as lifting baskets of laundry, running, and jumping. Pt. continues to wear two panty-liners daily as continued precaution to protect clothing.

O: **Status update:** Biofeedback reassessment was completed in supine with noted improvement in EMG activity levels for pelvic muscle contractions. Fair strength of pelvic floor muscle contraction, held 5 sec ×7 reps.

Rx: Pt. performed pelvic floor muscle contractions c̄ biofeedback program in the standing position. Pt. performed pelvic floor muscle contractions during a lunge to floor and back to standing, 3 reps each LE (practicing the movement for lifting a laundry basket). Practiced pelvic muscle contractions prior to a cough, 5 reps. Pt. ed: pelvic muscle contraction before coughing or lifting heavy objects to prevent incontinence. Revised HEP to ↑ pelvic muscle contractions in sitting for 20 1-sec contractions; followed by 20 min of 10-sec contractions in sitting.

A: Pt. reports a decrease in urinary losses over the past 3 days, which correlates with observed improvements in EMG activity levels for pelvic floor muscle contractions.

P: Continue PT 1×/wk. Progress with pelvic muscle strength trng and muscle reeducation during functional tasks, with instruction in progressive HEP to improve pt.'s level of ADLs.

CASE EXAMPLE 14.2 Session Note   Setting: Acute Hospital/Inpatient

Name: Wally Narcessian   **D.O.B.:** 3/7/51   **Gender:** Male   **Date of Eval.:** 6/20/23 (10:26:00 AM)

Current Condition
COPD/pneumonia

Goals
1. Pt. will demonstrate productive cough in a seated position, 3/4 trials.
2. Pt. will ambulate 150 ft with CS, no AD, on level indoor surfaces, within 45 sec (to enable in-home ambulation).

S: Pt. reports not feeling well today, "I'm very tired."
O: **Status update:** Auscultation findings: scattered rhonchi all lung fields.
Rx: Chest PT was performed in sitting (ant and post). Techniques included percussion, vibration, and shaking. Pt. performed a weak combined abdominal and upper costal cough that was nonbronchospastic, congested, and nonproductive. The cough/huff was performed with verbal cues. Pectoral stretch/ thoracic cage mobilizations performed in seated position. Pt. given towel roll placed in back of seat to open up ant chest wall. Strengthening exercises in standing—pt. performed hip flexion, extension, and abduction; knee flexion 10 reps ×1 set B. Pt. performs HEP with supervision (in evenings with wife). Pt. instructed to hold tissue over trach when speaking to prevent infection and explained importance of drinking enough water.

A: Pt. continues to present with congestion and limitations in coughing productivity. Pt. has been compliant with evening exercise program, which has resulted in increased tol. to ther ex. regimen and an increase in LE strength. Amb not attempted today 2° to pt. report of fatigue. Pt. should be able to tolerate short-distance amb within next few days.

P: Cont. current treatment plan including CPT; emphasize productive coughing techniques; increase strengthening exer reps to 15; attempt amb again tomorrow.

CASE EXAMPLE 14.3 Session Note   Setting: Outpatient

Name: Julie Jones   **D.O.B.:** 10/1/77   **Gender:** Female   **Date of Eval.:** 6/20/23

Current Condition Chronic left shoulder adhesive capsulitis.

Goal
To return to full-time work activities as an electrician including overhead wiring, pain-free in 4 wk.

S: Patient reports L shoulder pain localized over outer upper arm when performing overhead wiring at work.
O: **Status update:** Patient performs overhead fine motor tasks to simulate electrical work for 5 min before the onset of pain. **Rx:** Pt. received 5 min of manual L shoulder joint mobs, inferior and anterior glide grade 4. Followed by manual stretching to increase shoulder abduction and external rotation ROM. Strengthening exercises performed with green Theraband for int. rotation, ext. rotation, flex and ext of L shoulder: 3 sets of 10 reps for total 15 min. Pt. education: regarding proper posture when performing overhead work activities. (10 min). Total treatment time: 35 min.

A: Patient has been making slow gains in reducing L shoulder pain during her overhead work-related activities. She has been able to increase the length of time spent in overhead activities before the onset of pain.

P: Continue c̄ joint mobs and stretching to increase shoulder abduction and ER. Pt. HEP will be modified to add exercise for overhead activity endurance.

CASE EXAMPLE 14.4 **Session Note**   **Setting: Outpatient**

Name: Taylor Jones   **D.O.B.:** 3/25/02   **Gender:** Male   **Date of Eval:** 6/9/23
Treatment Date: 6/16/23

Current Condition
Post concussion syndrome with cervical pain following mild TBI on 5/12/23.

GOALS
1. 1. Pt. will be able to use laptop x1 hour during college classes without reports of headache within 4 wks.
2. Pt. will be able to drive x30 minutes without reports of dizziness to commute to their college campus within 4 wks.

Subjective
Pt. reports "I was able to shower this morning without getting dizzy, but my neck still hurt to tilt my head back when I washed my hair."

Objective
Segmental hypomobility noted with PAIVM from C3-C6 vertebral levels.

Rx: Today's treatment session included: manual SOR and soft tissue mobilization to cervical paraspinal musculature x10 min total to relieve tension in the musculature and reduce pain. Grade III/IV CPA mobilizations to C3-C6 x5 min total to improve segmental mobility. Oculomotor exercises for convergence using Brock string: 1 bead tracking moving arm's length along string x10 reps, 3 bead gaze transitions with 10 sec holds on each x5 total reps. VOR exercises to address gaze stability: VOR x1 exercises: seated with target held by pt. at eye level and arm's length distance, horizontal and vertical 3 x30 sec each with metronome at 80 beats per minute. VOR cancellation exercises with pt. focused on own thumb held at arm's length and eye level, standing horizontal 4 x30 sec with metronome at 80 beats per minute. Pt. experienced dizziness of 3/10 intensity with VOR cancellation exercise that fully resolved after 2 minutes of seated rest. Recumbent bike x15 min at 60% symptom threshold heart rate to improve exertional tolerance.

Assessment
Pt. had minimal symptom exacerbation during treatment session, resolving readily with rest break when encountered. Pt. was able to perform with increased in HR intensity on the recumbent bike without reports of dizziness or headache suggesting increasing exertional tolerance. Pt.'s headaches are likely stemming from a combination of upper to mid cervical spine mobility impairments, as well as VOR and convergence deficits. Rx to address these limitations will facilitate achievement of the pt.'s functional goals and return to their PLOF.

Plan
Continue with current stage of concussion treatment protocol at next visit. Anticipate progression to the next stage if pt. completes next session without symptoms. Coordinate with pt.'s college and physician regarding the possibility of granting temporary extended time for exams until concussion fully resolves.

CASE EXAMPLE 14.5 **Session Note**   **Setting: Outpatient**

Name: Timothy Barnes   **D.O.B.:** 3/10/19/82   **Gender:** Male   **Date of Eval:** 11/17/23
Treatment Date: 11/25/23

Current Condition s/p C4-C7 anterior cervical discectomy and fusion 8/13/23.

Goals (4 wk)
1. Pt. will be able to drive >1 hr without report of pain/fatigue (1-2/10).
2. Pt. will be able to perform work-related activity of lifting boxes up to 15 lb. without difficulty and no report of pain (1-2/10).
3. Pt. will be able to read/grade papers for 1 hr with pain level 1/10 and without fatigue.

Subjective
Pt. noted that they were not having a "good day" current pain level 4/10 at rest. Pt. also noted that they were sore after the last session.

Objective
Rx: Pt. received treatment as per flow sheet ×50 min. No complaint of increased pain with all activities.

Activity	Comments	Sets	Reps/Hold	Time	Current Procedural Terminology Code
Moist heat to cervical spine	Supine			10 min	97010
Soft Tissue Mob/Strain-Counterstarin	Traps & c/s in supine			15 min	97140
Manual subocciptal release				5 min	97140
Manual PROM—B sidebend, rotation, and flexion	c/s in supine			10 min	97140
Supine chin tucks	5-sec hold	2	10		97110
Theraband resisted rows—red band		2	10		97110
Chin tucks against wall	5-sec hold	2	10		97110
3-Way pec stretch standing		3	30		97110

Assessment
No further exercises were added to the program secondary to pt.'s report of soreness from the last session. Initiated today's session with manual therapy to improve ROM and decrease pain. Pt. noted reduction of symptoms following these interventions. Moderate muscle fatigue was noted during exercises but no increase in pain.

Plan
Tim will continue therapy as prescribed. Progress exercise program next session to include additional UE strengthening exercises.

CASE EXAMPLE 14.6 Session Note Setting: Acute Oncology

Name: John Rogers **D.O.B.:** 2/19/85 **Gender**: Male **Date of Eval.:** 8/9/23

Current Condition
38yo male patient with PMH of DM type 2, vitiligo, incidental right adrenal mass, recent diagnosed acute myelomonocytic leukemia.

Goal
Patient will ambulate > 250 feet modified independent with front-wheeled walker.

S: Pt. agreeable to PT. No reports of pain.

O: Able to perform 2 separate bouts of sit to stand, initially from slightly elevated surface and then from lowest bed surface (24"). Demonstrates ability to achieve full hip extension B in upright position, but requires use of BUE on FWW. Pt. benefitted from facilitation cues on distal R quadriceps to load through RLE and bear weight through both LE equally. Able to carry over that response for a few repetitions, but as fatigue increased, required minimal verbal cues to distribute weight evenly again.

During gait training, continues to present with excessive R hip ER, flat foot initial contact on RLE and decreased stride and step length, all due to decreased ankle DF ROM limiting ability to successfully complete swing phase of gait. With verbal cueing to perform greater knee and hip flexion to assist in clearing the foot during swing, pt able to achieve this task but reports that he is not used to that motion and therefore, fatigued quickly.

Pt. returned back to bed w/call button in reach and all needs met.

A: With tandem balance tasks, pt. demonstrates decreased stability overall, but greater deficits with LLE compared to RLE. Current self-selected gait speed is consistent with limited household ambulator status.

P: Assess ability to ascend/descend 1 or 2 steps using step stool to mimic shower set up at home; continue gait progression.

CASE EXAMPLE 14.7 Progress Note Setting: Outpatient

Name: Linda Smith **D.O.B.:** 5/12/87 **Gender**: Female **Date of Eval.:** 10/01/23

Current Condition
Thoracic pain, 2-wk reevaluation.

Goals
1. Change the diapers of their 6-month-old baby on changing table without pain (0/10).
2. Carry their 6-month-old baby for 20 min without pain (0/10).

S: Pt. reports: "I am able to get out of bed without pain." Pt. now reports ability to change diapers with pain rated as 2/10 and can carry child in carrier for 15 min, 2/10 pain.

O: Status update: Normal pelvic alignment with B ASIS, PSIS, and iliac crests all level. Correction of R posteriorly rotated innominate remains stable. Strength of abdominals 3+/5 and trunk extensors 4/5. Strength of B hip extensors and abductors: 4/5.

Rx: Interventions at today's session included: grade I/II P-A sacral mobs x5 min total to reduce pain; manual hold-relax stretching of B hamstrings x5 min total to improve muscle length; pt. education x10 min for proper standing posture and carrying techniques. Pt instruction in LE and trunk exercises x15 min consisting of hamstring and hip flexor stretch 3 x30 sec each, posterior pelvic tilt, bridging, bridging with marching, and dying bug exercise with abdominal draw-in maneuver all 2 sets of 15. Pt demonstrated proper technique and good understanding of exercises, as well as posture and carrying techniques.

A: Pt. is exhibiting steady progress with trunk strength and endurance since the initial evaluation, most likely due to enhanced neuromotor control. Further focus on core muscle strength, endurance, and coordination is needed for patient to achieve above-stated goals and to tolerate baby's continued weight gain. Patient independent with current HEP.

P: Continue current exercie regimen with progression of lumbosacral stabilization exercises as tolerated. Progress HEP as appropriate. Physical therapy sessions will continue 3×/wk for 2 more wks.

CASE EXAMPLE 14.8 Progress Note Setting: Outpatient

Name: Melissa Chau **D.O.B.:** 12/26/97 **Gender**: Female **Date of Eval.:** 10/01/23

Current Condition Patellofemoral dysfunction, 1 wk progress note.

Goals
1. Pt. will ascend and descend 2 flights of stairs, pain-free (4 wk).
2. Pt. will run on level surfaces 2 miles in 20 min, 2×/wk, pain-free (6 wk).

S: "My knee no longer hurts when I am sitting at my desk." (rated as 0/10)

O: Rx:: See flow sheet.

Status update: *Ambulation/stair-climbing.* Pt. able to walk 1/2 mile at comfortable speed without pain (65 m/min). Able to ascend 2 flights of stairs pain-free. Steady eccentric control observed without genu valgus when descending 1 flight of stairs, with pain rated as 4/10. *Running.* Pt. has not yet engaged in running activity. *Strength.* L hip abductors 4/5, R hip abductors 4/5, L quadriceps 4/5, L hamstrings 5/5; R quads and hamstrings 5/5. L unilateral stance time, static: 30 sec. R unilateral stance time, static: 60 sec.

A: Steady progress is being made toward the goal of pain-free stair negotiation. Pt. is exhibiting a steady improved eccentric quadriceps control when decreasing stairs with a decrease in reported pain. Patellar taping techniques used to recruit L vastus medialis have been successful. Balance deficits are still apparent as indicated by limited unilateral stance time on the LLE. Continued strength and balance gains are necessary for a patient to achieve the running goal.

P: Continue the current exercise program, with progression in intensity as tolerated. Home programs, consisting of SLRs, squats, step-ups, and patellar taping techniques, are to be completed daily. PT sessions will continue 2×/wk with the addition of low-impact activities. Eval. for orthotics next session.

CASE EXAMPLE 14.9   Progress Note   Setting: Outpatient Neurology Clinic

Name: Ralph Fisher   **D.O.B.:** 12/19/77   **Gender**: Male   **Date of Eval.:** 7/8/23

Current Condition
Huntington disease (HD) × 11 yr; 1 mo reevaluation.

Goals (12 wk)
1. Pt. will experience no falls during indoor or outdoor ambulation over 12-wk period.
2. Pt. will increase average outdoor walking speed on sidewalk with use of cane to 50 m/min, for distances >400 m.
3. Pt. will be independent with HEP, including walking program and completion of 35-min exercise video including ROM/flexibility, strengthening, and endurance trng.

S: Pt. reports that his balance "is getting better" and that he has had no falls in past 4 wk (since initial evaluation). He reports that he is not yet comfortable using the cane for outdoor ambulation. He reports having some difficulty keeping up with walking and turning exercises on exercise video.

O: Rx: Pt. has been seen 1×/wk for 4 wk to address balance impairments and ambulation difficulties related to HD. Intervention has consisted of (1) gait training on indoor and outdoor surfaces, including safety instruction and strategies to improve gait speed; (2) balance exercises and balance training in standing, emphasizing improving anticipatory balance; instruction in home program with exercise video (35 min in length)—exercises include ROM/flexibility, strengthening, and cardiovascular; discussion of home safety and recommendations made for grab bars in bathroom, removal of rugs, and supportive chair for mealtimes.

Status Update: *Activities:* Pt. is able to walk indoors s A; avg. walking speed 42 m/min. Pt. ambulates outdoors on sidewalk with a slower gait speed (35 m/

min) and is very cautious. Pt. avoids stairs and uneven surfaces whenever possible due to fear of falling; these activities have not yet been assessed in therapy. *Activities of Balance Confidence* remains at 80% (100% = complete confidence). Continues to demonstrate LOB (to the R and posteriorly) during indoor and outdoor ambulation but has I recovery. *Dystonia*: Unchanged; mod. trunk dystonia resulting in posturing into extension and R lateral flexion. *Chorea*: unchanged; mod. chorea ×4 extremities. *Balance*: Berg Balance Scale score increased from 39 to 44; pt. improved in tandem stance, turning in place, and picking up object from floor. Single-limb stance unchanged; limited to <2 sec B.

A: Pt. has demonstrated improvements in balance as measured by the Berg Balance Scale and has not had any falls in a 4-wk period. Pt. is able to perform HEP program independently with modifications. Pt. requires continued PT to address slow walking speed (goal 2) and standing balance impairments, focusing on single-limb stance to continue to minimize fall risk (goal 1).

P: Pt. will continue to be seen for skilled PT 1×/wk for 8 wk. Treatment focus on (1) gait training indoors and outdoors to address safety, speed, and balance (anticipatory and reactive); (2) balance training exercises, emphasizing single-limb stance activities; (3) revision of home program to modify walking and turning activities so pt. can keep up with recorded exercise program; (4) cont. education re: use of straight cane during outdoor ambulation; and (5) evaluate stair-climbing, curb negotiation, uneven surface ambulation, and initiate training for functional benefit, balance improvement, and strengthening.

CASE EXAMPLE: 14.10   Progress Note   Setting: Outpatient Hospital Clinic

Name: Chloe Schwartz   **D.O.B.:** 12/19/64   **Gender**: Female   **Date of Eval.:** 3/2/2023

Current Condition
ICD-10: M62.81 Muscle Weakness (generalized), U09.9: Post-COVID-19 condition unspecified.

Goals (4 wk)
1. Pt. will perform 6-minute walk test without standing rest breaks needed, to promote improved walking tolerance.
2. Pt. will be able to complete 12 sit-to-stands in 30 sec without symptoms.
3. Pt. will be able to complete household chores for 2 hr without reports of SOB and only mild fatigue noted.

S: History of Present Condition: Patient was diagnosed with COVID-19 in March 2020. They were very ill for about 10 days. Then when they were able to get the COVID-19 vaccine, they began to have severe fatigue, SOB, and increased anxiety. October 2022 had bacterial infection, November 2022 had potential flu-like symptoms, December 2022 had new high BP. Patient was seen in the ER for these symptoms and was referred to cardiologist and pulmonologist. They have had recent ECHO and stress testing which came back normal. Pt. reports being a very active person and has chickens at home. Pt. cleans daughter's home as well as her own. Pt. takes care of her grandkids.

Current Condition/Gains: Patient arrives with reports of improvements since start of PT. They still get fatigued after excessive activity, for example, yesterday they walked in the snow and needed to rest for the remainder of the day. They are compliant with HEP and remains active to their tolerance. They do still have intermittent dizziness that comes and goes based on how active they are.

Rx: Prescription (anxiety meds [2], depression medication)

O:
Incentive Spirometer: 2000, 1750, 1750 mL
PROMIS Global-10: 10
Duke Activity Status Index: 23.45

Outcome Measurement Tools
Berg Balance Test

3/2/23	2/1/23
49/56	45/56

30-Second Chair Stand

3/2/23	2/1/23
9 reps, without UE support with report of fatigue	6 reps, without UE support

6-Minute Walk Test

	SpO$_2$,%	HR	RR	BORG	Feet
Rest	97	63	16	4	
1 min					
2 min					
3 min					
4 min	95	70	17	8	680
5 min					
6 min	98	67	18	6	1030

Comments
BP pre: 137/81 mm Hg
BP post: 141/82 mm Hg
1 standing rest break taken ×2 min.

CASE EXAMPLE: 14.10   Progress Note   Setting: Outpatient Hospital Clinic—cont'd

MMT

	3/2/23 Right	3/2/23 Left	2/1/23 Right	2/1/23 Left
Upper Extremities				
Shoulder flexion	5/5	5/5	4+/5	4+/5
Shoulder extension	5/5	5/5	4+/5	4+/5
Elbow flexion	5/5	5/5	4+/5	4+/5
Elbow extension	5/5	5/5	4+/5	4+/5
Power grip	40 lb	45 lb	45 lb	45 lb
Lower Extremities				
Hip flexion	5/5	5/5	4+/5	4+/5
Knee flexion	4+/5	4+/5	4+/5	4+/5
Knee extension	4+/5	4+/5	4+/5	4+/5
Ankle dorsiflexion	5/5	4+/5	4+/5	4+/5

A: treatment sessions. Pt. has shown improvements in strength, balance, and endurance activities. They remain a good candidate for PT intervention.

Clinical Presentation: The clinical presentation is evolving with changing characteristics.

Pt. requires skilled therapy to restore prior level of function utilizing the treatment and modalities described in this plan of care.

P:

Management Plan
Pt. will be seen 2×/wk for 4 wk.

Medicaid Recertification
From: 3/2/2023
  To: 4/2/2023

Educational Instruction
Pt. will receive education on energy conservation techniques related to housework.

Procedural Intervention
Continue with current exercise program including Therapeutic Exercises, Therapeutic Activity, and Neuromuscular Rehabilitation. Progression with weight, reps, and time for endurance as tolerated.

EXERCISE 14.1

Identify whether the following statements belong in the Subjective (S) or Objective (O) section of either a session or progress SOAP note. Write a more appropriate statement in the space provided.

Statement	S or O	Rewrite
EXAMPLE: Mr. Jones reports that he has been unable to do anything.	S	Mr. Jones reports that he is unable to play the organ at church and give music lessons due to the pain in his L elbow.
1. Pt. states he hates using his walker.	_____	
2. Pt. has an awkward gait.	_____	
3. PROM at the knee is getting better.	_____	
4. Pt. is very confused.	_____	

Statement	S or O	Rewrite
5. Pt. reports that his son is concerned.	_____	_____
6. Pt. c/o fatigue after walking for 5 min.	_____	_____
7. Pt. complains of pain in left shoulder.	_____	_____
8. Pt. performed 10 reps of knee exercises.	_____	_____

EXERCISE 14.2

The following statements could be written as part of session SOAP notes. Using Table 14.1, classify each of the following statements into their appropriate category based on the SOAP format: G = Goal; S = Subjective; O = Objective; A = Assessment; P = Plan.

Statement	G, S, O, A, or P
1. Performed 10 reps SLR B.	_____
2. Pt. reports she was able to walk with her daughter to get the mail yesterday and did not experience any dizziness.	_____
3. Treatment next session will include progression to stationary bike ×10 min.	_____
4. Pt. walked 15 ft from bed to bathroom without SOB in 30 sec.	_____
5. Pt. states that she "felt sore" after the last treatment session.	_____
6. Pt. is progressing well with increasing repetitions of LE strengthening exercises and has achieved goal 1.	_____
7. Pitting edema noted in R ankle.	_____
8. Pt. was instructed to continue to maintain R leg in elevated position while sitting at desk during the day.	_____

Statement   **G, S, O, A, or P**

9. Pt. will transfer from bed to wheelchair independently, 4/5 trials within 2 wk.   _____

10. Pt. states she is anxious to return to work.   _____

11. Pt. will continue with daily walking program at home during off-therapy days, progressing to   _____
20 min each day by next week.

12. Pt. will stand $\overline{s}$ A for up to 1 min within 1 wk.   _____

13. Pt. reports pain in low back while walking as 5/10 and 8/10 while sitting at desk at work.   _____

14. Pt's. fear of falling is limiting his progress in improving his ability to ambulate in crowded   _____
environments and outdoors.

15. Pt. reports that she is going back to work on a trial basis next week.   _____

▌ EXERCISE 14.3[3]

You are a therapist in an outpatient practice and are working with a patient who has a diagnosis of lateral epicondylitis. Write a session SOAP note for your patient based on the case information provided below. You should create a plausible situation, including goals, subjective, objective, assessment, and plan. (NOTE: To complete this exercise accurately, it may be necessary to consult additional resources.) S. G. is a 40 y.o. woman who is a full-time receptionist. She has been referred to therapy with a diagnosis of lateral epicondylitis. S. G. reports of constant moderate to severe pain at her R lateral elbow that prevents her from playing tennis. The pain started about 1 mo ago, the morning after she spent a whole day pulling weeds and remained unchanged in severity or frequency until 3 days ago. She reports a slight decrease in pain severity over the last 3 days, which she associates with starting to take a nonsteroidal antiinflammatory drug prescribed by her physician. She has had similar symptoms previously after gardening or playing tennis, but these have always resolved within a couple of days without any medical intervention. Objective examination reveals tenderness and mild swelling at the right lateral epicondyle and pain without weakness with resisted wrist extension. All other tests, including upper extremity sensation, range of motion, and strength, are normal.

Goals:

_____

_____

_____

S:

_____

_____

_____

[3]There is no answer for this exercise in Appendix C

O:

_____

_____

_____

_____

_____

_____

_____

A:

_____

_____

_____

_____

_____

P:

_____

_____

_____

_____

_____

_____

_____

■ EXERCISE 14.4[4]

You are a therapist in an outpatient rehabilitation center, and you are working with a patient who has rheumatoid arthritis, primarily affecting her hands. Write a progress note (based on a 2-wsk time period, using a SOAP note format) for your patient based on the case information provided below. You should create a plausible situation, including goals, subjective, objective, assessment, and plan. (NOTE: To complete this exercise accurately, it may be necessary to consult additional resources.)

M. P. is a 62 y.o. woman with a diagnosis of rheumatoid arthritis of the hands. M. P. complains of stiffness and aching in all her finger joints, causing difficulties in gripping cooking utensils and performing other household tasks and pain with writing. The objective examination reveals stiffness and restricted flexion range of motion of the proximal interphalangeals to approximately 90 degrees and mild ulnar drift at the carpometacarpal joints bilaterally. The joints are not warm or edematous, and sensation is intact in both hands.

Goals:

_____

_____

_____

S:

_____

_____

_____

[4]There is no answer for this exercise in Appendix C

O:

_____

_____

_____

_____

_____

_____

A:

_____

_____

_____

_____

_____

P:

_____

_____

_____

_____

_____

_____

_____

Special Formats: Screening Evaluations, Discharge Summaries, Letters, and Patient Education Materials

LEARNING OBJECTIVES

After reading this chapter, the reader will be able to:
1. Describe the purpose of screening evaluation.
2. List the essential components of a discharge summary.
3. List the essential components of letters to third-party payers to justify the need for equipment or equipment purchases.
4. Identify the essential components of letters seeking to appeal denials or requesting continuation of services.
5. Discuss the patient-related and legal considerations for providing written patient education materials.

Physical therapy documentation can take many different forms. This book has focused on documentation of the initial evaluation as well as progress notes and session notes. However, physical therapists (PTs) are involved in many other types of documentation, including screening evaluations, discharge summaries, letters to third-party payers, and patient education materials. This chapter discusses specific issues related to some of the most common forms of specialized documentation and presents a framework for easy integration of a functional outcomes approach into each form.

SCREENING EVALUATIONS

Screening evaluations can take place in many patient settings and typically involve an abbreviated version of the initial evaluation. Screening evaluations involve the examination of someone who may have an undiagnosed condition or who may be at high risk for a particular condition. For example, a health and wellness screening is often performed before someone begins a new exercise program or regimen. A screening for falls risk is also a common type of screening evaluation, typically administered to elderly individuals or those who may be beginning to exhibit balance difficulties.

Documentation of screening evaluations should follow some of the same guidelines as initial evaluations. They will include the Reason for Referral, which will include any pertinent medical history, medications, social history, and current level of participation (e.g., work, home). The screening evaluation will include a brief overview of activities and impairments that are specific to the reason for the screening. Goals may or may not be included, but a summary of the assessment or impression after the screening should be included, as should specific recommendations (similar to a plan of care). *Case Example 15.1 provides an example of a health and wellness*

screening evaluation used before engagement in an exercise program, and Case Example 15.2 provides an example of a fall risk screening evaluation.

DISCHARGE SUMMARIES

At the completion of an episode of care, therapists are required to write a discharge summary. The American Physical Therapy Association's *Guidelines: Physical Therapy Documentation of Patient/Client Management* (BOD G03-05-16-41) state that "Documentation is required following conclusion of the current episode in the physical therapy intervention sequence, to summarize progression toward goals and discharge plans." The main purpose of a discharge summary is to document the status of the patient at the time he or she is discharged. A discharge summary does not require a complete reevaluation. However, therapists should report changes in the patient's participation, activities, and any limitations or impairments that are pertinent to the stated goals. These can be provided in a summary statement or in a table.

The following are essential components of a discharge summary:
- *Reason for Referral:* This should include a description of the patient's diagnosis and background information and can also include a description of the current Plan of Care. This section should also state a summary of the physical therapy intervention provided, including for what length of time and how many sessions the patient received physical therapy services. A brief summary of the interventions that were provided can be provided.
- *Current Status:* Summarize the patient's current status. This can include any impairments but should focus on the patient's functional abilities and any participation restrictions as appropriate.

- *Assessment:* A summary assessment should be given about the overall progress, the potential reasons for achieving/not achieving goals, and areas still needing to be addressed.
- *Goals:* It should be indicated whether the goals were achieved, partially achieved, or not achieved. If goals were not achieved or partially achieved, a brief explanation or justification is warranted. The goals can be combined with the Assessment section if appropriate.
- *Discharge/Discontinuation Plan:* The PT should list any recommendations for the patient at this point. This plan should include home-based instructions and follow-up or reevaluation instructions, caregiver training, or equipment recommendations. If the patient has moved to another facility (e.g., discharged from acute care to a skilled nursing facility), then any recommendations for continued therapy or other services should be provided.

Case Examples 15.3 and 15.4 are examples of discharge summaries written in outpatient settings.

LETTERS TO THIRD-PARTY PAYERS TO JUSTIFY EQUIPMENT OR SERVICES

Letters to third-party payers are frequently written by PTs. These letters are needed to provide justification for either continued services or equipment purchases. When writing such letters, it is important to consider that the reader may not be familiar with all medical terminology; thus it is essential to avoid medical jargon and abbreviations. The tone should be kept professional, without oversimplification. Therapists should not avoid using medical terminology; however, any uncommon words or terminology should be defined.

Therapists are frequently required to provide justification for the equipment that they plan to provide or wish to obtain for patients. Letters of medical necessity are often required by third-party payers for purchases of expensive medical equipment, such as customized wheelchairs, particularly those purchased through the Medicaid system. The purpose of these letters is to provide medical justification regarding the necessity of the equipment. It is also important to justify the cost. For example, the purchase of a certain piece of equipment now may reduce the need for surgery and/or extended hospital stays in the future. It is also important, when possible, to cite examples of research to back up your request. *Case Examples 15.5 and 15.6 provide sample letters used to justify purchase of a stander and a specialized wheelchair, respectively.*

The following list provides the essential components of a letter of medical necessity:

- **Patient Description:** This should include a description of the patient's diagnosis and background information and can also include a description of the current plan of care.
- **Current Status:** Summarize the patient's current status. This can include any impairments but should focus on the patient's level of participation and performance of activities as appropriate.
- **Equipment Description:** Describe the requested equipment in detail (provide a picture or other information if possible).

If special components or additions above and beyond standard equipment are required, each item should be separately and explicitly justified.

- **Medical Necessity of Equipment:** This is the most important component of the letter. The focus here should be on medical necessity. It should include the medical need for the equipment, specify benefits to the patient, and describe the patient's ability to use the equipment. It is important, when possible, to include evidence from the literature to support the need for the equipment. In addition, the inability of any alternatives (particularly cheaper ones) to meet the patient's medical needs should be discussed if appropriate. Cost benefits can be explained in detail as well.

Appealing Denials or Requesting Continued Services

PTs frequently write letters to request approval for additional physical therapy visits or payment for services after a claim has been denied. In these situations, PTs should include specific objective data outlining (1) the specific progress the patient has made in therapy to date, using objective and standardized test results when possible and (2) an overview of the specific skilled therapy intervention that the patient received (or will receive) and the rationale for each intervention. Tables, charts, grids, or bulleted lists are useful in demonstrating progress in therapy and are more readable for reviewers who see many files each day. *Case Example 15.7 provides a sample letter to a third-party payer requesting approval for additional visits for physical therapy intervention. Case Example 15.8 provides a sample letter written in response to a denial for payment of services.*

When available, therapists should provide reviewers and insurance companies with current literature or research reports to support the use of a particular intervention for a patient or patient population. This can be in the form of an entire article, which is sent with a detailed letter or a citation or summary of a research article in the body of the letter. Therapists must take care to ensure the letters are easy to read, use correct spelling and grammar, and avoid the use of jargon. Although these factors apply to all forms of documentation, they are particularly important for letters to third-party payers. Therapists should not oversimplify their documentation, but they should use terminology that can be relatively easily understood and should define any terminology that is unlikely to be known.

PATIENT EDUCATION MATERIALS

Patient education materials and home programs are some of the key components of most physical therapy plans of care (see *Case Example 15.9 for documentation of a home exercise program*). These materials are used in all types of settings and patient populations. If home exercise programs are to be used by a patient after discharge, then written handouts should be issued to patients individually. Instructions must be written carefully, with specific attention directed to the patient's educational level, language capabilities, and learning style. Many different types of patient education materials are available for purchase. Many can be tailored to individual patient needs. For example, there are online resources for exercise prescriptions that can be downloaded and given to patients. When possible, providing a visual representation of the information being conveyed can be helpful.

SUMMARY

- This chapter provides an overview of various kinds of specialized documentation in physical therapy, including screening evaluations, letters to third-party payers, discharge notes, and patient education materials.
- All forms of patient documentation should be concise, be free of jargon, and focus on the important aspects related to the patient's plan of care and improving the functional outcomes.
- Although formats and requirements change frequently, the principles related to the functional outcomes approach provide a consistent framework for all types of documentation.

CASE EXAMPLE 15.1 Health and Wellness Fitness Screening

This evaluation provides an example of a fitness screening evaluation, which can be conducted in preparation for a client beginning a new exercise program.

Name: Mark Jones	**Date of Birth:** 10/11/1961; 62 y.o.	**Gender:** Male	**Date of Eval:** 12/1/2023

Reason for Referral
You have self-referred for a health and wellness fitness screening before initiation of an exercise program. History reveals that you have several cardiovascular risk factors. They include being older than age 55 years, having blood pressure greater than 140/80 mm Hg, being more than 20 pounds overweight, and being physically inactive. Your cholesterol level is well controlled with lovastatin 20 mg daily. You take no other medication. History of smoking for 45 years; quit 8 months ago.

Cardiovascular/Cardiorespiratory Fitness (Part 1)
Resting heart rate (HR): 74 beats per minute—normal. Resting blood pressure: 154/84 mm Hg. This blood pressure is in the range of stage I hypertension. This puts you at higher risk for cardiovascular disease.

Musculoskeletal Alignment and Development
You have forward head posture with rounded shoulders and decreased lumbar lordosis (flattened low back); your neck is slightly side-bent to the right, and your right shoulder is lower. This posture may contribute to the development of low back, neck, and/or upper back pain.

Body Composition
Weight: 183 lb; height: 5'7"; body mass index (BMI): 28.7 kg/m²; waist circumference: 45".

This puts you in overweight category with high disease risk. You have increased risk of cardiovascular problems, diabetes mellitus, and certain cancers. This may also put more stress on your joints and increase your risk of developing joint pain.

Flexibility
- *Gross Range-of-Motion Screen:* Normal except for decreased hip internal rotation (L): 30° (normal is 45°) and slightly decreased trunk flexion (forward bending). This may indicate some osteoarthritis left hip.
- *Apley's Scratch Test (back scratch test):* Able to touch fingers at mid-back with (R) overhead, distance between fingertips (L) hand is 6 cm. Although you have less mobility with your right hand overhead, you are at low risk of having difficulty with activities of daily living (ADLs), such as dressing, grooming hair, and reaching back pants pocket.

- *Sit and Reach:* Your farthest distance reached was 10 in., which is in the 45th percentile for your age and gender. This indicates slight limitation of your lower body flexibility and decreased hamstring flexibility. You may be at risk of developing low back problems.

Muscular Strength and Endurance
- *Gross Manual Muscle Test:* No deficits in arm strength. Leg strength normal except for weakness (R) with knee extension (knee straightening) and weakness of your hips—lifting your leg behind you (extension) and out to the side (abduction). Your right hip is weaker than your left hip.
- *Handgrip Strength:* Best score (R) (dominant hand): 39 kg; best score (L): 34 kg. Combined score: 73 kg. This score is in poor category for your age and gender. This may indicate poor upper body strength.
- *Curl-up Test:* You were able to do 10 repetitions, which is between fair and good category, and in 40th percentile for your age and gender. Abdominal weakness may put you at risk for low back problems.
- *Push-up Test:* You were unable to do any push-ups. This puts you in the needs improvement category. With this score you may have difficulty lifting and/or carrying heavy things, especially over any distance.
- *Unilateral Step Down Test:* (R): 6; (L): 7. Poor category. This may indicate a decreased ability to do functional activities, such as squatting, lifting objects from the floor, or negotiating stairs. It also may indicate decreased muscular endurance.

Balance
- *Single Limb Stance:* 38 sec (L) leg; 35 sec (R) leg with eyes open, which is above normative value for your age and gender. With your eyes closed, you were able to maintain your balance for 2 sec, which is below normative value for your age and gender. This may indicate overreliance on vision or vestibular issues. You may be at risk of falls when there is poor lighting.
- *Upper Extremity Functional Reach Test:* Scores 15", 14.5", 15.5". Average score: 15", which is within normal range for your age and gender. This indicates low risk of losing your balance with reaching (e.g., into a shelf or closet).
- *Lower Extremity Functional Reach Test:* You rated in the good range in all directions tested. You should be able to step over obstacles without losing your balance.

Cardiovascular/Cardiorespiratory Fitness
- *Submaximal Bruce Protocol:* Test ended after first minute of stage 3 because your HR exceeded 85% of age-predicted maximum HR. Therefore VO₂max could not be calculated.

(Continued)

• *Heart rate end test:* 142 beats per minute; after 2 min: 115 beats per minute. Your HR recovery after exercise puts you in fair fitness category.

Impairments

1. Stage I hypertension, increased BMI, increased waist circumference
2. Poor posture: forward head posture with rounded shoulders, decreased lumbar lordosis.
3. Muscle weakness, especially core, upper body, lower extremities (hip extensors, abductors, quads).
4. Decreased muscle endurance.
5. Decreased balance with eyes closed.
6. Decreased flexibility hamstrings and trunk; decreased hip internal rotation (L).
7. Decreased aerobic capacity.

Recommendations

1. Consult with physician for management of your hypertension.
2. Consult with a nutritionist for education related to diet for weight loss and cholesterol management.
3. Complete postural and biomechanics education course.
4. Avoid walking in unlit places. Have a flashlight available for unlit parking lots, power outages, etc. Use a night-light in bathroom and hallways.
5. Participate in exercise program to address flexibility, muscle strength and endurance, postural problems, balance deficits, and decreased aerobic capacity. Exercise, along with diet, may also assist with weight loss and help control cholesterol.

Recommended Exercise Program

Flexibility

Frequency of 2-7×/wk. Daily best. Hold each stretch 30 sec. Repeat each stretch 2-4 repetitions. Avoid bouncing.

• Pectoral wall stretch, lying over foam roller to stretch pecs for 2-3 min, hamstring stretches, cat/camel back, hip internal rotation stretch using strap.

Strengthening

Each muscle group should be exercised 2-3×/wk, 8-12 reps each set, 2-4 sets. Rest 2-3 min between sets. Intensity should be at 60%-70% of 1 repetition max.

At this level, you can complete only between 8 and 12 repetitions before fatigue. When you can complete 12 repetitions of an exercise without difficulty completing the last repetition of the set, the exercise should be made more difficult by increasing resistance or performing on an unstable surface.

• Core stabilization/hip extensors/hip abductors: Focus on abdominal strength, esp. transverse abdominus, to decrease the risk of developing low back pain. Can initiate supine exercises with one leg on the surface and progress to an "unsupported" position. Can also progress to an unstable surface such as a Swiss ball or foam roller. Exercise in quadruped for spine extensors/posture. Planks as strength improves. Bridging sequence progressing to the use of Swiss ball under the lower leg. Side-lying leg lifts.
• Quadriceps: Wall slides, lunges, step-ups/step-downs of increasing heights.
• Upper body: W, Y's, I's in prone, progressing to over Swiss ball for unstable surface. Weight bearing onto upper extremities with weight shifting progressing to arm lifts. Wall push-ups progressing to modified push-ups to traditional push-ups. Planks as strength improves.

Balance

2-3×/wk, 20-30 min

• Feet in different positions: Romberg, modified tandem, tandem, single-leg stance with head turns and eyes closed. Increase challenge by adding non-compliant surface, such as foam or wobble board.
• Ambulation with head turns, nods, eyes closed.

Aerobic

Moderate intensity done at least 5 days/wk at target HR of 107 beats per minute to below 124 beats per minute (based on 40% to less than 60% of your HR reserve). You can progress to vigorous-intensity exercise 3 days/wk at target HR of 124-141 beats per minute (60%-80% HR). Your eventual goal is 3-5 days/wk of combination of moderate- and vigorous-intensity exercises.

You can choose any combination of aerobic exercise, including walking, swimming, treadmill, or stationary bicycle. Try to choose activities that you enjoy. Start with 20 min and progress to up to 60 min/session.

PATIENT: Jane Smith   **DOB:** 6/16/43   **GENDER:** Female   **DATE:** 4/20/23

Reason for Referral

Health Condition

Pt. is an 80 y.o. female who reports a gradual deterioration in functional independence over the past 2 years. Pt. defines the turning point in her health to be when she fell 2 years ago when getting into a cab, resulting in a (L) ankle fx. Pt. reports falling again with recurrent (L) ankle fx after a short course of rehabilitation. Pt. reports no further falls but notes an increased fear of falling. PMH significant for following: HTN, severe OA (B) hands, s/p 2 cataract surgeries, and NIDDM. Current medications include ibuprofen and Lopressor.

Social History and Participation

Pt. reports she lives alone in a one-storey senior residence center. She reports independence in ADLs using durable medical equipment (DME) and ambulation with an RW. Patient reports a relatively sedentary lifestyle since two reported falls, performing only those functions absolutely necessary throughout her day. Pt. reports volunteering in gift shop in White Plains over the past 7 years. Pt. reports she is able to sit at the gift shop the majority of her day. Results of SF-36 health status profile indicate a decline in health over the past year, limiting moderate to vigorous activities. Pt. reports difficulty with sit-to-stand transfers, bathing, dressing, lifting and carrying groceries, prolonged standing, climbing stairs, and ambulating greater than one block.

Functional Status

Ambulation: Pt. reports ambulating with an RW household and short community distances. Pt. is reliant on the RW for static and dynamic balance except in confined areas where pt. relies on furniture for stability.

Transfers: Sit-to-stand using (B) UE to pull up on table or push up from (B) armrests, requiring ≥5 sec to stabilize in standing using the walker for support.

Falls Efficacy Scale: Modified Falls Efficacy Scale showed this patient to be relatively confident of her functional abilities without falling, scoring an 8 on all activities except the following activities, which she scored all 7s: dressing, preparing a simple meal, taking a bath or shower, and walking around the inside of her home.

Impairments

Gait: Timed Up and Go Test: 32 sec with RW. Pt. demonstrated slow turns with multiple steps for 180° turn, decreased step length with (R) LE, and decreased (L) stance time. 10 m walk gait speed 0.84 m/sec.

CASE EXAMPLE 15.2   Falls Risk Assessment—cont'd

Balance: Postural Strategies: Pt. presents with absent ankle strategies, delayed use of hip strategies, and predominant use of stepping strategy with increased latency in response to perturbations. Berg Balance Scale = 14/56, placing patient at 100% risk for falls. Functional Reach Test = 3 in. (age-matched norm = 10.47 ± 3.53), placing pt. at significant risk for falls.

Posture: Pt. presents with forward flexed posture, bilateral rounded shoulders, increased thoracic kyphosis, and forward head posture.

Sensation/Skin Integrity: Light touch: Impaired sensation noted (B) LE distal to knee and (B) hands in stocking/glove distribution. Proprioception: Absent (B) great toe, impaired (B) ankle (2/5 correct), impaired (B) knee (3/5 correct), and intact (B) hips.

MMT/ROM: Not formally tested, but the patient appears to have generalized deconditioning (B) LE (distally > proximally) and below normal strength noted during sit-to-stand transfers, ambulation, and stair negotiation.

Assessment

Pt. presents with deconditioning, generalized weakness, impaired sensation, and balance that have all led to functional limitations and significant risk for falls with mobility skills and self-care activities.

Goals

Activity Goals

1. Patient will ambulate with a rolling walker independently on level indoor and outdoor surfaces without complaints of fatigue short community distances (300-500 feet) to allow for safe return to volunteering within 6 wk.

2. Patient will improve gait speed to 1.0 m/sec with RW for community ambulation.

3. Patient will be able to perform an ambulatory transfer in/out of car (cab) utilizing an RW safely and directing assistance needed independently within 6 wk.

Impairment Goals

1. Patient will stand unsupported for 5 min within 4 wk.

2. Patient will be able to reach 6 in. on functional reach test within 4 wk.

Plan of Care

Patient will be seen 3× per week for a 45-min treatment session. Patient will be reevaluated in 4 wk.

Educational Intervention

OT consultation for home safety evaluation and assistance with ADLs and self-care.

    Pt. will be instructed in home exercise program with emphasis on strengthening and flexibility of (B) LE. Patient will be instructed in performing safe and independent ADLs that are currently difficult and resulting in high risk for falls with appropriate DME and ambulatory equipment.

Procedural Intervention

Pt. will be given active and passive ROM therapeutic exercises (stretching proximal >distal musculature and strengthening) to improve trunk and lower extremity stability and function. Pt. will participate in balance and coordination training with specific incorporation into functional activities. Functional training will be initiated with focus on car transfers, sit-to-stand training, stair-climbing, curb negotiation, gait training on variable surfaces to improve endurance and safety, and functional reaching with object manipulation.

CASE EXAMPLE 15.3   Discharge Summary

Name: Suzie Sears   **DOB:** 5/20/64   **GENDER:** Female   **D/C Date:** 9/26/23

Reason for Referral

Suzie Sears was initially evaluated on 7/24/23 in our Outpatient PT Department due to a long-standing diagnosis of relapsing-remitting multiple sclerosis (RRMS), with recent exacerbation of symptoms. She has been treated 3×/wk for a total of 27 sessions over a period of 9 wk. She initially presented with lower extremity weakness and demonstrated deficits in sitting and standing balance, transfers and bed mobility, and ambulation and stair-climbing ability.

Current Status

Pt. has demonstrated the specific improvements in her functional ability:

	Initial Evaluation	Final Evaluation
Kurtzke Expanded Disability Status Scale (EDSS)	7.5 (unable to take more than a few steps)	6.0 (intermittent assistance to walk 100 m)
MS Impact Scale (MSIS): 29 (range, 0–145)	98	65
Standing ability	Stands for 10 sec with minimal assistance and walker	Stands for up to 5 min with walker independently
Transfers	Transfers with moderate assistance from walker to wheelchair	Transfers independently from walker to wheelchair within 10 sec

	Initial Evaluation	Final Evaluation
Bed mobility	Minimal assistance to position self in bed, including rolling bilaterally and coming to sit	Independent in all bed mobility
Ambulation	Able to ambulate approx. 5 steps with walker and minimal assistance before fatiguing; heart rate change from 78 to 104 beats per minute	Able to walk 100–150 m with walker and supervision on level surface in therapy gym; heart rate change from 82 to 96 beats per minute

Assessment

Pt. has made considerable progress over the past 9 wk, was able to make progress with her home exercise program tolerance, and is independent in performing a 30-min video-based routine aimed at improving flexibility, balance, and strength (summary of program is attached). Patient stated on 9/17/23 that she was happy to finally see some progress, and she is very pleased with her improved mobility. Pt. continues to struggle with muscle spasms and overall fatigue, and she has received education and written literature on managing her spasms and her fatigue levels.

(Continued)

CASE EXAMPLE 15.3   Discharge Summary—cont'd

Goals

Pt. has surpassed all goals set for this therapy period, and discharge from therapy is thus warranted.

Discharge Plan

Pt. has also been seen in consultation with the Outpatient OT Department for a custom wheelchair evaluation on 8/1/23. At the time of the evaluation, pt. was using a scooter that was broken beyond repair. After trials of several types of chairs, a midwheel power wheelchair was recommended, and the patient is currently awaiting its arrival. This chair will ultimately improve her safety and independence at home. The recommendation is to discharge the patient from therapy at this time. Continue with video-based home program for continued improvement of flexibility, balance, strengthening, and home walking program. Recommend reevaluation in 4 months.

Sandy Bower, PT, MS

CASE EXAMPLE 15.4   Discharge Summary

Name: Kimberly Miller   **D.O.B.:** 6/17/85   **Gender:** Female   **Eval Date**: 8/15/23   **Discharge Date**: 10/10/23

Diagnosis

8B93.Z	Radiculopathy, unspecified
ME84.0	Cervicalgia
FB3Z	Disorders of muscles, unspecified

Reason for Referral

Kimberly Miller is a 38 y.o. patient referred to physical therapy by Dr. Jones and evaluated on 8/15/23 for sudden onset of cervical pain radiating into BUEs. At the time of initial evaluation, the pt's chief complaints were difficulty dressing and grooming, waking from sleep due to pain, limitations in driving, difficulty grasping and lifting objects, and an inability to work as a registered nurse at the hospital. Pt. received physical therapy 2 to 3 times per week for 24 sessions over a 10-week period. PT interventions utilized at various points within the POC include: modalities, such as moist heat, e-stim, and mechanical cervical traction to reduce pain; therapeutic exercises and therapeutic activities for strength, ROM and improving functional abilities for ADLs and return to work; manual therapy to improve mobility and reduce pain, neuromuscular re-education for postural awareness and dynamic spinal stability. Pt. education was provided for proper body mechanics and the pt. demonstrated good awareness throughout treatment. The pt. was also instructed in an HEP and demonstrated good understanding and proper technique.

Current Status

Pt. reports full resolution of UE pain and neck pain now at 0/10 at best and 3/10 at worst (occurs with repetitive lifting), as compared to 5/10 at best and 9/10 at worst at the time of initial evaluation.

Neck Disability Index was completed today with a score of 18%, showing mild impairment compared with the score upon evaluation of 67%, showing severe impairment.

Range of Motion

Range of Motion

Cervical	Initial	Current	Comments
AROM	8-15-23	10-10-23	
Flexion	35°	70°	
Extension	25°	60°	
R rotation	45°	85°	
L rotation	40°	75°	1/10 pain at end range
R side bend	25°	45°	
L side bend	20°	40°	1/10 pain at end range

Upper Extremity

Upper Extremity	Initial	Current	Initial	Current	Comments
AROM	Right	Right	Left	Left	
Shoulder flexion	100°	175°	140°	175°	
Shoulder abduction	100°	175°	130°	180°	
Shoulder internal rotation	T8	T5	T10	T7	Discomfort on left
Shoulder external rotation	WNLs	WNLs	WNLs	WNLs	

CASE EXAMPLE 15.4 Discharge Summary—cont'd

Manual Muscle Test

Manual Muscle Test

Cervical	Initial	Current	Comments
Flexion	3	5	
Extension	3	5	
Right rotation	3	4	
Left rotation	3	4	1/10 pain with MMT
Right side bend	3	4	
Left side bend	3	4	1/10 pain with MMT

Upper Extremity

Upper Extremity	Initial	Current	Initial	Current	Comments
Right MMT	**Right**	**Right**	**Left**	**Left**	
Shoulder flexion	3+	4	4	5	
Shoulder abduction	3+	4	4	5	
Shoulder internal rotation	5	5	5	5	
Shoulder external rotation	4	5	5	5	

Grip Strength	Initial (R/L)	Current (R/L)
Grip dynamometer 1	22 lb/70 lb	58 lb/75 lb

Re-evaluation performed today with the findings noted above. Pt. then received treatment as per flow sheet with ther ex × 35 min and pt education for progression of HEP following discharge × 5 minutes. Total treatment time of 40 min.

Flow Sheet

Flow Sheet (Case Study 15.4)

Exercises	Comment	Sets	Reps	Band Color	Time
Tband Row/ext	Bilateral	3	15	Blue	
Tband PNF D1 flex/ext	Bilateral	3	10	Blue	
Tband PNF D2 flex/ext	Bilateral	3	10	Green	
Tband horiz abd/ B ER		3	10	Green	
Pecs doorway stretch	30 sec hold-3 way		2		
Prone cervical retractions	5 sec hold	2	10		5 min
UBE (backward)	120 rpm				
Theraputty gripping	Green putty × 3 minutes	2			
Prone B HABD	1 lb dumbbells	3	10		

Assessment

Pt. is a 38 y.o. initially referred to PT with dx of cervical radiculopathy and associated cervical and upper extremity weakness and pain. The pt.'s pain level has improved significantly and is no longer constant throughout the day. Kimberly is now independent in all ADLs and IADLs and can drive for greater than an hour with minimal discomfort. The pt.'s Neck Disability Index has improved from 67% to 18% functional impairment indicating improved ability to complete daily functional tasks. Kimberly demonstrates significant gains in strength and ROM, and has achieved nearly all PT goals. The pt. has returned to work with modified duty related to lifting restrictions when transferring patients. Minor residual deficits are still noted; however, these can continue to improve with regular pt. performance of an independent HEP. Kimberly is scheduled to see Dr. Jones in 2 weeks with release to full-duty work responsibilities likely at that time. Recommend discharge from skilled PT to HEP and follow up with physician as scheduled.

Goals	Time Frame	Result
Pt. will achieve B cervical rotation ROM of at least 60° to improve ease of driving.	4 wks	Goal met
Pt. will achieve B shoulder elevation AROM of at least 120° without pain to improve ability to dress and groom.	4 wks	Goal met
Pt. will increase B shoulder flexion strength to at least 4/5 for improved ability to lift objects during household tasks.	6 wks	Goal met
Pt. will report full resolution of B UE pain, indicating centralization of radiculopathy.	6 wks	Goal met
Pt will be able to don/doff clothing without pain > 1/10.	8 wks	Goal met
Pt will be able to drive x 30 min without pain > 1/10.	8 wks	Goal met
Pt will be able to return to all full-time work activities without restrictions.	8 wks	Partially met; pt. has returned to work with modified duty related to lifting restrictions. Anticipate MD release to full duty in 2 wks

Discharge Plan

Discharge patient from skilled physical therapy to independent HEP. Pt. to follow up with MD in 2 weeks.

CASE EXAMPLE 15.5 Equipment Justification

This is a sample letter to a third-party payer requesting specialized equipment. A synopsis of the patient's status is included, and the specific benefits to the patient are clearly delineated in the last few paragraphs.

Date: 03/17/23

Re: June Smith ID#:
TW51292R DOB: 1/4/10

Patient Description

The above equipment is being requested for June Smith. Ms. Smith is a 13 y.o. girl with a primary diagnosis of nemaline myopathy, status post T3 to pelvis posterior spine fusion for kyphoscoliosis 10/29/18. Medical history includes the following: osteopenia; left femur fracture ×2; restrictive lung disease; chronic respiratory failure; hypoxia following extubation 11/17; right pleural effusion; gastrostomy tube.

Current Status

Ms. Smith presents with low central tone resulting in decreased head and trunk control in sitting, limiting her ability to perform basic tabletop tasks and aid with her ADLs. She presents with decreased hip, knee, and ankle ROM; decreased trunk control/strength; decreased bilateral upper and lower extremity strength; and decreased sitting balance, limiting independence with all functional mobility. Ms. Smith presents with decreased bilateral hip and knee extension range of motion and strength, limiting her ability to bear weight through her lower extremities, resulting in the inability to perform stand pivot or squat pivot transfers. Ms. Smith has been nonambulatory since 2016 and is dependent on her personal wheelchair. Ms. Smith is receiving PT 2×/wk at Community Hospital.

Functional Status

Wheelchair to mat/bed: Via Beasy board transfer to various surfaces (including EasyStand Evolv Youth with shadow tray), Max A. Ms. Smith's sister demonstrated the ability to transfer Ms. Smith onto and off EasyStand Evolv Youth with shadow tray via Beasy board transfer.

Bed/mat mobility: Ms. Smith is able to roll from supine to side-lying with bed rails and minimal assistance. Supine ↔ side-lying, Min A; side-lying ↔ short sit, Max A.

Sitting Balance: Supported, with feet on ground and hands in lap Mod I. She is able to maintain balance against minimal perturbation; however, she presents with poor righting and protective reactions secondary to decreased trunk strength/control and UE weakness.

Standing Balance: Ms. Smith is able to stand in trial EasyStand Evolv Youth with shadow tray for 20-30 min without any skin irritation or redness. Ms. Smith's family demonstrates competency with appropriate positioning to optimize Ms. Smith's alignment before standing and verbalize safety concerns with tolerance to upright standing.

Impairments

Posture: Mid thorax rotation with multiple right rib humps

ROM: Ms. Smith presents with lower extremity PROM within normal limits except for the following limitations:

Left hip: 44°-96°
Right hip: 40°-96°
Left knee: 66°-132°
Right knee 78° 136°
Left ankle DF: 0°-10°
Right ankle DF: 0°-8°

Strength: Ms. Smith presents with poor to fair minus strength throughout her extremities.

Equipment Description

EasyStand Evolv Youth with shadow tray. This standing frame is required to implement a standing program as prescribed by Dr. Emans, which includes daily progressive weight bearing as tolerated. The goals of the standing program are (1) weight bearing to maintain and improve bone density, (2) improvement in hip and knee extension range of motion by 15 degrees bilaterally, and (3) improved independence with transfers.

Medical Necessity of Equipment

The above equipment would be of great benefit to Ms. Smith. The ability to stand would assist in improving current ROM limitation and prevent further shortening of hip flexors, hamstrings, and heel cords (maintaining available length of lower extremity muscles); maintaining bone strength through WB; maintaining respiratory function; regulating bowels; and promoting a sense of well-being and socialization. With the assistance of the tray, Ms. Smith will be able to perform tabletop tasks, including schoolwork.

In the long run it is projected that Ms. Smith will need fewer surgeries if a standing program is implemented.

In an attempt to find the most appropriate stander for home use, a few different standers, including the Grand Stand and Rifton Stander, were considered. Neither of these standers provided the adjustability or support of the EasyStand. Therefore the EasyStand Evolv Youth with shadow tray was chosen because of its unique features and ability to provide the best position and correction of postural malalignment.

One of the unique features is that the EasyStand Evolv with shadow tray allows Ms. Smith's family/caregivers to transfer her first to a sitting position and adjust her posture while sitting before placing her in a standing position. The stander will allow for weight bearing through the lower extremities even without complete extension range. The stander will allow Ms. Smith to achieve the most beneficial positioning with the aid of the shadow tray, secure foot straps, hip supports, lateral supports, independent knees, Velcro seat belt, and X-style chest vest. The adjustability and placement of the laterals and hip supports will aid in achievement and maintenance of the best upright position. Without these features, the postural deformities would be exaggerated with the downward pull of gravity.

The above equipment would be highly beneficial for Ms. Smith as discussed above. At this time, it is being requested that the EasyStand Evolv Youth with shadow tray be approved for Ms. Smith. If you have any further questions, please do not hesitate to contact me at 555-555-1243.

Sandy Jones, PT

CASE EXAMPLE 15.6 **Custom Wheelchair Justification**

This is a sample letter to provide medical justification for a customized wheelchair. A synopsis of the patient's status is included, and a detailed description of the specifications for the wheelchair is provided.

Patient Description

Name: Sarah Glass
Weight: 160 lb.
Height: 5′7″
Date of Birth: 01/18/1949
Date of Evaluation: 09/03/2023

Ms. Glass is a 74 y.o. female who sustained a severe R CVA on 6/5/23, with resultant dense hemiplegia throughout LUE and LLE, as well as her core musculature. Left limbs originally presented with total flaccidity but are now presenting with increased tone throughout.

Sensation is impaired throughout the entire left side. L side neglect is present, and visual field cuts are very obvious. PMH includes OA, RA, anemia, and HTN.

Current Status

Functional Status: Ms. Glass is able to assist with her upper body dressing and bathing, requiring moderate assistance for UB. She is dependent for all lower body bathing and dressing. She requires minimal assistance for grooming and self-feeding. Patient requires assistance for all bed mobility. She attempts to use her right extremities for rolling and scooting activities, but this is ineffective and she continues to need Mod assist ×1 for rolling and scooting activities. Patient requires Max assist ×1 to transition from supine to/from sitting position. She currently requires Max assist for stand pivot and sit-to-stand transitions from bed to/from w/c and w/c to/from secondary surfaces (car, couch, chair). Toilet transfers require the use of a Sabina Standing lift in order to allow for safe transfer as well as clothing management and hygiene.

Mobility: Ms. Glass is currently residing at the Pines of Poughkeepsie, a subacute rehabilitation facility, but will be D/C to home Friday, 9/12/23. While at the Pines, patient has required assistance for all functional mobility skills. She has a lot of shoulder pain when seated completely upright in a standard w/c and without proper LUE support. Thus she is currently in a high-backed recliner w/c, allowing slight recline with a specialized arm tray to support the subluxation at her left shoulder. She requires total assistance for w/c propulsion.

Home Environment: Ms. Glass lives with her husband in a cottage at an adult living facility. Her home is a one-storey structure without stairs. The home has ramps, wide doorways, wide bedrooms, and wide bathrooms. Patient will have an HHA around the clock to help her with her ADLs and wheelchair maintenance. Her son lives nearby and helps her with her medical appointments. He was present during the trial of the Tilt-in-Space wheelchair.

Functional/Sensory Processing Skills: Ms. Glass exhibits poor attention to her environment. Her motor planning skills and motor coordination and control are significantly limited. She is fully dependent on all her care needs. She is alert and oriented ×4; however, she is unable to communicate verbally due to apraxia. No receptive or expressive aphasia noted.

Sensation and Skin Issues: Ms. Glass presents with decreased awareness and sensation in the left upper and lower extremity. She is unable to discriminate between hot and cold or light and deep pressure. She is only aware of noxious stimulus and senses pain when the limb is placed in an uncomfortable position.

Posture: Ms. Glass is kyphotic with forward flexion of cervical and thoracic vertebrae with a posterior pelvic tilt and left lateral lean.

Sitting Balance: Ms. Glass's sitting balance is poor, requiring moderate assistance to sit upright unsupported. She requires Max A when performing dynamic balance activities at the edge of her base of support and beyond.

Standing Balance: Ms. Glass has poor standing balance, requiring Max A to stand with Max A to facilitate proper standing posture. Facilitation is required

at L quadriceps and gluteus muscles to encourage extension. She is unable to maintain standing without total assistance.

Ambulation: Ms. Glass is unable to ambulate and is dependent for all w/c mobility and parts management.

ADLs: Ms. Glass is able to assist with her UB dressing and bathing, requiring moderate assistance for UB. She is dependent for all LB bathing and dressing. She requires minimal assistance for grooming and self-feeding. Ms. Glass requires setup and supervision for self-feeding; she requires assistance to open containers and cut foods. She is currently eating a pureed diet with thin liquids. She currently requires Max A SPT and sit-to-stand activities. She requires total assistance with toileting for a standing lift in order for the caregiver to perform clothing management and hygiene tasks.

Strength and Range of Motion: Right UE ROM is WNL; however, she presents with weakness 3/5. Left UE initially was flaccid and has shown increased tone in the internal rotators of her shoulder, biceps, and supinators in her forearm with a fifth digit flexion contracture on her left hand. Her left UE has shown no functional or voluntary movements. Right LE ROM is WNL; however, she presents with weakness 3/5. Left LE initially was flaccid and has shown increased tone throughout. Flickers of volitional activity are noted but are not consistently reproducible. Head/neck WNL. Ms. Glass has asymmetric weakness in her abdominal and paraspinal muscles, resulting in the ability to maintain an erect sitting posture without assistance. She presents with left lateral lean, requiring moderate assistance to sit upright; however, she requires moderate assistance to flex forward for proper spinal alignment when seated.

Wheelchair Skills: Ms. Glass's disability prevents her from self-positioning. She cannot self-propel a manual wheelchair or use a powered mobility device to independently access her home environment. Therefore she will require a multitilt positioning wheelchair with customized seating whereby the caregiver can passively move her from her bed to other locations of her home and provide her with positioning as and when needed.

Mat Evaluation While Sitting

Shoulder width	17″	Seat to axilla	15″
Chest width	13″	Seat to shoulder	21″
Chest depth	6″	Seat to elbow	7″
Hip width	17″	Upper leg length	18″
Seat to top of head	28″	Lower leg length	17″
Foot length	11″		

Medical Necessity of Equipment

Ms. Glass was evaluated in an Invacare Solara 3G Adult Tilt-in-Space (16″ W × 17″ D) wheelchair and appeared to demonstrate improved sitting posture. This manual-tilt wheelchair is necessary to provide her with a safe mode of mobility. This chair will provide a durable and comfortable support system for Ms. Glass. Tilt is necessary to provide pressure relief since she is unable to weight shift independently. Ms. Glass is immobile, and her skin is exposed to moisture in the adult brief area. The ability to tilt in space is a requirement of postural control for this individual that cannot be achieved in any less expensive system.

Equipment Description

Standard and lightweight or even reclining wheelchairs are not appropriate for Ms. Glass's positioning needs. It will not allow for multiple positional changes throughout the day, as she is unable to self-correct her position independently. She requires multiple seat adjustments, which will provide her with optimal positioning using tilt adjustment for positioning, change in positioning of the seat-to-floor height, and tilt for pressure relief; adjustable back; and elevating leg rests for lower extremity positioning. The standard and lightweight wheelchairs cannot provide both custom seat and depth adjustable wheelbase and positional changes via tilt for postural alignment.

(Continued)

CASE EXAMPLE 15.6   Custom Wheelchair Justification—cont'd

The other components that are required are as follows:

1. A Comfort Acta-Back-Contoured Back with adjustable hardware 16″ W × 18″ is required to provide her optimal postural alignment, trunk support, lumbar/sacral support, and trunk in midline and maximum comfort. She presents with poor trunk control, low tone, and a curvature of the spine. Without this back, she will be unable to maintain an upright midline posture in her wheelchair. This back is required, as Ms. Glass's medical condition and resultant physical disability necessitate posterior trunk support to position her trunk in midline.

2. Adjustable comfort plus head support from Ottobock with detachable hardware is required to provide posterior head and neck support in all tilt positions and to improve visual orientation. The detachable hardware is required for removal of the headrest during transfers and positioning as needed.

3. Comfort M2 ATI 16W × 16D cushions are required to prevent breakdowns. Secondary to her left hemiplegia, she has impaired sensation throughout her left side. She is likely to be seated 8-10 hours a day and is at high risk for breakdowns.

4. T-post height adjustable full-length removable armrests are required to provide support for arms, with elbows at 90° and support for upper extremity support system.

   Removable feature is required for transfers and to enable to come close to a table/countertop for ADLs.

5. Elevating leg rests with Swing-Away footrests with angle adjustable footplates are required to provide lower extremity support. The Swing-Away option is required for transfers. Angle adjustable plates are required for optimal positioning of Ms. Glass's feet while in her wheelchair. Appropriate foot support will provide her with a weight-bearing surface through the feet to assist with maintaining a balanced pelvis for pressure distribution evenly along her thighs and the seat cushion. Elevating legs are required as she experiences pain and swelling in her LEs secondary to edema.

6. Sixteen-inch rear mag flat-free tires with 6 × 1″ casters are required for decreased maintenance, to prevent frequent flat tires, and to increase shock absorbency.

7. Standard auto seat belt is required for safety and to prevent slipping out of wheelchair when in an upright posture. It will also help maintain the alignment of the pelvis in a neutral position.

8. Foot-operated brakes required for safety during transport and transfers.

9. Antitippers for safety in preventing the chair from tipping back when in the tilted position.

10. Arm trough with palm extensor modular pad including associated swivel hardware from Ottobock is also required to adequately support Ms. Glass's left arm and hand. Ottobock has a specially contoured surface to correctly position her entire forearm and facilitate a passive stretch for all five digits (which flex into a loose fist if not supported). The swivel mounting mechanism is required to accommodate her arm position given the increased flexor tone. The strap is needed to hold her forearm in place despite frequent muscle spasms.

Physical Therapist Name
Laura Elmsworth, PT, DPT

Signature

Date: 9/10/23

I agree with the above findings of the Physical Therapist

Physician Name and Address:
Dr. Compo, General Hospital, Boston, Massachusetts

PHYSICIAN SIGNATURE

DATE

CASE EXAMPLE 15.7   Request to Third-Party Payer for Additional Visits

This is a sample letter to a third-party payer requesting approval for additional visits. The letter highlights the patient's quantitative improvements in functional performance, details the skilled intervention that was required to achieve these improvements, and provides evidence to support the benefits of physical therapy and the specific procedures used in this patient population.

In reply to: CBA Healthcare Inc.
Attention: Northeast Region Managed Care Division

To Whom It May Concern:

Subject: Request for Additional Physical Therapy Visits for Rupal Patel

Ms. Patel was referred for physical therapy evaluation and treatment on 6/15/2022, 2 wk s/p left ankle fracture with ORIF (DOS 6/1/2022). On initial evaluation, this patient presented with pain, edema, decreased LE ROM and strength, and limitations in transfers and ambulation. She has received 6/8 authorized physical therapy sessions to date, consisting of ultrasound, stretching/strengthening, standing balance training, gait training, and patient education in safety precautions and home exercise program activities. She has achieved the following progress:

Measurement	Initial Evaluation	Current Status
Activities		
Lower Extremity Functional Scale (range, 0-80; 80 = no functional limitations; clinically significant change = 9 points)	35	48
Ambulation	Amb 250 ft using toe-touch weight bearing on left leg, with bilateral axillary crutches, on level surfaces and stairs	Amb with straight cane, weight bearing as tolerated within home and outside up to 500 ft. Unable to amb longer distances (for recreational walking, walking in shopping mall)
Transfers	Transfers independently with B axillary crutches using toe-touch WB LLE	Transfers independently with straight cane and weight bearing as tolerated LLE
Impairments		
Pain	Left ankle pain reported as 8/10 on all standing/ambulatory activities	Pt. reports pain has subsided to 4/10 on standing/ambulatory activities
Anthropometric measurements (Figure 8)	L: 4l cm; R: 35 cm	L: 37.5 R: 35 cm; indicating decrease in L ankle edema|
AROM	PF: 0°-10°; DF: 0° Inversion: 0°-7°; eversion: 0°	PR 0°-20°; DF: 0°-5° Inversion: 0°-l5°; eversion: 0°-7°
Strength	PF: 2/5; DF 2/5 Supination: 2/5; pronation: 2/5	PR 3+/5; DF: 4/5 Supination: 4-/5; pronation: 4-/5

CASE EXAMPLE 15.7 Request to Third-Party Payer for Additional Visits—cont'd

Although significant progress has been achieved, Ms. Patel continues to present with the aforementioned impairments and activity limitations, limiting her ability to perform her normal ADLs. To date, manual therapy was not initiated due to her level of pain and discomfort. However, the pain levels have decreased substantially, and she would benefit from a more progressive treatment program including manual therapy. Research has demonstrated that manual therapy can improve ankle range of motion and mobility following ankle fracture, one which can have a significant impact on facilitating return to work and fully functioning within the home.

Ms. Patel requires continued PT treatment 2 ×/wk for 4 wk (8 sessions) as described to achieve the following updated PT goals:

1. Patient will return to normal activities of daily living within 2 wk, without restriction.
2. Patient will transfer independently without assistive device in 4 wk/8 sessions.
3. Patient will ambulate on level surfaces, ramps (to 15° incline), and stairs up to 1000 ft without assistive device to allow for community ambulation. Independently in 4 wk/8 sessions.
4. Patient's pain will be decreased to <2/10 in order to allow her to comfortably perform household chores in 4 wk/8 sessions.
5. Patient will be discharged from therapy and independent in a comprehensive home program.

Please do not hesitate to contact me if you have any questions. Thank you for your consideration.

Sincerely,
Jean Smythe, PT
Superior Physical Therapy Group Inc.
Courtesy James F. Ross

CASE EXAMPLE 15.8 Letter to Third-Party Payer Following Denial of Services

This sample letter to an insurance company is in response to the denial of payment for services. The letter highlights the patient's functional improvements, provides justification for the slow progress, and provides specific achievable functional goals for continued services.

November 15, 2022

ABC Insurance Co.
Re: Alicia Bremmer
Period: November 1, 2022 to December 31, 2022

To Whom It May Concern:
This letter is being offered to provide basis for support of medical necessity for restorative outpatient physical therapy services for Alicia Bremmer for the three visits attended to date beyond 10/31/2022 as well as four additional visits through 12/31/2022.

Ms. Bremmer was authorized for treatment at our facility for s/p lumbar fusion (DOS 8/15/2022) from 9/2/2022 to 10/31/2022 for 15 visits. Her progress was slow in a large part due to a left foot drop that occurred during the above-noted surgical procedure. Until recently, the patient continued to wear a Jewitt TLSO and is still using a cane for ambulation as well as an orthotic brace to compensate for left ankle weakness/instability.

Before injury/surgery, Ms. Bremmer was independent with all ADLs without the need for an assistance device. At present, she has not achieved her prior functional status, which has adversely affected her ability to perform her ADLs, such as squatting, descending stairs, and housework. Ms. Bremmer demonstrated significant improvement in her impairments since initiating therapy. Her range of motion has improved to 85% in all planes and strength improved to 4-/5 in her trunk and throughout her left lower extremity, except for dorsiflexion which is still 2+/5. The Back Index Score has improved from 71% on 9/2/2022, to 50% on 10/3/2022, to 33% on 10/31/2022. However, she continues to ambulate with a straight cane with decreased heel-strike and toe-off on the left, has difficulty descending stairs without a handrail, and feels unsteady/weak with daily activities.

Ms. Bremmer has responded well to manual therapy techniques as well as specific guided exercise prescriptions to help her achieve adequate hip/knee/foot/ankle strength and to optimize neural recruitment of the left ankle musculature.

Considering the consistent gains made with therapy to date as well as continued deficits with respect to her surgery and subsequent drop foot, I request authorization for the three visits attended to date (self-pay) as well as an additional four visits for a total of seven visits from 11/1/2022 to 12/31/2022 to address her remaining goals and improve her overall function. At that point, Ms. Bremmer will be discharged to a comprehensive home program to address any residual deficits.

Enclosed is a copy of the Ms. Bremmer's records including the evaluation/reevaluation findings, daily notes, and the treatment plan. If you have further questions regarding this case, please feel free to contact me at 555-555-5555.

Thank You,

Joe Jones, DPT
Community Hospital
Courtesy James F. Ross

CASE EXAMPLE 15.9 Home Exercise Program: Home Instructions

This case example provides a portion of a sample home program and instructions for activity following a total knee replacement. Simple, short sentences improve readability for patient-related instructions, and pictures with clear instructions are important to describe an exercise program.

Patient: Stefan Jones
Date: 2/5/23
Therapist: Laura Danforth

Activity
- Use your crutches as instructed, putting as much weight on the knee as you can comfortably tolerate. Take short walks (up to 10 min) often throughout the day. Do not sit for more than 45 min at a time.
- Wear shoes that fit well and have nonskid soles.

Precautions
- Do not twist or pivot your body when you are going to sit down or stand up from a sitting position.
- Do not climb up on a ladder or stepstool.
- Do not kneel down to pick up anything.
- When lying in bed, keep a pillow under your heel or ankle, NOT your knee. It is important to keep your knee straight. Try to stay in positions that do not bend your knee.
- Do not carry anything over 5 pounds.

Exercises
- Perform the following exercises 3×/day.
- Ice your knee 30 min before and 30 min after activity or exercises. Icing will decrease swelling.

(Continued)

CASE EXAMPLE 15.9   Home Exercise Program: Home Instructions—cont'd

Stretching Flexion

- Lie on your back with your legs straight and your back in neutral position (slightly arched).
- Lift the injured leg toward your chest, bending at the knee and hold it there with your hands as far as possible or until a gentle stretch is felt.
- Maintain the stretch and slowly return to initial position.
- Repetition: 5. No. of frequency: 2. Hold: 30 sec.
  (Fig. 15.1)

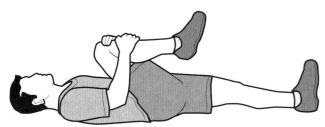

FIG. 15.1 Stretching flexion.

Knee Extension Stretch

- Sit (or lie down) with your involved leg straight out in front of you.
- Place the heel on a small, rolled-up towel with the knee unsupported.
- Optional: Place an ice pack on your knee while holding the position.
- Hold: 3 sec.
  (Fig. 15.2)

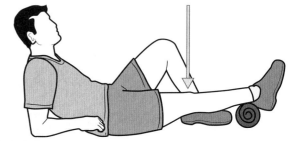

FIG. 15.2 Knee extension stretch.

Documentation in Pediatrics

Agnes McConlogue Ferro and Lori Quinn

LEARNING OBJECTIVES

After reading this chapter and completing the exercises, the reader will be able to:

1. Describe the laws governing documentation in early intervention and school-based settings in the United States.
2. Identify commonly used standardized assessments in early intervention and school-based settings.
3. Document components of early intervention evaluations and session notes, which are family-centered, child-specific, routines-based, and aligned with the natural environment.
4. Document components of school-based evaluations and session notes, which are child-centered and specific to the school setting.
5. Create goals with/for a pediatric client utilizing evidence-based resources and best practice standards, including child-centered, functional, within context, and relevant to participation within their natural environments of home/school.

OVERVIEW

Pediatric documentation is read by a wide range of health and non-health care team members, thus requiring a unique set of skills from the physical therapist (PT) to ensure effective communication. PTs must share their evaluation results, assessment, and goals in a way that maintains professional standards while providing jargon-free terminology so the non–health care team member is able to comprehend it with relative ease. The team member (parent, caregiver, teacher, administrator, and child as appropriate) is often unfamiliar with health care abbreviations and terms, and it is imperative that the reader have a clear understanding of such terms in order to accurately interpret any report. This typically results in lengthier narratives, with layperson terminology and parenthetical descriptions. The ability to create complete, comprehendible, and professional evaluative documentation is a critically important skill in pediatric settings and is an essential component in promoting optimal communication with all team members.

As a child progresses through the pediatric spectrum of service delivery, the scope of physical therapy documentation requires attention to the child, their family, and the associated performance expectations within their environment. The overriding principle for pediatric documentation, inclusive of evaluations, goals, and intervention plans, is the level of participation expected within their natural environment. The *natural environment* is typically defined by the child's age or stage of development and includes the routines of home (in early intervention) or school. Consideration of the unique needs of the child within their natural environment is paramount and must

be incorporated into the documentation and treatment process. In this chapter we will discuss documentation for the pediatric client as it pertains to two broad categories: early intervention (typically from birth to 3 years) and school aged (3-21 years).

EARLY INTERVENTION

Overview of Early Intervention Service Provision

The Program for Infants and Toddlers with Disabilities, also commonly known as Early Intervention or Part C of the Individuals with Disabilities Education Act (IDEA, 2004), is a federal program offering assistance to states to "maintain and implement a statewide, comprehensive, coordinated, multidisciplinary, interagency system of early intervention services for infants and toddlers with disabilities and their families" (IDEA, 2004, section 303.1 (a)). There is a clear focus on family involvement in the wording of IDEA (2004), throughout all phases of service delivery, most notably during the Early Intervention Program (EIP). Part C of IDEA (2004) requires that children who meet the criteria receive services from birth until no longer requiring them or when they reach their third birthday (Box 16.1). Related services provided during Early Intervention "are designed to meet the developmental needs of an infant or toddler with a disability, as identified by the individualized family service plan team" (IDEA, 2004, section 303.13(4)). In addition, these services are mandated to take place in the child's natural environment of home, daycare, playground, or locations where the family identifies barriers to their child's participation in expected routines.

Determining Eligibility

Early intervention encompasses children of ages 0-3 years who are deemed eligible to receive services in order to promote aspects of their development. Guidelines for determining eligibility for services, including physical therapy, differ from state to state because each state governs the specific eligibility criteria for developmental delay and at-risk children. Most states require scores from standardized outcome measures as the determinant of service implementation. Table 16.1 provides a listing of commonly used assessments in early intervention, and further information on standardized testing and outcome measures can be found in Chapter 4.

According to individual state requirements, a PT may be required to report findings for eligibility in terms of percent delay or as standard deviations from the normative values. For example, in certain states, for a child to receive services there must be a 33% delay or 2 standard deviations from the mean in one functional area or 25% delay or 1.5 standard deviations from the mean in each of two functional areas. PTs working in states that require specific criteria must therefore provide the results of standardized outcome measure(s) in their evaluation report, which will then be used to determine a child's eligibility for early intervention services. It is important to note again that although the results are reported as percentages and standard deviations, it must also be described in ways that would be comprehensible and meaningful to the parent or caregiver.

Family-Centered Planning

The focus on family-centered planning is an important component of EIPs. Family-centered planning, where the family lays the groundwork for the plan of care within their natural environment and daily routine, is not only considered the best practice (An & Palisano, 2014) but is incorporated in the law that governs the provision of related services through EIP (IDEA Part C, section 303.126). The ability of a PT, as a related service provider, to train and problem solve with the family directly is essential to the overall success of a child's rehabilitation plan. The child's role becomes even more important as they begin to self-determine personal needs and exploration within their own environment. The impact on future skill acquisition begins in infancy, and the PT and family's role in gross motor development cannot be more important than at this stage of development (Lobo et al., 2013; Morgan et al., 2021).

The ability to incorporate the family through a collaborative, team-based, problem-solving approach offers the maximal potential for success versus viewing the family and child

as passive recipients of individual services. Based on current research and best practice standards, early intervention therapists[1] should include the following as part of the initial discussion with the family: their concerns, their expectations, the child's strengths, and the family's daily routine (Farrell et al., 2009; Adams et al., 2013). If the therapist can obtain this information before the initial visit, the PT may be able to plan the assessment accordingly and have a greater chance of capturing the child's true abilities beyond the scope of standardized testing. In addition, infant/toddler development is a time of rapid changes with uniquely different trajectories for each aspect of growth: physical, emotional, and cognitive. In order to perform an evaluation that is truly representative of the child's current level of performance within the family's expected routines, the PT must incorporate the family into the assessment and treatment process.

According to IDEA, Part C, every child receiving an evaluation must have a "family-directed assessment of the resources, priorities, and concerns of the family and the identification of the supports and services necessary to enhance the family's capacity to meet the developmental needs of that infant or toddler" (303.321 (b)). There are many ways to incorporate the family into your assessment process; we describe two that are most commonly utilized in the pediatric population: routine-based and play-based assessments.

Routines-based assessments focus on identifying the child's specific routines and participation expectations throughout the day. PTs often adapt concepts of motivational interviewing to provide a full-scope representation of the child's expected routine and their performance capacity within those routines. This type of assessment allows the therapist and the family to easily identify areas of need along with opportunities for intervention and carryover. This is often referred to as *embedded intervention*: PT intervention plans are practiced within multicontextual aspects of the natural environment (home, playground, grocery store, etc.). The cornerstone of this approach is that of opportunity: allowing the child to practice a required skill throughout a typical day has obvious potential for a more timely impact on the child's ability to achieve that task as a learned skill.

Play-based assessments have been increasingly utilized over the past decade (O'Grady & Dusing, 2015). The strength of play-based assessments is in its simplicity: the functional expectation for infants and toddlers is the development of exploration, play, and interaction with their environment. At times, there is a misconception that early intervention practitioners are only comfortable with bringing their assessment and evaluation abilities framed through the medical model and strictly working at the impairment level, for example, obtaining measurements of range of motion and assessing strength. There is also a misconception that early intervention practitioners must have their toy bag! Although the toy bag carries opportunities that should not be dismissed, the more powerful option is the ability to truly observe the child's interaction within their expected

---

[1]The term *early interventionist* is being used in some states to facilitate a more generalized approach to early intervention services by all professionals.

TABLE 16.1 Commonly Used Standardized Tests to Assess Gross Motor and Functional Skills in Pediatric Clients

Test	Purpose	Target Population	Range	Description
Alberta Infant Motor Scale (AIMS) (Piper & Darrah, 1994; 2022)	Discriminative and evaluative	All infants except those with significant abnormal movement patterns	Birth to 18 mo or walking	Used to identify infants with motor delay and evaluate motor development over time
Bruininks-Oseretsky Test of Motor Proficiency, 2nd edition (BOT-2) (Bruininks & Bruininks, 2005)	Discriminative	All school-aged children	4.5–14.5 yr	Norm-referenced discriminative measure designed to assess the motor proficiency of all students (typically developing to those with moderate motor skill deficits)
Gross Motor Function Measure (GMFM) (Russell et al., 1989)	Evaluative	Children with cerebral palsy; also reliable for children with Down syndrome; osteogenesis imperfecta	6 mo–16 yr	Designed to evaluate change in gross motor function in children with cerebral palsy
Peabody Developmental Motor Scales-2 (PDMS-2) (Folio & Fewell, 2000) and PDMS (Folio & Fewell 2023)	Discriminative	Typically developing, suspected developmental delay	Birth to 5 yr 11 mo	Norm-referenced measure designed to assess gross and fine motor abilities of children from birth through age 5 yr
Pediatric Evaluation of Disability Inventory (PEDI; PEDI-MCAT) (Haley et al., 1992)	Discriminative and evaluative	Children with expected delays in functional performance	PEDI: 6 mo-7.5 yr; PEDI-MCAT: birth to 20 yr	Norm-referenced measure designed to evaluate functional capabilities and degree of caregiver burden performance in children with disabilities
School Functional Assessment (SFA) (Coster et al., 1998)	Evaluative	Children with disabling conditions	5-12 yr	Criterion-referenced measure that evaluates a student's performance of functional tasks and activities within the school environment
Test of Infant Motor Performance (TIMP) (Campbell et al., 2002)	Predictive	Infants born prematurely	34 wk' postconceptual age to 4 mo postterm	Test designed to predict long-term disability in infants
Test of Gross Motor Development-3 (TGMD-3) (Ulrich, 2016)	Discriminative	Preschool and school-age children who are significantly behind their peers in gross motor skill development	3-10 yr, 11 mo	Norm-referenced measure of common gross motor skills
Movement Assessment Battery for Children-3 (2023) (Handerson and Barnett, 2023)			3-25 years	

routines and with the resources that already exist within their environments.

Parents/caregivers and family members play the most important roles because they are the primary "facilitators" working with the child. Play-based assessments are as minimally intrusive as possible. Limited redirection may be used verbally or through environmental motivators. Assessments can be video recorded to allow for complete and thorough observation without requiring the child to repeat activities or tasks.

These routine and play-based assessments, along with the appropriate choice of standardized outcome measures, provide the PT with a comprehensive evaluation of the child's performance. In turn, the results allow for a true comparison of the child's current performance to that of the majority of their age-matched peers to determine if there is a delay. The determination to mandate physical therapy intervention is derived from the reporting of the PT evaluation results. A family-directed approach not only applies to involving the parent in the evaluation, goal setting, and interventions but should be taken into consideration in written reports (Nguyen et al., 2021). The need to provide meaningful

documentation is considered a crucial competency in the provision of early intervention physical therapy (Chiarello & Effgen, 2006; Weaver et al., 2018). Documentation of findings becomes as inherently important as the PT's ability to make observations, create goals, and implement plans for treatment.

Early Intervention Documentation
Individual Family Service Plan (IFSP) Evaluations

If services are mandated for the child, an *Individual Family Service Plan (IFSP)* is the multidisciplinary, documented plan that is created for provision of services for the child *and* the family (Lucas et al., 2014). This plan serves as the "contract" between the state governing agency and the family to outline the goals of early intervention for a child (McEwen, 2000). IDEA mandates a review of the IFSP every 6 months. PTs are expected to complete an assessment that involves the family, the child, and the multidisciplinary team (MDT) within the child's natural environment. The PT should consider communication with the entire MDT as important as their individual assessments/ interventions.

Early intervention evaluation reports are primarily read by individuals who are not health care professionals but are imperative to the growth and well-being of the child—most importantly, the child's parents. Best practice in early intervention report writing involves several key components (Box 16.2). The report should be free of jargon and easily interpreted by individuals outside the medical field. If medical terminology is required, it should be defined (often, parenthetically) whenever possible.

Case Example 16.1 provides an example of an early intervention physical therapy evaluation as part of an IFSP. As shown in this example, the headings for an early intervention evaluation can differ slightly from that typically written in a hospital or clinic setting but have the same general structure. As mentioned earlier, the results of standardized tests are frequently used in combination with a therapist's descriptive assessment to determine eligibility for services. The results of these tests should be documented in the evaluation report; however, the evaluation report should not focus *solely* on the results of the test nor on the child's performance on specific items.

As seen in Case Example 16.1 and Box 16.2, evaluations in early intervention should identify the problems or activities that the child *cannot* do but also on what he or she is *able* to do (otherwise known as *strengths-based*). Deficiencies can, and should, be highlighted in the report, but the overall tone of the evaluation should be centered on the child's abilities at the present time. The choice to highlight what is available allows the provider, and the reader, to find areas where those strengths serve as opportunities to foster areas that may be delayed. Strength-based report writing is not to be interpreted as curtailing the PT from using the terminology pertinent to the profession. It is crucial, however, that the parents, as the essential part of the family-centered planning, be able to understand and hopefully feel empowered by the therapist's assessment.

Goal Writing in Early Intervention

Collaboration with the family to identify goals that are participation-based is crucial during IFSP development. Collaborative goal setting is an essential component of family-centered care by engaging families actively in therapy services. Furthermore, there is some suggestion that effective use of goal setting is associated with improved outcomes (Brewer et al., 2014). Brewer et al. (2014) recommends setting an explicit goal-setting process. A critical component of goal setting requires taking time to interview parents and discuss together options for appropriate goals. Goals that are concrete, observable, contextualized, relevant, and set within a given time frame should then be formulated. Table 16.2 provides criteria for writing optimal IFSP

BOX 16.2 Strategies for Optimal Report Writing in Early Intervention

1. **Provide parenthetical definitions**.
   Joey was able to briefly maintain quadruped (on hands and knees) when placed there. While attempting to roll supine (on his back) to prone (on his stomach), he was observed to use an extensor pattern (use of primarily one muscle group) to complete the transition.
2. **Explain test results in plain language**.
   The scores on the standardized test of motor development indicate that Jane is currently performing at the third percentile. This means that the majority of her age-related peers are performing skills above her current level of performance, and based on parent report, scores, age equivalents, and discipline-specific assessment, Jane is eligible for early intervention services.
3. **Describe concepts functionally**.

Poor Example	Optimal Example
Annie presented with moderate hypotonia of the trunk.	Annie has a lower resting level of muscle stiffness than what is expected. This affects her posture and her ability to move against gravity with independence and efficiency.

4. **Eliminate negative reporting**.

Poor Example	Optimal Example
Nikki was resistant to handling and refused to participate in the evaluation process.	Nikki was self-directed in her play, preferring to follow her own agenda more exclusively than is typical for her age.

5. **Avoid deficit-focused language**.

Poor Example	Optimal Example
Mark has only fair strength of his abdominals and is unable to get into sitting independently.	Mark is able to maintain sitting when placed there. Strengthening his abdominal muscles to assist him in completing the transitions into and out of sitting will be a primary focus of physical therapy intervention.

6. **Lead with the child's competencies**.

Poor Example	Optimal Example
Sarina does not ascend/descend the stairs reciprocally.	Sarina is able to climb a flight of stairs. She is emergent in her ability to climb up and down the stairs using the mature pattern (step-over-step) expected of her age.

7. **Avoid "but/however" constructions**.

Poor Example	Optimal Example
Roberto can transition sit-to-stand but is unable to do it without help from his mother or holding onto the couch.	Roberto is able to transition from sit-to-stand when provided with external support from an adult or a stable surface.

Adapted from Towle PO, Farrel AF, Vitalone-Raccaro N. Report writing in early intervention: guidelines for user-friendly, strength-based writing. *Zero to Three*. 2008;28:53–60.

TABLE 16.2   Criteria for Optimal IFSP Outcomes

Criteria	Example
1. The outcome is necessary and functional for the child's and family's life.	*Jane will access her home environment to play with her toys.*
2. The outcome reflects real-life contextualized settings.	*Jane will maintain upright positions (sit, stand) to interact with her environment during food shopping, playground, and mealtime.*
3. The outcome integrates developmental domains and is discipline free.	*Jane will assist her mother with getting the mail.*
4. The outcome is jargon free and simple.	*"Jane will walk up and down the stairs" versus "Jane will ascend or descend the stairs with a step-to pattern."*
5. The outcome emphasizes the positive, not the negative.	*"Jane will sit with a posture that allows her to interact" versus "Jane will sit without requiring external assistance."*
6. The outcome uses active words rather than passive words.	*"Jane will independently walk" versus "Jane will improve her balance in order to walk."*

Adapted from Lucas A, Gillaspy K, Peters ML, Hurth J. *Enhancing Recognition of High Quality, Functional IFSP Outcomes.* Retrieved from: <http://www.ectacenter.org/~pdfs/pubs/rating-ifsp.pdf>; 2014.

outcomes, and Case Example 16.1 provides examples of goals written as part of an early intervention evaluation.

Session Notes in Early Intervention

There is considerable variation among states as to specific requirements for daily note documentation in early intervention. Regardless of state requirements, we recommend documentation of each session or contact point with a child and/or their family for several reasons. First, it provides a record of interventions and progress achieved toward goals, which is important for the therapist to continually reassess the intervention plan and guide clinical decision-making. Second, it is a useful resource for supporting collaboration with the parent/caregiver. Third, it serves as a legal record of the contact time between a therapist and a child and could be requested in the event of any disputes regarding provision of services.

Case Example 16.2 provides a sample daily note written for a child in early intervention. As shown in this example, daily notes do not need to be particularly long or detailed, but they should include important information such as the date, time, and location that the services were provided. The note should focus on the specific tasks or activities that were addressed and any progress that was achieved directly during the intervention session or that has occurred since the child was last seen. Language used in the session note is most effective when it is jargon free and strengths based. In addition, particular attention should be given to the support or training provided to the parent/caregiver during the session. This includes their feedback on

"what worked and what didn't" from the prior session and typically identifies the method of support provided to the parent/caregiver (e.g., observation, demonstration, and instructional feedback). The parent/caregiver is integral to the provision of services in early intervention, there is a shift from "family-centered" to "child-centered" when the child turns 3 and services, if still required, are provided through the local school district.

SCHOOL-BASED INTERVENTION

Overview of School-Based Service Provision

Children of ages 3-21 years with disabilities most commonly receive services in a school-based setting. Physical therapy is provided when the child is eligible as mandated under Part B of IDEA, and physical therapy intervention is required to "assist a child with a disability to benefit from special education" (IDEA, 2004, section 300.34). The shift from home and family-centered to that of school, the routines encountered there, and the providers who interact with the child is often a time of unique transition, particularly regarding provision of related services.

If a child continues to require related services to address developmental needs and aspects of performance after the age of 3 or if issues are identified for the first time at this age, the child is eligible to receive services under Part B of IDEA. This potentially encompasses children of ages 3-21. The lead agency typically changes from the county health department to the child's home school district. Subsequently, so do the documentation requirements.

The Committee on Preschool Education (CPSE) provides management of services for children of ages 3-5 years. The "CPSE" years are a time of transition, where the family is still strongly involved, but now the role of the child within expected routines of school becomes the central focus. The therapist takes into consideration that play is still an important component of the preschool child's expected routine throughout the day, but the shift toward function, skill performance, and meaningful interaction within the school environment begins to form. This has a direct impact on the choice of standardized outcome measures required to fully capture age-expected performance within the school-based environment.

The PT is now a part of a team that can include not just the family, as in early intervention, but anyone who interacts with that child, including but not limited to, the teacher, paraprofessional, physical education teacher, occupational therapist, and speech-language pathologist. This multidisciplinary team collaborates to create a framework of service evaluation and implementation referred to as the Individualized Education Plan (IEP).

Individualized Education Plans

As children enter elementary school, typically by the age of 5, the individual school districts are responsible for the services put in place for each child with a disability. Each student who receives physical therapy must have an IEP in place prior to the start of related services. The therapist, guided by state and specific district mandates, may be required to complete a full and appropriate evaluation to determine current functional status and goals.

IEPs are designed differently by each state. In most states, therapists are required to write "a statement of the child's present levels of academic achievement and functional performance" as they affect his or her performance in the school setting and "a statement of measurable annual goals, including academic and functional goals, designed to meet the child's needs that result from the child's disability to enable the child to be involved in and make progress in the general education curriculum" (IDEA, 2004 [§300.320(a)(4)]). The focus of IDEA (2004) within the school setting is on goal achievement; therapists must provide goals that are functional, measurable, and relevant to the educational setting.

IDEA mandates a review of the IEP on an annual basis. Thus therapists, educators, and other providers must write a new IEP with new goals for the upcoming year. Case Example 16.3 provides an example of an IEP written for child with cerebral palsy in a school-based setting.

In addition to the IEP, providers must assess goal achievement on a quarterly basis and provide a statement of how the identified goals will be measured. Another unique component of formulating the IEP is that it is child-centered, and the child becomes a member of the team, thus having a voice in creating his or her own goals.

Functional outcomes documentation is very important in the school setting. The purpose of a PT's evaluation and intervention within the school setting is to help the child function better within their school routine (e.g., in the lunchroom, classroom, playground). Case Example 16.4 provides an example of session note documentation in the school setting. In addition to writing on the IEP and documenting session notes, therapists may provide justification to obtain appropriate equipment required for the child to access the educational environment (see Case Example 16.5). The focus of this documentation should be on how limitations in physical functioning and gross motor skills affect the child's ability to participate in the school setting.

The International Classification of Functioning, Disability and Health (ICIDH-2) is a useful resource when observing and assessing function within the school setting. Fig. 16.1 offers an example of how the ICIDH-2 (ICIDH-2 is frequently referred to as the ICF model) can be used to describe and understand the components of a child's health and physical functioning in the school setting for a child who has cerebral palsy. This could relate to a child's ability to move within a classroom or between classrooms, to participate in gym class or on the playground, to climb stairs in the school, to get on and off the bus, or to participate in self-care skills such as dressing and toileting. This focus on function within the school setting can be challenging for the PT. The use of the ICF can be a useful tool for school-based PTs when utilized as a framework for goal setting and goal assessment (Nguyen et al., 2021).

For instance, when considering children diagnosed with cerebral palsy classified as level 5 on the Gross Motor Function Classification System (GMFCS) or considering a child with significant behavioral or cognitive issues, it can be less clear as to what "function" is for that individual child. Therapists, however, do have resources to assist them. The GMFCS offers guidance on functional expectations according to each classification level and across age spans, allowing for a loosely predictive guide to expectations as the child develops. Although not a predictive resource per se, therapists can use this classification system to assist them when formulating goals and considering treatment interventions that are within evidence-based parameters of realistic and relevant for the upcoming year, and potentially beyond. For example, in the case of the child classified as level

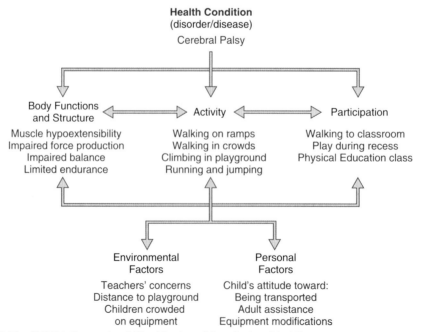

FIG. 16.1 The ICIDH-2 (International Classification of Functioning, Disability and Health) Framework can be used to describe the relationship of health condition and body functions/structure with a child's level of participation and activity as they relate to the school setting. Personal and environmental factors also influence functioning across the spectrum.

5, formulating goals that would have the child rise to stand with minimal assistance would not be realistic.

In addition, as often as possible, PTs are mandated to provide goals and interventions that are based upon "peer-reviewed research to the extent practicable" §300.320(a)(4). This leads the PT to be a constant consumer of research and current evidence-based practice. Resources that provide normative data are useful for comparison to age-matched peers but must be utilized appropriately. For example, the Timed Up and Go test (Itzkowitz et al., 2016) is an easy-to-use reference to provide goal attainment parameters as the PT seeks to complete assessments and create goals that are measurable, relevant, and realistic. This same test would not be an appropriate resource for children with complex diagnoses and presentations that may preclude ambulation as a realistic goal. The choice of standardized outcome measures plays an important role in the determination of meaningful goals, particularly within the school setting.

Use of Standardized Testing in the School Setting

One of the most important steps in delivering services that truly meet the mandate set by IDEA is the choice of standardized outcome measures. An overview of constructs related to standardized testing and outcome measures is provided in Chapter 4. Eligibility for services does not require scores from standardized outcome measures as the sole determining factor; however, standardized testing is important to provide a baseline of performance and to provide guidance in establishing that individualized plan for the upcoming year. The decision-making process when choosing the best outcome measure should take into consideration the child, the diagnosis, and the prognosis, but importantly, it should focus on expected performance of skills relevant to the school setting. Indeed, standardized testing is not always appropriate for pediatric clients for various reasons (Box 16.3).

Table 16.1 provides a list of some commonly used standardized tests for children, although by no means is this list exhaustive. Each test was designed with a specific purpose, and each has its own set of strengths and weakness, discussion of which is beyond the scope of this text. The pediatric therapist is required to have sufficient knowledge of multiple standardized assessments to choose the most appropriate for each individual

patient (Long & Toscano, 2002). However, some important considerations for choosing an appropriate measure are highlighted in Box 16.3. One example of a standardized outcome measure that supports the assessment of a broad spectrum of function within contextual parameters of the school environment is the School Function Assessment (Coster et al., 1998). The focus on function within the school setting often provides the PT with a clear idea of prioritized annual goals for the IEP.

Goal Writing in the School Setting
Writing Annual Goals on the IEP

The annual goals provide the foundation for the types of activities that should be addressed during the upcoming year. Goal writing on the IEP is mandated to address specific goals related to functioning in the school (see Case Example 16.3 for sample IEP goals). Therefore writing strictly impairment-related goals in this setting is not meaningful. Goals are read by parents and school personnel, who are often not familiar with medical terminology. Therapists should avoid jargon and define terms when necessary (see Chapter 2 for more detail on avoiding jargon).

In addition, it is important to discuss the relevance of *function* as it pertains to the child throughout his or her development. During early intervention services, *function* for the child refers to accessing his or her natural environments. During school-based services, *function* for the child refers to accessing his or her school-based environment, which of course can have direct carryover to their home environment. There must be a clear shift when formulating IEP goals, from isolated skill (standing on one leg) to that of functional task (stepping up onto bus).

Many standardized tests used by PTs focus on performance of gross motor tasks versus functional performance. It is important to clarify the difference because assessments should be viewed as a source of subsequent goals. *Gross motor tasks* can be composed of tasks such as ball manipulation, jumping, skipping, hopping, or standing on one leg. These tasks are expected at certain stages of development and may indicate areas of treatment intervention for the therapist. For example, a child who is not jumping by the age of 3 years may have issues related to strength, balance, or motor planning/coordination. These areas would be the focus of intervention strategies during treatment but should not be considered the *functional goal* for the child. A *functional goal* must address specific components or activities required to access or function efficiently within the child's environment (refer to Chapter 12 for additional discussion on functional goals). Using the example of the 3-year-old child who is unable to jump, if we hypothesize that, in addition to the inability to jump, the child is able to climb the stairs only with a step-to-step pattern using the handrail and hand-hold, then a potential functional goal could be to have the child use a more mature pattern to move independently from the parking lot up the stairs into the preschool. Focusing on the child's ability to jump independently is *not* the functional goal but may be a treatment intervention that the therapist works on to carry over to the goal of stair-climbing.

BOX 16.3 When Is Standardized Testing Not Appropriate?

Standardized testing is not appropriate in some cases. A child may not be able to follow directions to perform a specific test, or no test may be developed to measure the child's specific problems. In these cases, informed clinical opinion is warranted. Sometimes when children have severe motor impairments, the norms developed for a specific test may no longer be valid. Therapists therefore must provide compelling documentation to explain the nature of the child's problem and why and how it does (or may) result in delayed development. The therapist may find that combining sections of specific standardized tests allows for a baseline of information, which is commonly referred to as an *ecological assessment*. This type of assessment allows the therapist to report findings that reflect *aspects* of standardization, either criterion-referenced or norm-referenced, outside the parameters for true standardization.

Context Specificity and Use of Measurement Criteria

Writing goals within the school setting has two critical components. First, goals need to be context-specific, ideally defined by a relevant task that would enable the child to be involved in and make progress in the school setting. Second, goals need to be measurable so that goal attainment is quantified (McConlogue & Quinn, 2009, 2020). A goal analysis form, such as the GOALS checklist, can help therapists analyze their goals (annual, short-term, or benchmarks) to ensure that the goals are, in fact, functional and measurable as required by IDEA (McConlogue & Quinn, 2009, 2020).

Objective measurement criteria are required according to IDEA (2004). Therapists should use measurements that evaluate the degree of skill in performing functional tasks: consistency, efficiency, and flexibility. *Consistency* can be measured in the number of days per week or the number of consecutive observations. This can include the teacher, caregiver, parent, and/or other professionals. *Efficiency* in the simplest form can be reported as the amount of time for a task to be completed. *Flexibility* refers to the child's ability to perform the task in a variety of settings/environments. The following example includes all three optimal measurement criteria (see also Case Example 16.3 for examples of IEP goals).

> **Example:** *Sarah will climb 12 steps during transitions from class to cafeteria and 10 steps from cafeteria to outdoor recess (flexibility) within 3 min each (efficiency), as reported by her paraprofessional, a minimum of 3 days/wk (consistency).*

Measurement criteria would not have a lot of meaning if we did not know what we are comparing it to. For school-aged children, there are many normative values to refer to. The question then becomes: *Are the normative values useful?* In many ways, they are extremely useful, allowing comparison to what age-matched peers are doing and to help set the framework for expectations. The ability to use normative values as a form of objective measurement is clearly optimal. However, comparing children with known diagnoses who have extremely limited or no potential to achieve the skill within those normative parameters is not only unfair but unrealistic. Conversely, if the child has potential to complete the task in sync with his or her peers, using normative values can be useful to determine "finish lines." Once the goal has been set, the therapist should refer to the research literature and other resources to determine whether normative values exist and then to incorporate the findings into the measurement criteria.

Goal attainment scaling (GAS) is a useful tool in creating and analyzing IEP goals (Effgen et al., 2016; King et al., 1999; Mailloux et al., 2007). The GAS is a 5-point scale used to quantify individual goal achievement. It can be particularly useful when creating goals for a child with multiple handicapping conditions. In such a case, it may be difficult for the PT to define functional tasks for the child if the child is dependent for all activities of daily living. Furthermore, the evaluation may be limited due to lack of available standardized assessments to address the unique performance levels of a child with severe

---

> ### BOX 16.4   Example of Goal Attainment Scale for Child with GMFCS Level 5
>
> Goal: Child will participate during transfers into and out of wheelchair.
> −2: Dependent throughout transfer.
> −1: Lifts head away from headrest for >3 sec.
> 0: Maintains upper trunk erect for >3 sec when supported at the pelvis/lower trunk.
> +1: Maintains trunk erect when given support at the pelvis for >5 sec.
> +2: Actively brings trunk forward to scoot forward in wheelchair given assist at the pelvis.

---

limitations in function. The GAS allows the therapist to identify the most basic components of a task and to chart the progress of the child as he or she works toward achieving the task one component at a time. The use of the GAS is not limited to patients with severe limitations and can be used to chart intervention efficacy for any child. Box 16.4 shows how the GAS can be used for a pediatric client.

Writing Collaborative and Shared IEP Goals

Related service providers should encourage school-aged children to be active participants when developing their goals and intervention plans. The impact of self-determination and goal setting even for young children is critically important in the success of their intervention plans (Pritchard-Wiart et al., 2019, 2022). Furthermore, pediatrics often involves multidisciplinary collaboration, perhaps even more so than in other patient populations. IEP goals should be formulated with the child, teacher, family, and providers directly involved in the child's daily routine (Brewer et al., 2014; Pritchard et al., 2022). This can include paraprofessionals, bus drivers, cafeteria attendants, and any other individuals who are directly involved in a child's daily functioning. This shared and collaborative approach allows the therapist the ability to create optimal goals that address all aspects of expected function within the school. This can include activities such as transfers onto/off of the bus, ability to feed, dress, and safely complete transfers during toileting, or carry a cafeteria tray in an open environment.

Shared goals are often viewed as a form of collaboration, wherein the related service providers work together on a common annual goal and the goals are identified as being meaningful to the child. Individual disciplines (e.g., physical therapy, occupational therapy) remain unique by creating individual benchmarks required to achieve the common goal. For example, a shared goal that states "*the child will eat lunch with his peers*," could have the same goal across domains but different components requiring individual related service: physical therapy—working on carrying the tray through the line and to the cafeteria table; speech therapy—requesting luncheon items in an audible voice and with accuracy; and occupational therapy—eating, drinking, and cleaning up after the meal. In this way, all disciplines are focused on the same outcome: *The child will eat lunch with his peers*, but with attention to the components of that activity that require the unique attention of each of those related services.

II. <u>GOALS checklist</u>

1. <u>**Generate**</u> – the goal: _____
   - ☐ Input from team members (TM): child, parent, teacher, staff
   - ☐ Addresses identified skill-based needs
   - ☐ Addresses school-based function/performance/participation
   - ☐ Identifies context in which the targeted skill will be occurring
   - ☐ Provides consistent measurement criteria

2. <u>**Observe**</u> – performance of projected goal
   - ☐ Observed within natural context(s) of routine
   - ☐ Objective data collected within routine
   - ☐ Unable to observe, data collected by:_____.

3. <u>**Align**</u> – cannot be done in isolation!! Must be aligned with school routine.
   - ☐ Goal is aligned with school-based routine (context)
   - ☐ Goal is required for performance/participation (relevant)
   - ☐ Goal is defined within expected parameters of success (realistic)
   - ☐ Goal is **NOT** a treatment intervention or an impairment-based remediation.

4. <u>**Link**</u> – objective findings to measurement criteria. Imperative for goal-mastery.
   - ☐ 2-3 components of skill acquisition is represented:
     - _____consistency (# of trials)
     - _____flexibility (variety of contexts)
     - _____efficiency (time)
   - ☐ Normative values/baseline data utilized as parameters

5. <u>**Set**</u> – goal and intervention plan
   - ☐ Goal will be regularly assessed within specific context/routine
     - ____Service Provider and/or TM: _____
   - ☐ Reviewed for required components:
     - ___ school-based function/participation
     - ___ context specific
     - ___ measurement criteria
   - ☐ Intervention roadmap established: your plan to achieve goal-mastery
     - _____1-2 treatment frameworks per goal
     - _____evidence or practice based
     - _____ Goal Attainment Scaling is matched to interventions(s)

FIG. 16.2 IDEA to GOALS checklist.

Framework for Writing Goals in the School Setting

To assist therapists in reviewing the basic components required for optimal goal setting, the goal formulation format of ABCDE (see Chapter 12) should be used. However, for the pediatric population and specifically within school settings, there are goal-setting resources available. The American Physical Therapy Association has created an extensive Fact Sheet on Collaborative IEP goals that may provide useful information for school-based related service providers (American Physical Therapy Association, 2021). In addition, we have created a goal-setting framework for school-based therapists to utilize when assessing and creating IEP goals (McConlogue & Quinn, 2020).

The IDEA (Identify, Define, Expand, and Assess) to GOALS (McConlogue & Quinn, 2014, 2020) framework allows the therapist to go step by step through the identification, planning, and implementation of assessment and goal setting for the child within the context of the child's daily school routine. Importantly, it also includes opportunity for the therapist to identify collaborative team members (TMs) who have the potential to carry over the task/activity throughout the school day. One of the most important sections of this framework is that of communication: with the child, family, and TMs from the school.

IDEA TO GOALS FRAMEWORK

IDEA (Identify, Define, Expand, and Assess)

I: Identify the targeted skill(s) that need to be addressed for that child to participate more fully in his or her daily routine. To do this successfully, the PT must have communication with TMs for specific feedback on performance needs throughout the day in a variety of contexts. For example, if the PT has identified a sit-to-stand transfer as a targeted skill, he or she needs to talk to people who might be involved in observing or assisting with that skill: there are assumed TMs (e.g., paraprofessional, teacher), but there also other TMs who may play a significant role (e.g., physical education teacher, nurse, librarian, bus driver).

Within the identification process is also the step of determining the Two Rs: Is it relevant? Is it realistic? A targeted skill is proved to be **relevant** if it is necessary for *functional* performance within the school environment. PTs need to identify the context in which the activity is occurring to make it relevant. For example, a child who is performing the activity of sit-to-stand with the PT during the individual session looks quite different than one who is performing that same activity from the cafeteria bench during a crowded lunch period. A targeted skill is thought to be **realistic** when all the influencing factors—age, diagnosis, and personal/environmental factors—are taken into consideration and the potential for improvement within the school year exists.

D: Define the specific components required to perform specific activities. Using parameters of the ICIDH-2, the PT should analyze and define the limiters to performance: body functions and structure (range of motion, strength, posture, gait); personal

factors (age, coping skills, education level); environmental factors (affordances from the school environment, products/technology); and participation level (full or limited).

E: Expand upon findings by observing the targeted skill/activity within the context of the daily routine. Often, this is not possible, especially for the transient PT going from school to school. In these instances, the PT identifies the TM who would report on specific performance components. The ability to do this also allows the PT to obtain baseline measurements of functional performance: How is the skill performed in an open environment and within context? In addition, the PT can expand the targeted skill to a variety of school-based contexts, allowing the relationship of *skill–context–TM* to be readily apparent. The more opportunities for collaboration and carryover, the quicker the potential for skill acquisition.

A: Assess the individual skills in a standardized manner. The skills have been identified, defined, and observed throughout the day and are now ready for assessment. By identifying the skill(s) and gathering the information before making the choice of standardized outcome measure, you allow the child's unique needs within the true context of his or her daily routine to make the choice for you. Recommendations and the outline for your plan of intervention are formed as goal areas are identified. The individual goal-setting process is a natural next step.

GOALS (Generate, Observe, Align, Link, Set)

To assist pediatric therapists in optimal goal setting, a GOALS checklist was created and found to be useful by school-based PTs (McConlogue & Quinn, 2014, 2020; Fig. 16.2). This checklist can be used to review the goal once it is created *or* to refer to as the goal is being set. This can also be used programmatically, across disciplines, and for shared/collaborative goals.

G—Generate the goal.
O—Observe performance of the projected goal.
A—Align the goal with the school routine.
L—Link objective findings to measurement criteria.
S—Set the goal and review for required components.

■ SUMMARY

- This chapter provides an overview of the specialized documentation involved for the pediatric client. Sample evaluations, letters of justification, IFSPs, and IEPs are provided to assist therapists in incorporating functional outcomes assessment with this population.
- All documentation in pediatrics should be concise, free of jargon, and focused on improving functional outcomes.
- The pediatric therapist is required to have sufficient knowledge of multiple standardized assessments to choose the most appropriate for each individual patient.
- Goal writing for the pediatric patient must be done in collaboration with the child whenever possible and with other TMs. Goals should be functional in nature and context-specific and should include measurement criteria.

CASE EXAMPLE 16.1 Early Intervention Evaluation Suzanne Jones, DPT, Jones Pediatric Therapy

Name: Jane Johnson   **D.O.B.:** 4/5/21   **Date of Eval.:** 10/15/22

Jane is an 18-month-old girl diagnosed with developmental delay. Birth history was typical. Jane was evaluated in her home during play and snack time with her mother and brother, age 5, present. She has a vocabulary of 4-6 words and enjoys music/singing.

Activity/Participation (Assessment of Child's Ability to Function Within His or Her Natural Environment)

Jane enjoys playing with toys in her lap when ring sitting (knees bent with soles of the feet touching) on the floor. She consistently achieves this by flexing her trunk forward and pushing herself back over her pelvis with her arms. Jane has begun pulling at the couch or in the crib to stand. Jane is able to creep on hands and knees for approximately 2 ft. Primary mobility is to scoot across the floor in a ring-sit position, using her legs to pull herself, with her trunk flexed forward. She enjoys using her push toy to take 4-5 steps (exhibiting a wide base of support). She has difficulty climbing the stairs; her mother reports she prefers to carry her up and down.

During mealtime, she uses a high-chair without footrest. She is starting to eat finger foods and maintains puree diet. Her mother reports that she must reposition Jane throughout the meal. In addition, when she is food shopping or pushing her on a swing, she will often reposition Jane as she "slumps" typically to the right side.

Jane is involved in an organized playgroup, and her mother reports that she is extremely motivated to be with her peers. She enjoys trying to pop the bubbles from a seated position, while her peers prefer standing. She will request assistance to "march" during music play.

Body Functions and Structure (Assessment of Child's Strength and Mobility)

Jane is able to complete a pull to sit after a diaper change, with slight head lag (exhibits need for abdominal strengthening). She can lift, bang, throw, and squeeze toys of light weight (stuffed animals, small blocks/balls) within her base of support. There is evidence of emergent strength of the lower extremities as she pulls to stand through half-kneel and take steps when given support at the upper extremities.

Standardized Assessments (These are Tests That Measure A Child's Performance on Certain Tasks To That of Their Peers or as Specific Levels for Individual Task Performance)

1. *Pediatric Evaluation of Disability Inventory (PEDI):* Scored as follows: Self-Care: 40.4, Mobility: 20.3, and Social Function: 50.8. (Reported to allow comparison to peers. Children are expected to function within 2 standard deviations of the mean [which is where 50% of the population would perform the same task]. Therefore a range of functional skill scores between 30 and 70 is expected.) This indicates that Jane is within expected ranges for Self-Care and Social Function and exhibits a lower level of functioning in the category of Mobility.
2. *Alberta Infant Motor Scale:* This is a developmental mobility assessment that indicates that Jane is currently performing at the fifth percentile, supporting the findings from the PEDI that Mobility is a domain that requires assistance.

Assessment/Plan of Care

It is recommended that Jane receive physical therapy 2 times per week for 45-min sessions.

Goals for intervention, identified by the family, will focus on assisting Jane to achieve her expected motor milestones within the next 6 months:

1. Jane will sit with a posture that allows her to interact with her environment during mealtime, food shopping, or at the playground as reported by her mother, a minimum of 3 times per day.
2. When called by her mother, Jane will independently walk to access family area or kitchen, at least once a day, within 2 min.
3. Jane will climb the stairs with her mother when retrieving the mail or going to the car, a minimum of 2 times per day.

If you have any questions, please do not hesitate to contact me.

Sincerely,

Suzanne Jones, DPT, License #53093484

CASE EXAMPLE 16.2 Session Note Early Intervention

Jane climbed 6 steps with 1 rail hold, using a step-to-step pattern, when entering the house with her mother. She now prefers to climb the steps without adult assistance. Today we introduced dual-task activities: She was able to climb 1 step while holding her doll in the other hand; she will continue to use this strategy for safe, efficient stair-climbing. Reviewed cues and body placement with the mother to promote more activation and independence for Jane.

Suzanne Jones DPT, Lic #——, 1/14/22, 9:30 AM-10:00 AM, home

CASE EXAMPLE 16.3 Sample Annual IEP Used in a School Setting

IEP: present level of academic achievement and functional performance

School District #: 1   **Student ID #:** 456   **Class:** Regular education, Kindergarten
Name of student: Katy McKenna   **Date of Birth:** 5/13/17
Diagnosis: Cerebral palsy, GMFCS Level 3, spastic diplegia   **Name of Physical Therapist:** Martina Smith, DPT

Describe the Student's Strengths and Ability to Participate in the Educational Program

Katy is determined to participate in all class activities and insists on peer interaction throughout the school day. She is extremely motivated and eager to learn. Katy requires adult assistance to navigate within her school environment, particularly during activities in the open environments of recess, physical education, lunchtime, and classroom transitions. She is currently using a manual wheelchair, requiring assistance to propel for long distances (>200 ft).

She requires occasional assistance for wheelchair manipulation within her environment, for example, she will often ask a classmate to help her push her chair in under her desk or cafeteria table. Katy is an eager and active participant in physical education and recess, requiring intermittent assistance for navigation and rest periods. She recently is showing a preference to ambulate with a gait trainer or walker and is having great success. Currently, she is training with a posterior walker and can complete in class navigation with distant supervision.

(Continued)

CASE EXAMPLE 16.3   Sample Annual IEP Used in a School Setting—cont'd

Describe the Student's Present Level of Academic Achievement or Functional Performance

According to the Gross Motor Classification System, Katy is classified as a level 3, indicating potential for her to be an independent ambulator. Katy is learning to rise to stand using the posterior walker for assistance after completing "morning meeting" or "read aloud" units. Her daily classroom job is to take messages to the front office, a distance of 300 ft, which she achieves within 7 min, given assistance from paraprofessional or therapist for manipulation of the walker in tight spaces. Returning to her class takes up to 10 min and requires rest periods due to fatigue. She is extremely motivated to participate during physical education and recess when using the walker. She is now able to complete 20 min of the 30-min period before asking to sit back in her wheelchair.

Measurable Annual or Functional Goal to Enable the Student to Be Involved in and Progress in the General Education Curriculum

1. Katy will use her walker to complete her job of bringing messages to/from the office (distance of 300 ft) without rest periods or assistance, within 3 min, 5×/week.

2. Katy will rise to stand, using her walker for support, after completing "floor time" units in her classroom and after floor stretches during physical education, given stand by assistance from paraprofessional or teacher, within 8 sec to keep pace with her peers.

3. Katy will complete a 30-min physical education class or recess period each day without requesting to use her wheelchair and exhibiting an exercise heart rate of 130 beats per minute.

4. Katy will use her posterior walker for self-care activities 2×/day to increase her independence, including toileting, drinking from the fountain, and eating with peers; a goal attainment scale will be utilized and monitored by paraprofessional or therapist.

Procedures for Observing the Student's Progress Toward Meeting the Annual Goal

PT, teacher, paraprofessional, child, and daily progress chart

Measurement and Reports of Student's Progress Toward Annual Goal

PT, provided quarterly along with report card

CASE EXAMPLE 16.4   Session Note in a School-Based Setting

1/16/15, 9:30 AM-10:00 AM, class

Per her request, Katy used the posterior walker to go to the bathroom today. She required assistance, physical and verbal prompts, in order to navigate the walker, manipulate clothing, and manipulate the faucet when washing her hands. She completed all of this within 5 min and is eager to use this as her new toileting strategy (vs. being pushed or "walked" into the bathroom). Completed strengthening therapeutic exercise for lower extremities and trunk rotators in order to assist with the transitions required in the bathroom. Part practice activities within the bathroom to ensure safe navigation and manipulation of the walker.

Martina Smith, DPT

CASE EXAMPLE 16.5   Letter of Medical Justification for Equipment

This shows a sample letter of justification written to a school district to request a specific piece of equipment that is necessary for the child's optimal functioning in the school setting. In addition to this letter, therapists would typically include up to three quotes for equipment costs from different vendors. For example, additional letters of justification written to insurance companies, see Chapter 15.

Jump Ahead Physical Therapy (555) 555-5555

Child's Name: Katy McKenna   **D.O.B.:** 5/13/16   **Diagnosis:** Cerebral palsy

Date: 9/15/22

To whom it may concern,

This letter is to request a posterior walker for Katy McKenna, a 6-year-old girl currently enrolled in a kindergarten class at her local school. She has a diagnosis of cerebral palsy, classified as spastic diplegia and categorized on the Gross Motor Function Classification as a level 3. (This indicates that she has the potential to be an independent ambulator with an assistive device.)

She is currently receiving physical therapy 3 times a week, 45 min each session, to assist her to maximize her ability to participate throughout the school day. Katy is motivated to participate in all school-based activities with her peers.

When ambulating without an assistive device, she exhibits limited postural control, experiences frequent loss of balance, and requires adult assistance throughout all standing and waking activities. She uses bilateral hinged ankle-foot orthotics to assist with maintaining alignment. Katy is able to navigate a "loaner" posterior walker throughout her classroom with independence. Katy is learning to stand up from the ground using her walker and is independently able to transfer from her classroom chair to the posterior walker. She is now utilizing the walker to participate during physical education class and is able to perform the classroom job of going to the main office for messages. In addition, her teacher has commented that she is now keeping pace with her peers when utilizing the walker during classroom transitions.

Katy has exhibited success with the loaner walker. We are therefore requesting a posterior walker to address the following goals: independent ambulation using the posterior walker in a variety of contexts, given distant supervision, to achieve the full independence she needs to participate safely and without assistance. Katy's ability to improve her independence and her ability to function within her school environment require her to use a posterior walker. If you have any questions, please do not hesitate to contact me.

Sincerely,

Martina Smith, DPT

EXERCISE 16.1

Identify the errors in the following statements that could be found in an early intervention evaluation report, which will be read by other service providers and the child's parents. Rewrite a more appropriate statement in the space provided.

Statement	Rewrite Statement
1. The child was uncooperative.	
2. John has poor strength.	
3. Lucy has spasticity of B hamstrings and gastrocsoleus.	
4. Kelly cannot walk and is currently wheelchair bound.	
5. Tommy can climb stairs but can only do so with one hand held by his mother.	
6. ROM R knee ✓ 100°.	
7. Samantha sits in W-sitting with excessive kyphotic posture.	
8. Timmy performed very poorly on the PEDI with a standard score of 20.	

EXERCISE 16.2

Based on the following case scenario, write three plausible IEP goals that would be appropriate for this child. Use Fig.16.2 to assist with optimal goal-writing.

Tim is an 8 y.o. boy with diagnosis of spina bifida. *Activity/Participation:* He is able to walk in school, on flat tile surface, with Lofstrand crutches. He is slower than his peers (avg. gait speed 0.8 m/sec) and is having difficulty managing his books to travel between classes this year. He prefers taking the elevator in the school versus using the stairs. He utilizes a wheelchair for long-distance mobility, including any outdoor activities at school. *Impairments:* Mild L thoracic C-curve scoliosis; PROM limited R ankle dorsiflexion −5°; weakness knee flexion R 2+/5; L 3−/5; ankle dorsiflexion R 2/5, L 2+/5; ankle PF R 0/5, L 1/5; hip extension 0/5 B. Impaired sensation L4-S2 dermatomes.

Goals

1. _____

_____

2. _____

_____

3. _____

_____

RECOMMENDED RESOURCES

Websites

- American Physical Therapy Association, Pediatric Section (APTA)
  http://pediatricapta.org/
- Can Child: Center for Childhood Disability Research McMaster University
  http://www.canchild.ca
- Gross Motor Function Classification Scale (GMFCS)
  http://www.canchild.ca
- Individuals with Disabilities Education Act (IDEA)
  http://idea.ed.gov/

REFERENCES

*Items noted with an asterisk (*) are important resources for further information pertinent to functional outcomes and documentation.

ADA. *Guidelines for Reporting and Writing About People With Disabilities.* 7th ed. RTCIL Publications; 2008.

Adams J. The purpose of outcome measurement in rheumatology. *Br J Occup Ther.* 2002;65(4):172–174.

Adams MA, Mannion AF, Dolan P. Personal risk factors for first-time low back pain. *Spine.* 1999(23):2497–2505.

Adams R, Tapia C. Council on children with disabilities. Early intervention, IDEA part c services, and the medical home: collaboration for best practice and best outcomes. *Pediatrics.* 2013;132(4):1073–1088.

Alrwaily M, Timko M, Schneider M, et al. Treatment-based classification system for patients with low back pain: the movement control approach. *Phys Ther.* 2017 Dec 1;97(12):1147–1157. https://doi.org/10.1093/ptj/pzx087. PMID: 30010971.

APTA Guide to Physical Therapist Practice 4.0. American Physical Therapy Association, 2023. https://guide.apta.org/

*APTA Guide to Physical Therapist Practice 4.0. American Physical Therapy Association. *The Guide to Physical Therapist Practice.* 3rd ed. American Physical Therapy Association; 2014. Available at: <http://guidetoptpractice.apta.org/>. Accessed 03.05.15.

APTA Guide to Physical Therapist Practice 4.0. American Physical Therapy Association. *Guidelines: Physical Therapy Documentation of Patient/Client Management.* American Physical Therapy Association; 2008. http://www.apta.org/uploadedFiles/APTAorg/About_Us/Policies/BOD/Practice/DocumentationPatientClientMgmt.pdf.

APTA Guide to Physical Therapist Practice 4.0. American Physical Therapy Association. Improving your clinical documentation: reflecting best practice. 2011. https://www.apta.org/your-practice/documentation.

An M, Palisano RJ. Family-professional collaboration in pediatric rehabilitation: a practice model. *Disabil Rehabil.* 2014;36(5):434–440.

Barber-Westin SD, Noyes FR, McCloskey JW. Rigorous statistical reliability, validity, and responsiveness testing of the Cincinnati knee rating system in 350 subjects with uninjured, injured, or anterior cruciate ligament-reconstructed knees. *Am J Sports Med.* 1999;27(4):402–416.

Berg KO, Wood-Dauphinee SL, Williams JI, Maki B. Measuring balance in the elderly: validation of an instrument. *Can J Public Health.* 1992;83(suppl 2):S7–S11.

Bergner M, Bobbitt RA, Carter WB, et al. The sickness impact profile: development and final revision of a health status measure. *Med Care.* 1981;19:787–805.

Bernstein NA, ed. *The Co-ordination and Regulation of Movements.* Pergamon Press; 1967:15–59.

Bickley LS, Hoekelman RA. *JG Bates' Guide to Physical Examination & History Taking.* 7th ed. Lippincott Williams & Wilkins; 1999.

Binkley JM, Stratford PW, Lott SA, Riddle DL. The Lower Extremity Functional Scale (LEFS): scale development, measurement properties, and clinical application. North American Orthopaedic Rehabilitation Research Network. *Phys Ther.* 1999;79(4):371–383.

Bohannon RW. Manual muscle testing: does it meet the standards of an adequate screening test? *Clin Rehabil.* 2005;19:662–667.

Booher LD, Hench KM, Worrell TW, et al. Reliability of three single leg hop tests. *J Sport Rehabil.* 1993;2:165–170.

Bovend'Eerdt T, Botell R, Wade D. Writing SMART rehabilitation goals and achieving goal attainment scaling: a practical guide. *Clin Rehabil.* 2009;23:352–361.

Bowman S. Impact of electronic health record systems on information integrity: quality and safety implications. *Perspect Health Inf Manag/AHIMA.* 2013;10:1c.

Borg G, Linderholm H. Exercise performance and perceived exertion in patients with coronary insufficiency, arterial hypertension and vasoregulatory asthenia. *Acta Med Scand.* 1970;187:17–26.

Brewer K, Pollock N, Wright FV. Addressing the challenges of collaborative goal setting with children and their families. *Phys Occup Ther Pediatr.* 2014;34(2):138–152.

Brooks R, Rabin R, de Charro F, eds. *The Measurement and Valuation of Health Status Using EQ-5D: An European Perspective.* Springer Netherlands: Evidence from the EuroQol BIOMED Research Programme; 2003.

Bruininks RH, Bruininks BD. *Bruininks-Oseretsky Test of Motor Proficiency (BOT-2).* 2nd ed. American Guidance Center; 2005.

Budassi-Sheehy S. *Emergency Nursing: Principles and Practice.* 3rd ed. Mosby; 1992.

Campbell SK, Wright BD, Linacre JM. Development of a functional movement scale for infants. *J Appl Meas.* 2002;3:190–204.

Carr JH, Shepherd R. *Neurologic Rehabilitation: Optimizing Motor Performance.* Butterworth Heinemann; 1998.

Carr JH, Shepherd RB, et al. Investigation of a new motor assessment scale for stroke patients. *Phys Ther.* 1985;65:175–180.

Chiarello L, Effgen SK. Updated competencies for physical therapists working in early intervention. *Pediatr Phys Ther.* 2006;18(2):148–158.

Cole AB. *Physical Rehabilitation Outcomes Measures.* Canadian Physiotherapy Association; 1995.

Constant CR, Murley AH. A clinical method of functional assessment of the shoulder. *Clin Orthop Relat Res.* 1987;214:160–164.

Coster WJ, Deeney T, Haltiwanter J, et al. *School Function Assessment.* The Psychological Corporation; 1998.

Craig CL, Marshall AL, Sjöström M, et al. International physical activity questionnaire: 12-country reliability and validity. *Med Sci Sports Exerc.* 2003;35(8):1381–1395.

Crawford L, Maxwell J, Colquhoun H, et al. Facilitators and barriers to patient-centred goal-setting in rehabilitation: a scoping review. *Clin Rehabil.* 2022 Dec;36(12):1694–1704. https://doi.org/10.1177/02692155221121006. Epub 2022 Aug 25. PMID: 36017567; PMCID: PMC9574028.

Csuka M, McCarty DJ. Simple method for measurement of lower extremity muscle strength. *Am J Med.* 1985;78:77–81.

Daley K, Mayo N, et al. Reliability of scores on the Stroke Rehabilitation Assessment of Movement (STREAM) measure. *Phys Ther.* 1999;79(1):8–19, quiz 20-13.

Davies GJ, Wilk A, Ellenbecker TS. Assessment of strength. In: Malone TR, McPoil TG, Nitz AJ, eds. *Orthopedic and Sports Physical Therapy.* 2nd (ed.). Mosby; 1996.

Davis P. *The American Heritage Dictionary of the English Language.* 4th ed. Houghton Mifflin; 2000.

Davis NM. *Medical Abbreviations: 55,000 Conveniences at the Expense of Communications and Safety 16th ed. Edition.* Neil M. Davis Associates; 2019.

Delitto A, George SZ, Van Dillen LR, et al. Low back pain. *J Orthop Sports Phys Ther.* 2012;42(4):A1–A57. https://doi.org/10.2519/jospt.2012.42.4.A1.

*Delitto A, Snyder-Mackler L. The diagnostic process: examples in orthopedic physical therapy. *Phys Ther.* 1995;75:203–211.

Dittmar SS, Gresham GE. *Functional Assessment and Outcome Measures for the Rehabilitation Health Professional.* Aspen Publishers, Inc; 1997.

Doran GT. There's a S.M.A.R.T. way to write management's goals and objectives. *Management Review (AMA FORUM).* 1981;70(11):35–36.

El-Kareh R, Gandhi TK, Poon EG, et al. Trends in primary care clinician perceptions of a new electronic health record. *J Gen Intern Med.* 2009;24:464–468.

Enright PL. *The six-minute walk test.* Respir Care. 2003. Aug;48(8):783-5. PMID: 12890299.

Escolar DM, Henricson EK, Mayhew J, et al. Clinical evaluator reliability for quantitative and manual muscle testing measures of strength in children. *Muscle Nerve.* 2001;24(6):787–793.

Fairbank JC, Pynsent PB. The Oswestry Disability Index. *Spine.* 2000;25(22):2940–2952.

Farrell A, O'Sullivan C, Quinn L. Parent perspectives on early childhood assessment: a focus group inquiry. *Early Childhood Services.* 2009;3(1):61–76.

Fearon H., Levine S.M., Lee G.R. APTA audio conference presentation. 2009.

Feuerstein M, Berkowitz SM, Huang GD. Predictors of occupational low back disability: implications for secondary prevention. *J Occup Environ Med.* 1999;41(12):1024–1031.

Ferro AM, Quinn L. A structured goal-setting process to promote functional and measurable outcomes in school-based physical therapy: a knowledge translation study. *Pediatr Phys Ther.* 2020 Jul;32(3):211–217. https://doi.org/10.1097/PEP.0000000000000707. PMID: 32604362.

Fisk JD, Ritvo PG, Ross L, et al. Measuring the functional impact of fatigue: initial validation of the fatigue impact scale. *Clin Infect Dis.* 1994;18(suppl 1):S79–S83.

Folio MR, Fewell RR. *Peabody Developmental Motor Scales (PDMS-2).* 2nd ed. Riverside Publishing; 2000.

Folio M.R, Fewell R.R. Peabody Developmental Motor Scales *(PDMS-3).* 2024.

Folstein MF, Robins LN, Helzer JE. The mini-mental state examination. *J Psychiatr Res.* 1975;12:189–198.

Franchignoni F, Vercelli S, Giordano A, et al. Minimal clinically important difference of the disabilities of the arm, shoulder and hand outcome measure (DASH) and its shortened version (QuickDASH). *J Orthop Sports Phys Ther.* 2014;44(1):30–39.

Frese E, Brown M, Norton BJ. Clinical reliability of manual muscle testing: middle trapezius and gluteus medius muscles. *Physiotherapy.* 1987;67(7):1072–1076.

Fritz JM, Brennan GP. Preliminary examination of a proposed treatment-based classification system for patients receiving physical therapy interventions for neck pain. *Phys Ther.* 2007;87(5):513–524.

Fugl-Meyer A, Jaasko L, Leyman I, et al. The post-stroke hemiplegic patient: a method for evaluation of physical performance. *Scand J Rehabil Med.* 1975;6:13–31.

Gandek B, Sinclair SJ, Jette AM, et al. Development and initial psychometric evaluation of the participation measure for post-acute care (PM-PAC). *Am J Phys Med Rehabil.* 2007;86:57–71.

Gans BM, Haley SM, Hallenborg SC, et al. Description and inter-observer reliability of the Tufts assessment of motor performance. *Am J Phys Med Rehabil.* 1988;67:202–210.

Gentile AM. Skill acquisition: action, movement, and neuromotor processes. In: Shepherd R, Carr J, eds. *Movement Science: Foundations for Physical Therapy in Rehabilitation.* 2nd ed. Aspen Publishers; 2000.

Goldstein LB, Bertels C, Davis JN. Interrater reliability of the NIH stroke scale. *Arch Neurol.* 1989;46:660–662.

Goldston SE, ed. *Concepts of primary prevention: A framework for program development.* California Department of Mental Health; 1987.

Goodman CC, Synder TK. *Functional Gait Assessment: Concurrent, Discriminative, and Predictive Validity in Community-Dwelling Older Adults.* Saunders; 2012.

Gordon J, Quinn L. Guide to physical therapist practice: a critical appraisal. *Neurol Report.* 1999;23(3):122–128.

Green SD, Thomas JD. Interdisciplinary collaboration and the electronic medical record. *Pediatr Nurs.* 2008;34:225–229.

Greenhalgh J, Long AF, Brettle AJ, Grant MJ. Reviewing and selecting outcome measures for use in routine practice. *J Eval Clin Pract.* 1998;4(4):339–350.

Guccione A. Physical therapy diagnosis and the relationship between impairment and function. *Phys Ther.* 1991;71:499–504.

Guccione AA, Mielenz TJ, Devellis RF, et al. Development and testing of a self-report instrument to measure actions: outpatient physical therapy improvement in movement assessment log (OPTIMAL). *Phys Ther.* 2005;85(6):515–530.

Gummesson C, Ward MM, Atroshi I. The shortened disabilities of the arm, shoulder and hand questionnaire (Quick DASH): validity and reliability based on responses within the full-length DASH. BMC musculoskeletal disorders. 2006 Dec 1;7(1):44.

Guralnik JM, Simonsick EM, Ferrucci L, et al. A short physical performance battery assessing lower extremity function: association with self-reported disability and prediction of mortality and nursing home admission. *J Gerontol.* 1994;49:M85–M94.

Guyatt GH, Sullivan MJ, Thompson PJ, et al. The 6-minute walk: a new measure of exercise capacity in patients with chronic heart failure. *Can Med Assoc J.* 1985;132:919–923.

Hakes B, Whittington J. Assessing the impact of an electronic medical record on nurse documentation time. *Comput Inform Nurs.* 2008;26:234–241.

Haley S, Faas R, Coster W, et al. *Pediatric Evaluation of Disability Inventory.* New England Medical Center; 1992.

Heick J & Lazaro R. Goodman and Snyder's Differential Diagnosis for Physical Therapists Screening for referral. 7th Edition. Elsevier. 2022.

Herbold JA, Bonistall K, Blackburn M, et al. Randomized controlled trial of the effectiveness of continuous passive motion after total knee replacement. *Archiv Phys Med Rehabil.* 2014;95(7):1240–1245.

Ho YX, Gadd CS, Kohorst KL, Rosenbloom ST. A qualitative analysis evaluating the purposes and practices of clinical documentation. *Appl Clin Inform.* 2014 Feb 26;5(1):153-68. https://doi:10.4338/ACI-2013-10-RA-0081. PMID: 24734130; PMCID: PMC3974254.

Hoffmann T, Bakhit M, Michaleff Z. Shared decision making and physical therapy: What, when, how, and why? *Braz J Phys Ther.* 2022 Jan-Feb;26(1):100382. https://doi:10.1016/j.bjpt.2021.100382. Epub 2022 Jan 1. PMID: 35063699; PMCID: PMC8784295.

Hudak PL, Amadio PC, Bombardier C. Development of an upper extremity outcome measure: the DASH (disabilities of the arm, shoulder and hand) [corrected] The Upper Extremity Collaborative Group (UECG). Am J Ind Med. 1996;29(6):602-608. *Am J Ind Med.* 1996;30(3):372.

Individuals with Disabilities Education Act. 20 u.s.c.1400. <http://idea.ed.gov/>; 2004.

Itzkowitz A, Kaplan S, Doyle M, et al. Timed up and go: reference data for children who are school age. *Pediatr Phys Ther.* 2016;28(2):239–246.

Jebsen RH, Taylor N, Trieschmann RB, et al. An objective and standardized test of hand function. *Arch Phys Med Rehabil.* 1969;50:311–319.

Jelles F, Van Bennekom CA, Lankhorst GJ, et al. Inter- and intra-rater agreement of the rehabilitation activities profile. *J Clin Epidemiol.* 1995;48:407–416.

Jennett B, Teasdale G. Aspects of coma after severe head injury. *Lancet.* 1977;23(1):878–881.

Jensen MP, Karoly P, Braver S. The measurement of clinical pain intensity: a comparison of six methods. *Pain.* 1986;27:117–126.

*Jette AM. Physical disablement concepts for physical therapy research and practice. *Phys Ther.* 1994;74(5):380–386.

Jette AM, Tao W, Haley SM. Blending activity and participation sub-domains of the ICF. *Disabil Rehabil.* 2007;29:1742–1750.

Jiandani MP, Mhatre BS. Physical therapy diagnosis: How is it different? *J Postgrad Med.* 2018 Apr-Jun;64(2):69-72. https://doi:10.4103/jpgm.JPGM_691_17. PMID: 29692395; PMCID: PMC5954814.

Kaiser Family Foundation. Snapshots: health care spending in the United States & selected OECD countries. <http://kff.org/health-costs/issue-brief/snapshots-health-care-spending-in-the-united-states-selected-oecd-countries/>; 2011.

Keith RA, Granger CV, Hamilton BB, et al. The functional independence measure: a new tool for rehabilitation. *Adv Clin Rehabil.* 1987;1:6–18.

Kelley MJ, Shaffer MA, Kuhn JE, et al. Shoulder pain and mobility deficits: adhesive capsulitis. *J Orthop Sports Phys Ther.* 2013;43(5):A1–A31. https://doi.org/10.2519/jospt.2013.43.1.A1.

*Kettenbach G. *Writing SOAP Notes.* 3rd ed. FA Davis; 2003.

King G, McDougall J, Palisano RJ, et al. Goal attainment scaling: Its use in evaluating pediatric therapy programs. *Phys Occup Ther Pediatr.* 1999;19:30–52.

Kolobe TH, Bulanda M, Susman L. Predicting motor outcome at preschool age for infants tested at 7, 30, 60, and 90 days after term age using the Test of Infant Motor Performance. *Phys Ther.* 2004;84(12):1144–1156.

Kopec JA, Esdaile JM, Abrahamowicz M, et al. The Quebec Back Pain Disability Scale: measurement properties. *Spine.* 1995;20(3):341–352.

Kowalski K, Rhodes R, Naylor PJ, et al. Direct and indirect measurement of physical activity in older adults: a systematic review of the literature. *Int J Behav Nutr Phys Act.* 2012;9:148. https://doi.org/10.1186/1479-5868-9-148.

Kuhn T, Basch P, Barr M, Yackel T; Medical Informatics Committee of the American College of Physicians. Clinical documentation in the 21st century: executive summary of a policy position paper from the American College of Physicians. *Ann Intern Med.* 2015 Feb 17;162(4):301-3. https://doi:10.7326/M14-2128. PMID: 25581028.

Kuster SP, Ruef C, Bollinger AK, et al. Correlation between case mix index and antibiotic use in hospitals. *J Antimicrob Chemother.* 2008;62:837–842.

Lamb SE, Guralnik JM, Buchner DM, et al. Factors that modify the association between knee pain and mobility limitation in older women: the Women's Health and Aging Study. *Ann Rheum Dis.* 2000;59(5):331–337.

Law M. Appendix 2: outcome measures rating form guidelines. In: Law M, Baum C, Dunn W, eds. *Measuring Occupational Performance: Supporting Best Practice in Occupational Therapy.* Slack; 2001.

Lawton MP, Brody EM. Assessment of older people: self-maintaining and instrumental activities of daily living. *Gerontologist.* 1969;9:179–186.

Levack W.M. Ethics in goal planning for rehabilitation: a utilitarian perspective. Clin Rehabil. 2009;23:345–351.

Lobo MA, Harbourne RT, Dusing SC, McCoy SW. Grounding early intervention: physical therapy cannot just be about motor skills anymore. *Phys Ther.* 1 January 2013;93(1):94–103. https://doi.org/10.2522/ptj.20120158.

Long T, Toscano K. *Handbook of Pediatric Physical Therapy.* 2nd ed. Lippincott Williams & Wilkins; 2002.

Lucas A., Gillaspy K., Peters M.L., Hurth J. Enhancing recognition of high quality, functional IFSP outcomes. <http://www.ectacenter.org/~pdfs/pubs/rating-ifsp.pdf>; 2014.

Macy MG, Bricker DD, Squires JK. Validity and reliability of a curriculum-based assessment approach to determine eligibility for part C services. *J Early Interv.* 2005;28:1–16.

Mager R.F. Preparing Instructional Objectives: A Critical Tool in the Development of Effective Instruction. Center for Effective Performance; 3rd edition (May 1, 1997).

Mahoney F, Barthel D. Functional evaluation: the Barthel index. *Md State Med J.* 1965;14:61–65.

Mailloux Z, et al. Goal attainment scaling as a measure of meaningful outcomes for children with sensory integration disorders. *Am J Occup Ther.* 2007;61:254–259.

Malone TR, McPoil TG, Nitz AJ, eds. *Orthopedic and Sports Physical Therapy.* 2nd ed. Mosby; 1996.

Martin S. Language shapes thought. *PT Magazine.* 1999:44–46.

McCaffery M, Beebe A, et al. *Pain: Clinical Manual for Nursing Practice.* Mosby; 1989.

McConlogue A, Quinn L. Analysis of physical therapy goals in a school-based setting: a pilot study. *Phys Occup Ther Pediatr.* 2009;29:156–171.

McConlogue A., Quinn L. Goals that drive intervention. Course at annual therapies in the school conference. Education Resources; 2014.

McDougal J, King G. *Goal Attainment Scaling: Descriptions, Utility And Applications In Pediatric Therapy Services.* Thames Valley Childrens Centre; 2007.

McEwen I. *Providing Physical Therapy Services Under Parts B & C of the Individuals With Disabilities Education Act (IDEA).* American Physical Therapy Association; 2000.

McGough JJ, Faraone SV. Estimating the size of treatment effects: moving beyond P values. *Psychiatry.* 2009;6(10):21–29.

Melin J, Nordin A, Feldthusen C, Danielsson L. Goal-setting in physiotherapy: exploring a person-centered perspective. *Physiother Theory Pract.* 2021;37(8):863–880. https://doi.org/10.1080/09593985.2019.1655822.

Morgan, C;, Fetters, L., Adde L, et al., Early Intervention for Children Aged 0-2 Years With or at High Risk of Cerebral Palsy: International Clinical Practice Guideline Based on Systematic Reviews. *JAMA Pediatrics.* 2021; 175(8): 846 858. https://doi:10.1001/jamapediatrics.20210878

Nagi S. Some conceptual issues in disability and rehabilitation. In: Sussman M, ed. *Sociology and Rehabilitation.* American Sociological Association; 1965.

Nguyen L, Cross A, Rosenbaum P, Gorter JW. Use of the International Classification of Functioning, Disability and Health to support goal-setting practices in pediatric rehabilitation: a rapid review of the literature. *Disabil Rehabil.* 2021;43(6):884–894.

Norton BJ. Harnessing our collective professional power: diagnosis dialog. *Phys Ther.* 2007;87(6):635–638.

O'Grady MG, Dusing SC. Reliability and validity of play-based assessments of motor and cognitive skills for infants and young children: a systematic review. *Phys Ther.* 2014;95(1):25–38.

O'Sullivan SB, Schmidt TJ, Fulk G. *Physical Rehabilitation.* Elsevier; 2013.

Perenboom RJ, Chorus AM. Measuring participation according to the International Classification of Functioning, Disability and Health (ICF). *Disabil Rehabil.* 2003;25:577–587.

Piper MC, Darrah J. *Motor Assessment of the Developing Infant.* WB Saunders; 1994.

Playford ED, Siegert R, Levack W, Freeman J. Areas of consensus and controversy about goal-setting in rehabilitation: a conference report. *Clin Rehabil.* 2009;23:334–344.

Podsiadlo D, Richardson S. The timed "up & go": a test of basic functional mobility for frail elderly persons. *J Am Geriatr Soc.* 1991;39:142–148.

Portney LG, Watkins MP. *Foundations of Clinical Research.* 3rd ed. Prentice Hall; 2008.

Purtilo RB. Applying the principles of informed consent to patient care. *Phys Ther.* 1984;64(6):934–937.

Pritchard-Wiart L, Thompson-Hodgetts S, McKillop AB. A review of goal setting theories relevant to goal setting in paediatric rehabilitation. *Clin Rehabil.* 2019;33(9):1515–1526.

Quinn L, Debono K, Dawes H, et al. Task-specific training in Huntington disease: a randomized controlled feasibility trial. *Phys Ther.* 2014;94(11):1555–1568.

Quinn L, Riley N, Tyrell CM, et al. A framework for movement analysis of tasks: recommendations from the Academy of Neurologic Physical Therapy's movement system task force. *Phys Ther.* 2021 Sep 1;101(9):pzab154. https://doi.org/10.1093/ptj/pzab154. PMID: 34160044.

Randall KE, McEwen IR. Writing patient-centered functional goals. *Phys Ther.* 2000;80:1197–1203.

Research and Training Center on Independent Living, 8th ed. <http://rtcil.org/sites/rtcil.drupal.ku.edu/files/images/galleries/Guidelines%208th%20edition.pdf>; 2013. Accessed 17.09.15.

Roach KE. Measurement of health outcomes: reliability, validity and responsiveness. *J Prosthet Orthot.* 2006;18(suppl 1):S8–S12.

Rodrigues-Rodrigues P, Jiménez-Garcia R, Hernández-Barrera V, et al. Prevalence of physical disability in patients with chronic obstructive pulmonary disease and associated risk factors. *COPD.* 2013;10(5):611–617.

Roland M, Jenner J. A revised Owestry disability questionnaire. In: Hudson-Cook N, Tomes-Nicholson K, Breen A, eds. *Back Pain: New Approaches to Rehabilitation and Education.* Manchester University Press; 1989.

Roland M, Morris R. A study of the natural history of back pain. Part I: development of a reliable and sensitive measure of disability in low-back pain. *Spine.* 1983;8(2):141–144.

Russell DJ, Rosenbaum PL, Cadman DT, et al. The gross motor function measure: a means to evaluate the effects of physical therapy. *Dev Med Child Neurol.* 1989;31(3):341–352.

Sackett DL, Haynes RB. The architecture of diagnostic research. *BMJ.* 2002;324(7336):539–541.

Sackett DL, Haynes RB, Tugwell P. *Clinical Epidemiology: A Basic Science for Clinical Medicine.* Little, Brown; 1985.

Sahrmann SA. The human movement system: our professional identity. *Phys Ther.* 2014;94(7):1034–1042. https://doi.org/10.2522/ptj.20130319.

Shirley Sahrmann, Defining Our Diagnostic Labels Will Help Define Our Movement Expertise and Guide Our Next 100 Years, *Physical Therapy*, Volume 101, Issue 1, January 2021, pzaa196, https://doi.org/10.1093/ptj/pzaa196.

Sahrmann S, Azevedo DC, Dillen LV. Diagnosis and treatment of movement system impairment syndromes. *Braz J Phys Ther.* 2017 Nov-Dec;21(6):391–399. https://doi.org/10.1016/j.bjpt.2017.08.001. Epub 2017 Sep 27. PMID: 29097026; PMCID: PMC5693453.

Sahrmann SA. The human movement system: our professional identity. *Phys Ther.* 2014 Jul;94(7):1034–1042. https://doi.org/10.2522/ptj.20130319. Epub 2014 Mar 13. Erratum in: Phys Ther. 2014 Dec;94(12):1828. PMID: 24627430.

Sallis JF, Haskell WL, Wood PD, et al. Physical activity assessment methodology in the Five-City Project. *Am J Epidemiol.* 1985;121(1):91–106.

Scheets PK, Sahrmann SA, Norton BJ. Use of movement system diagnoses in the management of patients with neuromuscular conditions: a multiple-patient case report. *Phys Ther.* 2007;87:654–669.

Schlessman, PT, DPT, DHS (chair); Jessica Barreca, PT, DPT; Karen Sivils, PT, DPT; Sharon Galitzer, PT, DSc, PT, MS, CIMI; Benita Hodges, PT, MAE, PCS, ATP; Chelsea Hovis, PT, DPT; Sara McGuff, PT, DPT; Jennifer Stevens, PT, DPT, PCS. Supported by the Fact Sheet Committee of APTA Pediatrics.

Scott RW. *Legal, Ethical, and Practical Aspects of Patient Care Documentation: A Guide for Rehabilitation Professionals.* 4th ed. Jones and Bartlett Publishers; 2011.

Smith LA. *Brunnstrom's Clinical Kinesiology.* F.A. Davis; 1996.

Stedman's. Abbreviations, Acronyms & Symbols Stedman's. 5th ed.; 2012.

Stewart AL, Hays RD, Ware Jr JE. The MOS shot general health survey: reliability and validity in a patient population. *Med Care.* 1988;26:724–735.

Stewart AL, Mills KM, King AC, et al. CHAMPS physical activity questionnaire for older adults: outcomes for interventions. *Med Sci Sports Exerc.* 2001;33(7):1126–1141.

Stewart DL, Abeln SH. *Documenting Functional Outcomes in Physical Therapy.* Mosby; 1993.

Stokes E. *Rehabilitation Outcome Measures.* Elsevier; 2010.

Stratford P, Gill C, Westaway M, Binkley J. Assessing disability and change on individual patients: a report of a patient specific measure. *Physiother Can.* 1995;47:258–263.

Stuck AE, Walthert JM, Nikolaus T, et al. Risk factors for functional status decline in community-living elderly people: a systematic literature review. *Soc Sci Med.* 1999;48:445–469.

Sullivan GM, Feinn R. Using effect size—or why the p value is not enough. *J Grad Med Educ.* 2012;4(3):279–282.

Tinetti ME. Performance-oriented assessment of mobility problems in elderly patients. *J Am Geriatr Soc.* 1986;34:119–126.

Topolski TD, LoGerfo J, Patrick DL, et al. The rapid assessment of physical activity (RAPA) among older adults. *Prev Chronic Dis.* 2006;3(4):A118.

Ulrich D. Test of gross motor development. <http://www.proedinc.com/customer/productView.aspx?ID=1776>.

Uniform Data System for Medical Rehabilitation. <http://www.udsmr.org/>.

United States Department of Health & Human Services. *Summary of the HIPAA Privacy Rule.* Office of Civil Rights; 2003.

Van Dillen LR, Roach KE. Reliability and validity of the acute care index of function for patients with neurologic impairment. *Phys Ther*. 1988;68(7):1098–1101.

Van Straten A, de Haan RJ, Limburg M, et al. A stroke-adapted 30-item version of the sickness impact profile to assess quality of life (SA-SIP30). *Stroke*. 1997;28:2155–2161.

Wade DT. Goal setting in rehabilitation: an overview of what, why and how. *Clin Rehabil*. 2009;23(4):291–295.

Ware JE, Sherbourne CD. The MOS 36-item short-form health survey (SF-36): I. Conceptual framework and item selection. *Med Care*. 1992;30:473.

Washburn RA, Smith KW, Jette AM, Janney CA. The physical activity scale for the elderly (PASE): development and evaluation. *J Clin Epidemiol*. 1993;46:153–162.

Weaver P, Cothran D, Dickinson S, Frey G. Physical therapists' perspectives on importance of the early intervention competencies to physical therapy practice. *Infants Young Child*. 2018;31(4):261–274.

APTA Pediatric Physical Therapy, American Physical Therapy Association. FactSheet_DevelopingCollaborativeIEPGoals_2021.docx©2021 <http://www.pediatricapta.org>; 2021. Developed by a volunteer workgroup of the APTA Pediatric Physical Therapy's School-Based Special Interest Group (chaired by Laurie Ray, PT, PhD). Special thanks to expert contributors: Amy.

Weed LL. The problem oriented record as a basic tool in medical education, patient care and clinical research. *Ann Clin Res*. 1971;3(3):131–134.

Whiteneck GG, Charlifue SW, Gerhart KA, et al. Quantifying handicap: a new measure of long-term rehabilitation outcomes. *Arch Phys Med Rehabil*. 1992;73:519–526.

WHOQOL Group Development of the WHOQOL-BREF quality of life assessment. *Psychol Med*. 1998;28:551–558.

Wolf SL, Catlin PA, Gage K, et al. Establishing the reliability and validity of measurements of walking time using the Emory functional ambulation profile. *Phys Ther*. 1999;79:1122–1133.

Wong DL, Baker CM. Pain in children: comparison of assessment scales. *Okla Nurse*. 1988;33:8.

World Health Organization. *International Classification of Functioning, Disability, and Health*. World Health Organization; 2001.

World Health Organization. *World Health Organization Disability Assessment Schedule II (WHODAS II)*. World Health Organization; 2001.

Wrisley DM, Kumar NA. Functional gait assessment: concurrent, discriminative, and predictive validity in community-dwelling older adults. *Phys Ther*. 2010;90(5):761–773.

Wu RC, Straus SE. Evidence for handheld electronic medical records in improving care: a systematic review. *BMC Med Inform Decis Mak*. 2006;6:26.

American Physical Therapy Association Position on Documentation

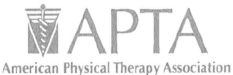

Last Updated: 05/19/14
Contact: nationalgovernance@apta.org

__GUIDELINES: PHYSICAL THERAPY DOCUMENTATION OF PATIENT/CLIENT MANAGEMENT__ BOD G03-05-16-41 (Amended BOD 02-02-16-20; BOD 11-01-06-10; BOD 03-01-16-51; BOD 03-00-22-54; BOD 03-99-14-41; BOD 11-98-19-69; BOD 03-97-27-69; BOD 03-95-23-61; BOD 11-94-33-107; BOD 06-93-09-13; Initial BOD 03-93-21-55) (Guideline)

PREAMBLE

The American Physical Therapy Association (APTA) is committed to meeting the physical therapy needs of society, to meeting the needs and interests of its members, and to developing and improving the art and science of physical therapy, including practice, education, and research. To help meet these responsibilities, APTA's Board of Directors has approved the following guidelines for physical therapy documentation. It is recognized that these guidelines do not reflect all the unique documentation requirements associated with the many specialty areas within the physical therapy profession. Applicable for both handwritten and electronic documentation systems, these guidelines are intended to be used as a foundation for the development of more specific documentation guidelines in clinical areas while at the same time providing guidance for the physical therapy profession across all practice settings. Documentation may also need to address additional regulatory or payer requirements.

Finally, be aware that these guidelines are intended to address the *documentation* of patient/client management, not to describe the provision of physical therapy services. Other APTA documents, including APTA Standards of Practice for Physical Therapy, Code of Ethics and Guide for Professional Conduct, and the Guide to Physical Therapist Practice, address provision of physical therapy services and patient/client management.

APTA POSITION ON DOCUMENTATION

Documentation Authority for Physical Therapy Services

Physical therapy examination, evaluation, diagnosis, prognosis, and plan of care (including interventions) shall be documented, dated, and authenticated by the physical therapist who performs the service. Interventions provided by the physical therapist or selected interventions provided by the physical therapist assistant under the direction and supervision of the physical therapist are documented, dated, and authenticated by the physical therapist or, when permissible by law, the physical therapist assistant.

Other notations or flowcharts are considered a component of the documented record but do not meet the requirements of documentation in or of themselves.

Students in physical therapist or physical therapist assistant programs may document when the record is additionally authenticated by the physical therapist, or when permissible by law, documentation by physical therapist assistant students may be authenticated by a physical therapist assistant.

OPERATIONAL DEFINITIONS

Guidelines
APTA defines a "guideline" as a statement of advice.

Authentication
The process used to verify that an entry is complete, accurate, and final. Indications of authentication can include original written signatures and computer "signatures" on secured electronic record systems only.

The following describes the main documentation elements of patient/client management: (1) initial examination/evaluation, (2) visit/encounter, (3) reexamination, and (4) discharge or discontinuation summary.

Initial Examination/Evaluation
Documentation of the initial encounter is typically called the "initial examination," "initial evaluation," or "initial examination/evaluation." Completion of the initial examination/evaluation is typically completed in one visit but may occur over more than one visit. Documentation elements for the initial examination/evaluation include the following:

Examination

Includes data obtained from the history, systems review, and tests and measures.

Evaluation

Evaluation is a thought process that may not include formal documentation. It may include documentation of the assessment of the data collected in the examination and identification of problems pertinent to patient/client management.

Diagnosis

Indicates level of impairment, activity limitation, and participation restriction determined by the physical therapist. May be indicated by selecting one or more preferred practice patterns from the *Guide to Physical Therapist Practice*.

Prognosis

Provides documentation of the predicted level of improvement that might be attained through intervention and the amount of time required to reach that level. Prognosis is typically not a separate documentation element, but the components are included as part of the plan of care.

Plan of care

Typically stated in general terms, this includes goals, interventions planned, proposed frequency and duration, and discharge plans.

Visit/Encounter

Documentation of a visit or encounter, often called a progress note or daily note, documents the sequential implementation of the plan of care established by the physical therapist, including changes in patient/client status and variations and progressions of specific interventions used. It may also include specific plans for the next visit or visits.

Reexamination

Documentation of reexamination includes data from repeated or new examination elements and is provided to evaluate progress and to modify or redirect intervention.

Discharge or Discontinuation Summary

Documentation is required following the conclusion of the current episode in the physical therapy intervention sequence to summarize progress toward goals and discharge plans.

GENERAL GUIDELINES

- Documentation is required for every visit/encounter.
- All documentation must comply with the applicable jurisdictional/regulatory requirements.
- All handwritten entries shall be made in ink and will include original signatures. Electronic entries are made with appropriate security and confidentiality provisions.
- Charting errors should be corrected by drawing a single line through the error and initialing and dating the chart or through the appropriate mechanism for electronic documentation that clearly indicates that a change was made without deletion of the original record.
- All documentation must include adequate identification of the patient/client and the physical therapist or physical therapist assistant:
  - The patient's/client's full name and identification number, if applicable, must be included on all official documents.
  - All entries must be dated and authenticated with the provider's full name and appropriate designation:
    - Documentation of examination, evaluation, diagnosis, prognosis, plan of care, and discharge summary must be authenticated by the physical therapist who provided the service.
    - Documentation of intervention in visit/encounter notes must be authenticated by the physical therapist or physical therapist assistant who provided the service.
    - Documentation by physical therapist or physical therapist assistant graduates or other physical therapists and physical therapist assistants pending receipt of an unrestricted license shall be authenticated by a licensed physical therapist, or when permissible by law, documentation by physical therapist assistant graduates may be authenticated by a physical therapist assistant.
    - Documentation by students (student physical therapist/student physical therapist assistant) in physical therapist or physical therapist assistant programs must be additionally authenticated by the physical therapist, or when permissible by law, documentation by physical therapist assistant students may be authenticated by a physical therapist assistant.
- Documentation should include the referral mechanism by which physical therapy services are initiated. Examples include:
  - Self-referral/direct access
  - Request for consultation from another practitioner
- Documentation should include indications of no shows and cancellations.

INITIAL EXAMINATION/EVALUATION

Examination (History, Systems Review, and Tests and Measures)
History

Documentation of history may include the following:
- General demographics
- Social history
- Employment/work (job/school/play)
- Growth and development
- Living environment
- General health status (self-report, family report, caregiver report)
- Social/health habits (past and current)
- Family history
- Medical/surgical history
- Current condition(s)/chief complaint(s)

- Functional status and activity level
- Medications
- Other clinical tests

Systems Review

Documentation of systems review may include gathering data for the following systems:
- Cardiovascular/pulmonary
  - Blood pressure
  - Edema
  - Heart rate
  - Respiratory rate
- Integumentary
  - Pliability (texture)
  - Presence of scar formation
  - Skin color
  - Skin integrity
- Musculoskeletal
  - Gross range of motion
  - Gross strength
  - Gross symmetry
  - Height
  - Weight
- Neuromuscular
  - Gross coordinated movement (e.g., balance, locomotion, transfers, and transitions)
  - Motor function (motor control, motor learning)

Documentation of systems review may also address communication ability, affect, cognition, language, and learning style:
- Ability to make needs known
- Consciousness
- Expected emotional/behavioral responses
- Learning preferences (e.g., *education needs*, *learning barriers*)
- Orientation (person, place, time)

Tests and Measures

Documentation of tests and measures may include findings for the following categories:
- Aerobic Capacity/Endurance
  Examples of examination findings include:
  - Aerobic capacity during functional activities
  - Aerobic capacity during standardized exercise test protocols
  - Cardiovascular signs and symptoms in response to increased oxygen demand with exercise or activity
  - Pulmonary signs and symptoms in response to increased oxygen demand with exercise or activity
- Anthropometric Characteristics
  Examples of examination findings include:
  - Body composition
  - Body dimensions
  - Edema
- Arousal, Attention, and Cognition
  Examples of examination findings include:
  - Arousal and attention
  - Cognition
  - Communication

- Consciousness
- Motivation
- Orientation to time, person, place, and situation
- Recall

- Assistive and Adaptive Devices
  Examples of examination findings include:
  - Assistive or adaptive devices and equipment use during functional activities
  - Components, alignment, fit, and ability to care for the assistive or adaptive devices and equipment
  - Remediation of impairments, activity limitations, and participation restrictions with the use of assistive or adaptive devices and equipment
  - Safety during use of assistive or adaptive devices and equipment
- Circulation (Arterial, Venous, Lymphatic)
  Examples of examination findings include:
  - Cardiovascular signs
  - Cardiovascular symptoms
  - Physiological responses to position change
- Cranial and Peripheral Nerve Integrity
  Examples of examination findings include:
  - Electrophysiological integrity
  - Motor distribution of the cranial nerves
  - Motor distribution of the peripheral nerves
  - Response to neural provocation
  - Response to stimuli, including auditory, gustatory, olfactory, pharyngeal, vestibular, and visual
  - Sensory distribution of the cranial nerves
  - Sensory distribution of the peripheral nerves
- Environmental, Home, and Work (Job/School/Play) Barriers
  Examples of examination findings include:
  - Current and potential barriers
  - Physical space and environment
- Ergonomics and Body Mechanics
  Examples of examination findings for *ergonomics* include:
  - Dexterity and coordination during work
  - Functional capacity and performance during work actions, tasks, or activities
  - Safety in work environments
  - Specific work conditions or activities
  - Tools, devices, equipment, and workstations related to work actions, tasks, or activities

  Examples of examination findings for *body mechanics* include:
  - Body mechanics during self-care; home management; work; community; or leisure actions, tasks, or activities
- Gait, Locomotion, and Balance
  Examples of examination findings include:
  - Balance during functional activities with or without the use of assistive, adaptive, orthotic, protection, supportive, or prosthetic devices or equipment
  - Balance (dynamic and static) with or without the use of assistive, adaptive, orthotic, protective, supportive, or prosthetic devices or equipment

- Gait and locomotion during functional activities with or without the use of assistive, adaptive, orthotic, protective, supportive, or prosthetic devices or equipment
- Gait and locomotion with or without the use of assistive, adaptive, orthotic, protective, supportive, or prosthetic devices or equipment
- Safety during gait, locomotion, and balance
- Integumentary Integrity
  Examples of examination findings include:
  Associated skin
  - Activities, positioning, and postures that produce or relieve trauma to the skin
  - Assistive, adaptive, orthotic, protective, supportive, or prosthetic devices and equipment that may produce or relieve trauma to the skin
  - Skin characteristics
- Wound
  - Activities, positioning, and postures that aggravate the wound or scar or that produce or relieve trauma
  - Burn
  - Signs of infection
  - Wound characteristics
  - Wound scar tissue characteristics
- Joint Integrity and Mobility
  Examples of examination findings include:
  - Joint integrity and mobility
  - Joint play movements
  - Specific body parts
- Motor Function
  Examples of examination findings include:
  - Dexterity, coordination, and agility
  - Electrophysiological integrity
  - Hand function
  - Initiation, modification, and control of movement patterns and voluntary postures
- Muscle Performance
  Examples of examination findings include:
  - Electrophysiological integrity
  - Muscle strength, power, and endurance
  - Muscle strength, power, and endurance during functional activities
  - Muscle tension
- Neuromotor Development and Sensory Integration
  Examples of examination findings include:
  - Acquisition and evolution of motor skills
  - Oral motor function, phonation, and speech production
  - Sensorimotor integration
- Orthotic, Protective, and Supportive Devices
  Examples of examination findings include:
  - Components, alignment, fit, and ability to care for the orthotic, protective, and supportive devices and equipment
  - Orthotic, protective, and supportive devices and equipment use during functional activities

- Remediation of impairments, activity limitations, and participation restrictions with use of orthotic, protective, and supportive devices and equipment
- Safety during use of orthotic, protective, and supportive devices and equipment
- Pain
  Examples of examination findings include:
  - Pain, soreness, and nocioception
  - Pain in specific body parts
- Posture
  Examples of examination findings include:
  - Postural alignment and position (dynamic)
  - Postural alignment and position (static)
  - Specific body parts
- Prosthetic Requirements
  Examples of examination findings include:
  - Components, alignment, fit, and ability to care for prosthetic device
  - Prosthetic device use during functional activities
  - Remediation of impairments, activity limitations, and participation restrictions with use of the prosthetic device
  - Residual limb or adjacent segment
  - Safety during use of the prosthetic device
- Range of Motion (ROM; Including Muscle Length)
  Examples of examination findings include:
  - Functional ROM
  - Joint active and passive movement
  - Muscle length, soft tissue extensibility, and flexibility
- Reflex Integrity
  Examples of examination findings include:
  - Deep reflexes
  - Electrophysiological integrity
  - Postural reflexes and reactions, including righting, equilibrium, and protective reactions
  - Primitive reflexes and reactions
  - Resistance to passive stretch
  - Superficial reflexes and reactions
- Self-care and Home Management (Including Activities of Daily Living and Instrumental Activities of Daily Living)
  Examples of examination findings include:
  - Ability to gain access to home environments
  - Ability to perform self-care and home management activities with or without assistive, adaptive, orthotic, protective, supportive, or prosthetic devices and equipment
  - Safety in self-care and home management activities and environments
- Sensory Integrity
  Examples of examination findings include:
  - Combined/cortical sensations
  - Deep sensations
  - Electrophysiological integrity
- Ventilation and respiration
  Examples of examination findings include:
  - Pulmonary signs of respiration/gas exchange
  - Pulmonary signs of ventilatory function
  - Pulmonary symptoms

- Work (Job/School/Play), Community, and Leisure Integration or Reintegration (Including Instrumental Activities of Daily Living)
  Examples of examination findings include:
  - Ability to assume or resume work (job/school/plan), community, and leisure activities with or without assistive, adaptive, orthotic, protective, supportive, or prosthetic devices and equipment
  - Ability to gain access to work (job/school/play), community, and leisure environments
  - Safety in work (job/school/play), community, and leisure activities and environments

Evaluation

- Evaluation is a thought process that may not include formal documentation. However, the evaluation process may lead to documentation of impairments, activity limitations, and participation restrictions using formats, such as:
  - A problem list.
  - A statement of assessment of key factors (e.g., cognitive factors, comorbidities, social support) influencing the patient/client status.

Diagnosis

- Documentation of a diagnosis determined by the physical therapist may include impairment, activity limitation, and participation restrictions. Examples include:
  - Impaired joint mobility, motor function, muscle performance, and ROM
  - Associated with localized inflammation (4E)
  - Impaired motor function and sensory integrity associated with progressive disorders of the central nervous system (5E)
  - Impaired aerobic capacity/endurance associated with cardiovascular pump
- Dysfunction or failure (6D)
  - Impaired integumentary integrity associated with partial-thickness skin involvement and scar formation (7C)

Prognosis

- Documentation of the prognosis is typically included in the plan of care. See below.

Plan of Care

- Documentation of the plan of care includes the following:
  - Overall goals stated in measurable terms that indicate the predicted level of improvement in functioning
  - A general statement of interventions to be used
  - Proposed duration and frequency of service required to reach the goals
  - Anticipated discharge plans

VISIT/ENCOUNTER

- Documentation of each visit/encounter shall include the following elements:
  - Patient/client self-report (as appropriate).
  - Identification of specific interventions provided, including frequency, intensity, and duration as appropriate. Examples include:

- Knee extension, three sets, 10 repetitions, 10# weight
- Transfer training bed to chair with sliding board
- Equipment provided
- Changes in patient/client impairment, activity limitation, and participation restriction status as they relate to the plan of care.
- Response to interventions, including adverse reactions, if any.
- Factors that modify frequency or intensity of intervention and progression goals, including patient/client adherence to patient/client-related instructions.
- Communication/consultation with providers/patient/client/family/ significant other.
- Documentation to plan for ongoing provision of services for the next visit(s), which is suggested to include, but not be limited to:
  - The interventions with objectives
  - Progression parameters
  - Precautions, if indicated

REEXAMINATION

- Documentation of reexamination shall include the following elements:
  - Documentation of selected components of examination to update patient's/client's functioning, and/or disability status.
  - Interpretation of findings and, when indicated, revision of goals.
  - When indicated, revision of plan of care, as directly correlated with goals as documented.

DISCHARGE/DISCONTINUATION SUMMARY

- Documentation of discharge or discontinuation shall include the following elements:
  - Current physical/functional status.
  - Degree of goals achieved and reasons for goals not being achieved.
  - Discharge/discontinuation plan related to the patient/client's continuing care. Examples include:
    - Home program
    - Referrals for additional services
    - Recommendations for follow-up physical therapy care
    - Family and caregiver training
    - Equipment provided

Relationship to Vision 2020: Professionalism (Practice Department, ext 3176)

EXPLANATION OF REFERENCE NUMBERS

BOD P00-00-00-00 stands for Board of Directors/month/year/page/vote in the Board of Directors Minutes; the "P" indicates that it is a position (see below). For example, BOD P11-97-06-18 means that this position can be found in the November 1997 Board of Directors minutes on Page 6 and that it was Vote 18. P: Position | S: Standard | G: Guideline | Y: Policy | R: Procedure.

Rehabilitation Abbreviations

This list provides abbreviations most commonly used by rehabilitation professionals. It is divided into the categories of general, professional, medical diagnosis, and symbols. In addition, the entire list is organized alphabetically by name. Online resources for abbreviations include the following:

Open MD: https://openmd.com/dictionary/medical-abbreviations

Taber's Medical Dictionary: http://www.tabers.com/

The Joint Commission has an official "do not use" list for abbreviations that should be avoided. These include q.d. (daily) and q.o.d. (every other day). For these abbreviations, the full words should be written instead. (See https://www.jointcommission.org/resources/news-and-multimedia/fact-sheets/facts-about-do-not-use-list/.)

GENERAL

A or Ⓐ	assistance
A	assessment
AAA	abdominal aortic aneurysm
AAFO	articulating ankle-foot orthosis
AAROM	active assistive range of motion
Abd or ABD	abduction
ABG	arterial blood gases
abn	abnormal
AC	alternating current
ACA	anterior cerebral artery
ACL	anterior cruciate ligament
AD	assistive device
Add or ADD	adduction
ADL	activities of daily living
ad lib	at discretion
Afib	atrial fibrillation
AFO	ankle-foot orthosis
AG	against gravity
AK	above knee
amb	ambulatory, ambulation
ant	anterior
AP	anteroposterior
approx	approximate, approximately
appt	appointment
A&O	alert and oriented
AROM	active range of motion
ASIA	American Spinal Injury Association
ASIS	anterior superior iliac spine
assist	assistant, assistance
ATNR	asymmetric tonic neck reflex
AV	atrioventricular

B or Ⓑ	bilateral
B&B	bowel and bladder
bal	balance
BE	below elbow
b.i.d.	twice a day
bil	bilateral
b.i.w.	biweekly
BK	below knee
BM	bowel movement
BNL	below normal limits
BOS	base of support
BP	blood pressure
bpm	beats per minute
BS	breath sounds
c̄	with
CA	cancer, cardiac arrest
cap	capsule
CICU	cardiac intensive care unit
CG	contact guarding
cm	centimeter
CNS	central nervous system
c/o	complained of, complains of
cont'd	continued
CO_2	carbon dioxide
COM	center of mass
COP	center of pressure
CPAP	continuous positive airway pressure
CPT	chest physical therapy
CS	close supervision
CSF	cerebrospinal fluid
CT	computed tomography
d	day
D or Ⓓ	dependent
DAI	diffuse axonal injury
DBE	deep breathing exercise
D/C	discharge; discontinue
dep	dependent
desat	desaturation
DF	dorsiflexion
DIP	distal interphalangeal (joint)
dist	distance, distant
DME	durable medical equipment
DS	distant supervision
DTR	deep tendon reflex
dx	diagnosis
ECF	extended care facility
ECG	electrocardiogram
EEG	electroencephalogram
EMG	electromyogram

ENT	ear, nose, throat	LBP	lower back pain
EOB	edge of bed	LBQC	large-based quad cane
equip	equipment	LE	lower extremity
ER	emergency room; external rotation; extended release	LLB	long leg brace
		LLE	left lower extremity
ESRD	end-stage renal diseas	LLL	left lower lobe
e-stim	electrical stimulation	LLQ	left lower quadrant
eval	evaluation	lig(s)	ligament(s)
ex	exercise	LOA	level of assistance
exam	examination	LOB	loss of balance
ext	external; extension; extremities	LOC	loss of consciousness
ext rot, ER	external rotation	L/min	liters per minute
F	fair (muscle grade); female	LTC	long-term care
FES	functional electric stimulation	LTG	long-term goal(s)
FiO$_2$	fraction of inspired oxygen	LTM	long-term memory
flex	flexion	LUE	left upper extremity
FOS	flight of stairs	LUL	left upper lobe
freq	frequently, frequency	LUQ	left upper quadrant
FT	full-time	LVH	left ventricular hypertrophy
F/U	follow-up	m	meters
FWB	full weight bearing	M	male
fx	function, fracture	MAP	mean arterial pressure
G	good (muscle grade)	max	maximal, maximum
GCS	Glasgow Coma Scale	MCA	middle cerebral artery
GE	gravity eliminated	MCP	metacarpophalangeal (joint)
GI	gastrointestinal	med	medical or medicine
G-tube	gastrostomy tube	MH	moist heat
h or hr	hour	min	minute(s), minimal
HA	headache	ml	milliliter
HD	hemodialysis	MMT	manual muscle test
HEP	home exercise program	mod	moderate
HHA	home health aide	mo	month
H/O	history of	MRI	magnetic resonance imaging
HOB	head of bed	MVA	motor vehicle accident
HOH	hard of hearing	mvt	movement
HPI	history of present illness	N	normal (muscle grade)
HR	heart rate	N/A	not applicable, not available
HS	heel strike	NBQC	narrow-based quad cane
HTN	hypertension	NC	nasal cannula
hx	history	Neg	negative
H$_2$O	water	NG	nasogastric
Ind or I or Ⓘ	independent	NICU	neonatal intensive care unit
I&O	intake and output	NPO	nothing by mouth
ICU	intensive care unit	NS	normal saline
IM	intramuscular	N/T	not tested
inf	inferior	NWB	non–weight bearing
int	internal	O$_2$	oxygen
int rot, IR	internal rotation	OOB	out of bed
IP	inpatient	OP	outpatient
IQ	intelligence quotient	OR	operating room
IV	intravenous	ORIF	open reduction internal fixation
jt	joint	p̄	after
J-tube	jejunostomy tube	P	poor (muscle grade)
K	potassium	PA	posteroanterior
KAFO	knee-ankle-foot orthosis	PCA	posterior cerebral artery
kcal	kilocalorie	PET	positron emission tomography
kg	kilogram(s)	PF	plantar flexion
L or Ⓛ	left	PIP	proximal interphalangeal (joint)
L	liter	PLOF	prior level of function
lat	lateral	PLS	posterior leaf splint
lb	pound	PMH	past medical history

PO	by mouth
post	posterior
postop	postoperative
PRE	progressive resistive exercise(s)
prn	as needed
PROM	passive range of motion
prox	proximal
PRW	platform rolling walker
PSH	past surgical history
PSIS	posterior superior iliac spine
pt	patient
PT	part-time
PTA	prior to admission
P&V	percussion and vibration
PWB	partial weight bearing
q	every
quads	quadriceps
R or ®	right
re	concerning, regarding
rehab	rehabilitation
rep(s)	repetition(s)
RLE	right lower extremity
RLL	right lower lobe
RLQ	right lower quadrant
RML	right middle lobe
R/O	reports of, rule out, ruled out
ROM	range of motion
RR	respiratory rate
RROM	resisted range of motion
R/T	related to
RUE	right upper extremity
RUL	right upper lobe
RUQ	right upper quadrant
RW	rolling walker
Rx	prescription; treatment; orders
S or Ⓢ	supervision
s̄	without
SAQ	short arc quads
sat	saturation
SB	sliding board
SBA	standby assistance
SBQC	small-based quad cane
SBT	sliding board transfers
SC	straight cane
SCM	sternocleidomastoid muscle
sec	second(s)
sig	significant
SLR	straight-leg raise
SNF	skilled nursing facility
S/O	standing order
SOB	shortness of breath
SOS	step-over-step (stair-climbing)
s/p	status post
SpO₂	pulse oxygen saturation (pulse oximetry)
SPT	stand pivot transfers
staph	*Staphylococcus*
stat	immediately, at once
STG	short-term goal(s)
STM	short-term memory
STNR	symmetric tonic neck reflex
str cane	straight cane
strep	*Streptococcus*

STS	sit to stand; step-to-step (stair-climbing)
supp	supported
surg	surgical, surgery
sx	symptoms
symm	symmetric, symmetry
T	trace (muscle grade)
tab	tablet
TBA	to be assessed
TBE	to be evaluated
TDWB	touch-down weight bearing
temp	temperature
TENS	transcutaneous electrical nerve stimulation
ther ex	therapeutic exercise
t.i.w.	three times per week
TMJ	temporomandibular joint
TO	toe off
T/O	throughout
tol	tolerate(s)
trach	tracheostomy
trans	transverse, transferred
trng	training
TTWB	toe-touch weight bearing
Tx	treatment
UE	upper extremity
U/L	unilateral
unsupp	unsupported
URI	upper respiratory infection
US	ultrasound
UTI	urinary tract infection
VAS	visual analog scale
VC	verbal cues, vital capacity, vocal cord
V/O	verbal order
VS	vital signs
Vtach	ventricular tachycardia
WB	weight bearing
WBAT	weight bearing as tolerated
WBQC	wide-based quad cane
W/C	wheelchair
WFL	within functional limits
WNL	within normal limits
WS	weight shift
wk	week(s)
×	times (e.g., 6 × d = six times daily); for (e.g., ×5 yr = for 5 years); of (e.g., 3 sets ×10 reps)
x̄	except
y/o or y.o.	year old

PROFESSIONAL

ATC	Athletic Trainer Certified
CCC-A	Certificate of Clinical Competence–Audiology
CCC-SLP	Certificate of Clinical Competence–Speech-Language Pathology
CDN	Certified Dietician Nutritionist
CFY-SLP	Clinical Fellowship Year–Speech-Language Pathology
CNA	Certified Nursing Assistant
CNS	Clinical Nurse Specialist
COTA	Certified Occupational Therapy Assistant
CSW	Certified Social Worker
CTRS	Certified Therapeutic Recreation Specialist

CRTT	Certified Respiratory Therapy Technician
DC	Doctor of Chiropractic
DO	Doctor of Osteopathic Medicine
DPM	Doctor of Podiatric Medicine
DPT	Doctor of Physical Therapy
DTR	Registered Dietetic Technician
GYN	Gynecologic, gynecology
HHA	Home Health Aide
LPN	Licensed Practical Nurse
MD	Medical Doctor
MSW	Master of Social Work
NP	Nurse Practitioner
OB	Obstetrics
OT	Occupational Therapy
OTOL	Otolaryngology
OTR	Occupational Therapist Registered
OTR/L	Occupational Therapist Registered/Licensed
PED	Pediatrics, pediatrician
PA	Physician's Assistant
PT	Physical Therapist, physical therapy
PTA	Physical Therapist Assistant
RD	Registered Dietitian
RN	Registered Nurse
RRT	Registered Respiratory Therapist
SLP	Speech-Language Pathologist
ST	Speech Therapist
TR	Therapeutic Recreation

MEDICAL DIAGNOSIS

ADD	attention deficit disorder
ADHD	attention deficit–hyperactivity disorder
AIDS	acquired immunodeficiency syndrome
AKA	above-knee amputation
ALS	amyotrophic lateral sclerosis
ASD	atrial septal defect
ASHD	arteriosclerotic heart disease
AVM	arteriovenous malformation
BKA	below-knee amputation
CA	carcinoma
CABG	coronary artery bypass graft
CAD	coronary artery disease
CFS	chronic fatigue syndrome
CHF	congestive heart failure
CHI	closed head injury
COPD	chronic obstructive pulmonary disease
CVA	cerebrovascular accident
DVT	deep vein thrombosis
DJD	degenerative joint disease
GBS	Guillain-Barré syndrome
GSW	gunshot wound
HD	Huntington disease
HIV	human immunodeficiency virus
IDDM	insulin-dependent diabetes mellitus (type 1)
MI	myocardial infarction
MS	multiple sclerosis
NIDDM	non–insulin-dependent diabetes mellitus (type 2)
OA	osteoarthritis
OBS	organic brain syndrome
PD	Parkinson disease

PSP	progressive supranuclear palsy
PVD	peripheral vascular disease
RA	rheumatoid arthritis
SAH	subarachnoid hemorrhage
SCI	spinal cord injury
TB	tuberculosis
TBI	traumatic brain injury
THA	total hip arthroplasty
THI	traumatic head injury
THR	total hip replacement
TIA	transient ischemic attack
TKA	total knee arthroplasty
TKR	total knee replacement
TSR	total shoulder replacement

SYMBOLS

1°	initial, primary, first degree
2°	secondary, second degree
3°	tertiary, third degree
=	equal
≠	not equal
−	negative, minus, inhibitory
+	positive, plus, facilitatory
>	greater than
<	less than
/	extension, extensor
✓	flexion, flexor
♀	female
♂	male
‖	parallel
@	at
Δ	change
↓	decrease, down, decline
↑	increase, up, improve
↔	to and from
#	pound, number

ABBREVIATIONS BY WORD

abdominal aortic aneurysm	AAA
abduction	Abd or ABD
abnormal	abn
above the knee	AK
above-knee amputation	AKA
acquired immunodeficiency syndrome	AIDS
active assistive range of motion	AAROM
active range of motion	AROM
activities of daily living	ADL
adduction	Add or ADD
after	$\bar{p}$
against gravity	AG
alert and oriented	A&O
alternating current	AC
ambulatory, ambulation	amb
American Spinal Injury Association	ASIA
amyotrophic lateral sclerosis	ALS
ankle-foot orthosis	AFO
anterior	ant
anterior cerebral artery	ACA

anterior cruciate ligament	ACL
anterior superior iliac spine	ASIS
anteroposterior	AP
appointment	appt
approximate, approximately	approx
arterial blood gases	ABG
arteriosclerotic heart disease	ASHD
arteriovenous malformation	AVM
articulating ankle-foot orthosis	AAFO
as needed	prn
assessment	A
assistance	A or Ⓐ
assistant, assistance	assist
assistive device	AD
asymmetric tonic neck reflex	ATNR
at	@
at discretion	ad lib
Athletic Trainer Certified	ATC
atrial fibrillation	Afib
atrial septal defect	ASD
atrioventricular	AV
attention deficit disorder without hyperactivity	ADD
attention deficit–hyperactivity disorder	ADHD
balance	bal
base of support	BOS
beats per minute	bpm
below normal limits	BNL
below the elbow	BE
below the knee	BK
below-knee amputation	BKA
bilateral	bil, B, or Ⓑ
biweekly	b.i.w.
blood pressure	BP
bowel and bladder	B&B
bowel movement	BM
breath sounds	BS
by mouth	PO
cancer	CA
capsule	cap
carbon dioxide	CO_2
carcinoma	CA
cardiac arrest	CA
cardiac intensive care unit	CICU
center of mass	COM
center of pressure	COP
centimeter	cm
central nervous system	CNS
cerebrovascular accident	CVA
cerebrospinal fluid	CSF
Certificate of Clinical Competence–Audiology	CCC-A
Certificate of Clinical Competence–Speech-Language Pathology	CCC-SLP
Certified Dietitian	CDN
Certified Nursing Assistant	CNA
Certified Occupational Therapy Assistant	COTA
Certified Respiratory Therapy Technician	CRTT
Certified Social Worker	CSW
Certified Therapeutic Recreation Specialist	CTRS
change	Δ
chest physical therapy	CPT
chronic fatigue syndrome	CFS
chronic obstructive pulmonary disease	COPD
Clinical Fellowship Year–Speech-Language Pathology	CFY-SLP
Clinical Nurse Specialist	CNS
close supervision	CS
closed head injury	CHI
complained of, complains of	c/o
computed tomography	CT
congestive heart failure	CHF
contact guarding	CG
continued	cont'd
continuous positive airway pressure	CPAP
coronary artery bypass graft	CABG
coronary artery disease	CAD
day	d
decrease, down, decline	↓
deep breathing exercise	DBE
deep tendon reflex	DTR
deep vein thrombosis	DVT
degenerative joint disease	DJD
dependent	dep or D or Ⓓ
desaturation	desat
diagnosis	dx
diffuse axonal injury	DAI
discharge	D/C
discontinue	D/C
distal interphalangeal (joint)	DIP
distance, distant	dist
distant supervision	DS
Doctor of Chiropractic	DC
Doctor of Osteopathic Medicine	DO
Doctor of Physical Therapy	DPT
Doctor of Podiatric Medicine	DPO
dorsiflexion	DF
durable medical equipment	DME
ear, nose, throat	ENT
edge of bed	EOB
electrical stimulation	e-stim
electrocardiogram	ECG
electroencephalogram	EEG
electromyogram	EMG
emergency room	ER
end-stage renal disease	ESRD
equal	=
equipment	equip
evaluation	eval
every	q
examination	exam
except	x̄
exercise	ex
extended care facility	ECF
extended release	ER
extension	ext, /
extensor	/
external	ext
external rotation	ext rot, ER
extremities	ext
facilitatory	+

fair (muscle grade)	F	large-based quad cane	LBQC
female	♀, F	lateral	lat
first degree	1°	left	L or Ⓛ
flexion, flex	✓	left lower extremity	LLE
flexor	✓	left lower lobe	LLL
flight of stairs	FOS	left lower quadrant	LLQ
follow-up	F/U	left upper extremity	LUE
for (e.g., ×5 yr = for 5 years)	×	left upper lobe	LUL
fraction of inspired oxygen	fiO₂	left upper quadrant	LUQ
fracture	fx	left ventricular hypertrophy	LVH
frequently, frequency	freq	level of assistance	LOA
full weight bearing	FWB	less than	<
full-time	FT	Licensed Practical Nurse	LPN
function	fx	ligament(s)	lig(s)
functional electric stimulation	FES	liters	L
gastrointestinal	GI	liters per minute	L/min
gastrostomy tube	G-tube	long leg brace	LLB
Glasgow Coma Scale	GCS	long-term care	LTC
good (muscle grade)	G	long-term goal(s)	LTG
gravity eliminated	GE	long-term memory	LTM
greater than	>	loss of balance	LOB
Guillain-Barré syndrome	GBS	loss of consciousness	LOC
gunshot wound	GSW	lower back pain	LBP
gynecology	GYN	lower extremity	LE
hard of hearing	HOH	magnetic resonance imaging	MRI
head of bed	HOB	male	♂, M
headache	HA	manual muscle test	MMT
heart rate	HR	Master of Social Work	MSW
heel strike	HS	maximal, maximum	max
hemodialysis	HD	mean arterial pressure	MAP
history	hx	medical	med
history of	H/O	medical doctor	MD
history of present illness	HPI	medicine	med
home exercise program	HEP	metacarpophalangeal (joint)	MCP
home health aide	HHA	meters	m
hour	h or hr	middle cerebral artery	MCA
human immunodeficiency virus	HIV	milliliter	mL
Huntington disease	HD	minus	–
hypertension	HTN	minute(s), minimal	min
immediately, at once	stat	moderate	mod
increase, up, improve	↑	moist heat	MH
independent	Ind or I or Ⓘ	month	mo
inferior	inf	motor vehicle accident	MVA
inhibitory	–	movement	mvt
initial	1°	multiple sclerosis	MS
Inpatient	IP	myocardial infarction	MI
insulin-dependent diabetes mellitus (type 1)	IDDM	narrow-based quad cane	NBQC
		nasal cannula	NC
intake and output	I&O	nasogastric	NG
intelligence quotient	IQ	negative	–, neg
intensive care unit	ICU	neonatal intensive care unit	NICU
internal	int	non–insulin-dependent diabetes mellitus (type 2)	NIDDM
internal rotation	int rot, IR		
intramuscular	IM	non–weight bearing	NWB
intravenous	IV	normal (muscle grade)	N
improve	≠	normal saline	NS
jejunostomy tube	J-tube	not applicable, not available	N/A
joint	jt	not equal	≠
kilocalorie	kcal	not tested	N/T
kilogram(s)	kg	nothing by mouth	NPO
knee-ankle-foot orthosis	KAFO	number	#

Nurse Practitioner	NP	repetition(s)	rep(s)
obstetrics	OB	reports of	R/O
Occupational Therapy	OT	resisted range of motion	RROM
Occupational Therapist Registered	OTR	respiratory rate	RR
Occupational Therapist Registered/ Licensed	OTR/L	rheumatoid arthritis	RA
		right	R or ®
of (e.g., 3 sets ×10 reps)	×	right lower extremity	RLE
open reduction internal fixation	ORIF	right lower lobe	RLL
operating room	OR	right lower quadrant	RLQ
orders	Rx	right middle lobe	RML
organic brain syndrome	OBS	right upper extremity	RUE
osteoarthritis	OA	right upper lobe	RUL
otolaryngology	OTOL	right upper quadrant	RUQ
out of bed	OOB	rolling walker	RW
Outpatient	OP	rule out, ruled out	R/O
oxygen	O_2	saturation	sat
parallel	//	second(s)	sec
Parkinson disease	PD	secondary, second degree	2°
partial weight bearing	PWB		
part-time	PT	short arc quads	SAQ
passive range of motion	PROM	shortness of breath	SOB
past medical history	PMH	short-term goal(s)	STG
past surgical history	PSH	short-term memory	STM
patient	pt	significant	sig
pediatrics	ped	sit to stand	STS
percussion and vibration	P&V	skilled nursing facility	SNF
peripheral vascular disease	PVD	sliding board	SB
Physician's Assistant	PA	sliding board transfers	SBT
Physical Therapist, physical therapy	PT	small-based quad cane	SBQC
Physical Therapist Assistant	PTA	Speech Therapist	ST
plantar flexion	PF	Speech-Language Pathologist	SLP
platform rolling walker	PRW	spinal cord injury	SCI
poor (muscle grade)	P	standby assistance	SBA
positive, plus	+	stand pivot transfers	SPT
posterior	post	standing order	S/O
posteroanterior	PA	*Staphylococcus*	staph
posterior cerebral artery	PCA	status post	s/p
positron emission tomography	PET	step-over-step (stair-climbing)	SOS
posterior leaf splint	PLS	step-to-step (stair-climbing)	STS
posterior superior iliac spine	PSIS	sternocleidomastoid muscle	SCM
postoperative	postop	straight cane	str cane or SC
potassium	K	straight-leg raise	SLR
pound	lb, #	*Streptococcus*	strep
prescription	Rx	subarachnoid hemorrhage	SAH
primary	1°	supervision	S or ⑤
prior level of function	PLOF	supported	supp
prior to admission	PTA	surgical, surgery	surg
progressive resistive exercise(s)	PRE	symmetric, symmetry	symm
progressive supranuclear palsy	PSP	symmetric tonic neck reflex	STNR
proximal	prox	symptoms	sx
proximal interphalangeal (joint)	PIP	tablet	tab
pulse oxygen saturation	SpO_2	temperature	temp
quadriceps	quads	temporomandibular joint	TMJ
range of motion	ROM	tertiary	3°
regarding, concerning	re	therapeutic exercise	ther ex
Registered Dietetic Technician	DTR	therapeutic recreation	TR
Registered Dietitian	RD	third degree	3°
Registered Nurse	RN	three times per week	t.i.w.
Registered Respiratory Therapist	RRT	throughout	T/O
rehabilitation	rehab	times (e.g., 6 × d = six times daily)	×
related to	R/T	to and from	↔

to be assessed	TBA	upper extremity	UE
to be evaluated	TBE	upper respiratory infection	URI
toe off	TO	urinary tract infection	UTI
toe-touch weight bearing	TTWB	ventricular tachycardia	Vtach
total hip arthroplasty	THA	verbal cues	VC
total hip replacement	THR	verbal order	V/O
total knee arthroplasty	TKA	visual analog scale	VAS
total knee replacement	TKR	vital capacity	VC
total shoulder replacement	TSR	vital signs	VS
touch-down weight bearing	TDWB	vocal cord	VC
trace (muscle grade)	T	water	H_2O
tracheostomy	trach	week(s)	wk
training	trng	weight bearing	WB
transcutaneous electrical nerve stimulation	TENS	weight bearing as tolerated	WBAT
		weight shift	WS
transient ischemic attack	TIA	wheelchair	W/C
transverse, transferred	trans	wide-based quad cane	WBQC
traumatic brain injury	TBI	with	$\bar{c}$
traumatic head injury	THI	within functional limits	WFL
treatment	Tx, Rx	within normal limits	WNL
tuberculosis	TB	without	$\bar{s}$
twice a day	b.i.d.	year old	y/o or y.o.
ultrasound	US		
unilateral	U/L		
unsupported	unsupp		

Answers to Exercises

CHAPTER 1

Exercise 1-1

1. **I**—Range of motion is an impairment at the level of body structures and function. Musculoskeletal flexibility is measured in units of joint rotation.
2. **A**—A person's ability to walk is generally measured at the activity level.
3. **HC**—A tear of the anterior cruciate ligament is a medical diagnosis specifying the location and type of tissue damage.
4. **P**—The ability to fulfill occupational role is at the level of participation.
5. **I**—Strength is measured at the level of body structures and function.
6. **A**—Dressing is a functional activity.
7. **HC**—This is a medical diagnosis that specifies the location and nature of tissue damage.
8. **A**—Climbing stairs is an activity. Could potentially be included in I as heart rate is a measure of circulation/respiration.
9. **HC**—Multiple sclerosis describes a type of disease. This is a medical diagnosis.
10. **A**—Eating is a functional activity. Here, the word *independently* is used, specifying how the performance is achieved.
11. **I**—Lateral pinch strength represents a body function of the musculoskeletal system.
12. **A**—Transfers are functional activities, described here in terms of goal attainment and with the use of adaptive equipment (sliding board).
13. **I**—Passive range of motion represents a body function of the musculoskeletal system.
14. **A**—Crawling is an activity of locomotion for a child.
15. **A**—Reaching and grasping a cup is an activity.
16. **A**—Standing at a kitchen sink is an important functional activity.
17. **I**—A straight-leg raise reflects the performance of a body system (musculoskeletal). This is a way of specifying an active range of motion.
18. **I**—Pain is considered an impairment. A functional activity is not mentioned.
19. **P**—Daily household chores describe a range of activities that encompass a person's participation related to his or her personal roles in life.
20. **A**—Cooking and preparing dinner are specific functional activities.
21. **A**—Getting in and out of a wheelchair is an important functional activity for a person who uses a wheelchair for mobility.
22. **HC**—A spinal cord injury is a specific pathologic condition; the motor vehicle accident specifies the mechanism of injury.
23. **P**—Accessibility to a person's community encompasses that person's participation in society. It is a global measure rather than specifically identifying his or her functional skill in wheelchair mobility, for example.
24. **HC**—A rotator cuff tear is a pathologic condition of the shoulder.
25. **P**—Work represents a component of a person's participation (occupational role).

CHAPTER 2

Exercise 2-1

1. Manual muscle test 3/5 right quadriceps.
2. Patient can stand without assistance for 30 seconds without loss of balance.
3. Patient can transfer from bed to wheelchair with moderate assistance using a sliding board.
4. Patient instructed in performing right short arc quads, 3 sets of 10 repetitions.
5. Passive range of motion of right ankle dorsiflexion is 5 degrees.
6. Received order from (or prescription from) medical doctor for weight bearing as tolerated on left lower extremity.
7. Patient was instructed to perform a home exercise program twice a day, with 10 repetitions of each exercise.
8. Patient was admitted to the emergency room on 10/12/23 with a Glasgow Coma Scale score of 4.
9. Medical diagnosis: right hip fracture with open reduction, internal fixation.
10. Active range of motion in bilateral lower extremities is within normal limits.
11. Patient instructed in the use of transcutaneous electrical nerve stimulator unit on an as-needed basis.
12. Chest physical therapy for 20 minutes, percussion and vibration to the right lower lobe.
13. Patient was discharged from the neonatal intensive care unit on 3/3/23.

14. Past medical history: insulin-dependent diabetes mellitus for 5 years, high blood pressure for 10 years.
15. Magnetic resonance imaging revealed moderate left middle cerebral artery cerebral vascular accident.

Exercise 2-2

1. Pt. underwent CABG 3/17/21; *or* Pt. s/p CABG 3/17/21.
2. PT to coordinate ADL training c̄ OT and RN staff.
3. Pt.'s HR Δ'd from 90 to 120 bpm for 3 min of amb. at a comfortable speed.
4. Pt.'s OB/GYN reported pt. had LBP t/o pregnancy.
5. Pt.'s daughter reports pt. has had recent ↓ in fx abilities and h/o falls.
6. BS ↓ B. Pt. instructed in DBE b.i.d.
7. Pt.'s wife reports pt. has h/o chronic LBP ×15 yr.
8. Pt.'s LTG is to walk using only SC; *or* Pt.'s LTG is to amb. using only str cane.
9. DTR R biceps 2+.
10. Pt. can ↑↓ 1 flight of stairs I, 1 hand on railing.
11. Rx received for PT: ther ex and gait trng.
12. 82 y.o. 1° med dx of CHF.
13. ECG revealed Vtach.
14. Pt. s/p CVA c̄ hemiplegia R UE & LE.
15. HHA instructed to assist pt. in AAROM exer: SLR and hip abd in supine.

Exercise 2-3*

1. *A person with quadriplegia will often require help with transfers.*
   Quadriplegic is a label that reduces an individual to a disability or physical condition. Terms such as *quad* or *para* (or *paraplegic*) should never be used to refer to a person.
2. *The patient was diagnosed with multiple sclerosis when she was in her 20s.*
   Expressions such as *afflicted with*, *suffers from*, or *is a victim of* sensationalize a person's health status and may be considered patronizing. Simply say the patient was first diagnosed with multiple sclerosis in her 20s or that the condition developed in the patient.
3. *Many PTs are involved in foot clinics for people with diabetes.*
   Here again, the problem is a label.
4. *Have you finished the documentation for Mrs. Jones, who had a shoulder injury?*
   Unbelievable as it may seem, some health care providers still can be heard referring to patients as body parts. This question could easily be reworded as, "Have you finished the documentation for the patient with shoulder pain in room 316?"
5. *The patient reported pain in the right upper extremity.*
   Complaining of may suggest that the patient is overreacting to his or her symptoms or is difficult to work with.
6. *OK*

---

*Some answers are adapted with permission from Martin S. Language shapes thought. *PT* Magazine. 1999;44–46.

7. *Although this computer program was designed for users with disabilities, users without disabilities will also find it helpful.*
   In this sentence, the term *disabled* has the effect of grouping individuals into a distinct "disability class." Again, focus on the person and not on the disability.
8. *Because of a spinal cord injury, the patient used a wheelchair for mobility.*
   To a person who lives an active, full life with the use of a wheelchair, *confined to* can have a patronizing tone.
9. *OK*
10. *The patient stated he was not doing his home exercises because they were not helping "at all."*
   This has a negative connotation and is derogatory. Statements should be kept to objective facts (e.g., stating what the patient's behavior was, rather than interpreting it).
11. *Which therapist is treating Mr. Smith, the patient in room 216 with a brain injury?*
   People-first language should be used.
12. *A person who has had a stroke can often return to work.*
   Patients are not victims.
13. *After a discussion of heel height, the patient reported that she believed it wasn't necessary to modify her heel height choice.*
   Refused may be too strong a word.
14. *Mr. Johnson will first go on the bike for 10 minutes; then Ms. Glaser will receive moist heat.*
   Patients have names, and it is important to use them or at least refer to patients as people.
15. *The patient has a diagnosis of Parkinson disease.*
   The original wording implies that people with Parkinson disease (or any other disease) suffer in some way, which is not always the case.

CHAPTER 7

EXERCISE 7-1

1. **G**—This sentence states that the child "will" be able to do something; this reflects a goal and thus belongs in the expected outcomes section.
2. **I**—Limitation in range of motion is a common impairment.
3. **I**—Blood pressure and heart rate also are impairments; they represent the "organ" level of impairments.
4. **R**—A seizure represents a health condition (damage to the cellular process or homeostasis); thus it belongs in Reason for Referral, where health condition information is listed.
5. **PC**—Patient education is an important component of the Plan of Care.
6. **R**—Describing a patient's work status or occupation information is a component of his or her participation and is listed in Reason for Referral.
7. **Ac**—Stair-climbing is a functional activity.
8. **As**—This statement links impairments (poor expiratory ability) with activity (ineffective cough and lowered endurance for daily care activities). The link provides the

foundation for a diagnosis and is stated in the Assessment section of a report.

9. **R**—Describing a patient's profession or occupation is listed in Reason for Referral.
10. **G**—This sentence states that the patient "will" be able to stand at the bathroom sink; this reflects a goal and thus belongs in the Goals section.
11. **PC**—Therapeutic exercise is a commonly used intervention by physical therapists, which is described in the Plan of Care.
12. **I**—Muscle strength is a measure of impairments.
13. **As**—This statement links impairments (ineffective right toe clearance; weak R hip musculature) with function (slow and unsafe ambulation indoors). The link is related to a PT diagnosis and is stated in the Assessment section of a report.
14. **Ac**—Lifting a box is an activity.
15. **PC**—Coordinating intervention with other professionals (OT and nursing staff) is documented in the Plan of Care.

CHAPTER 8

Exercise 8-1

1. PMH
2. N/A—strength would be documented in Impairments.
3. CC
4. MED
5. N/A—this information is not pertinent to an evaluation report.
6. OTHER
7. CC
8. CC
9. PLF
10. PMH
11. SOC
12. N/A—this would be listed in the Goal section
13. D
14. D
15. CC

Exercise 8-2

Example	What Is Wrong?	Rewrite Statement (Examples)
1. Pt. had heart surgery yesterday.	DP—Type of surgery not described. Also best to indicate date of surgery rather than *yesterday*.	Pt. underwent L total hip replacement (posterior approach) 7/2/23.
2. Pt. reports pain starting 5/10/23.	L—Location of pain is not described in detail; does not provide meaningful information about the health condition.	Pt. reports pain in central low back, radiating into left buttock, starting 5/10/23 after a slip near her pool.
3. Pt. had a right-sided stroke.	L—Location of stroke not specified. TC—Date of stroke occurred needs to be included.	Pt. s/p R MCA stroke on 12/5/21.
4. Pt. is an amputee.	L—Location and type of amputation are not included. TC—Date of amputation n eeds to be included; avoid use of *amputee*; statement is labeling; person-first terminology is not used.	Pt. is an 18 y.o. male s/p R transtibial amputation 5/12/24.
5. Pt. has typical problems related to aging.	DP—Describe specific problems the patient is experiencing. TC—How long has problem existed?	Pt. reports general forgetfulness of short-term events over the past 2 mo but does not report any problems with long-term memory.
6. Pt. complains of fatigue.	DP—Type of fatigue needs to be included. TC—Time course needs to be included. *Complains of* have a negative connotation and should be avoided.	Pt.'s primary problem is general fatigue, which has been constant for the past 3 wk and does not change based on activity level or time of day.
7. Pt. has a broken leg.	L—Specific bone needs to be specified. Also, fracture is more appropriate terminology than broken leg. TC—Date of fracture occurred needs to be included.	Pt. fractured his R femur (comminuted) on 1/23/22 after skiing accident.
8. Pt. diagnosed with cancer NOV. 2020.	L—Location of cancer not specified. More specifics of cancer could be included (e.g., stage of cancer, primary or secondary site).	Pt. was diagnosed c̄ stage II colon cancer on NOV. 2020.

Exercise 8-3

Past Medical History and Medications	Rewrite Statement (Examples)
1. Pt. has h/o cardiac problems.	Pt. has h/o coronary artery disease with stable angina, dx in 2020.
2. Pt. has h/o several surgeries.	Pt. had C-section 6/6/17 and appendectomy 12/2/23.
3. Pt. is a diabetic.	H/o IDDM ×10 yr.
4. Pt. is taking multiple medications for various medical conditions.	Pt. is currently taking 2.0 mg Haldol daily to minimize involuntary movements; 20 mg Paxil for depression.
5. Pt. is taking antispasticity meds.	Pt. is currently taking baclofen 20 mg t.i.d. to reduce upper extremity spasticity.
6. Pt. takes Flexeril once a day.	Pt. has been taking Flexeril 5 mg, 1×/day for the past week.

Exercise 8-4

Statement	What Is Wrong?	Rewrite Statement
1. Pt. is confined to a wheelchair.	This statement could be more descriptive about the type of wheelchair and what the patient uses the wheelchair for. Also, *confined to* has a negative connotation.	Pt. uses a lightweight W/C with gel seat cushion for primary means of indoor and outdoor mobility.
2. Has poor motivation to return to work.	*Poor motivation* has a negative connotation and reflects an opinion rather than an objective finding. Stick to objective findings about a patient's participation in rehabilitation program.	Pt. reports that he is "not interested in returning to work."
3. Works on a loading dock.	Not enough detail. Patient's general responsibilities and level of physical activity required on the job need to be included.	Pt. works on a loading dock lifting boxes as heavy as 50 lb, up to 8 hr/day.
4. Client enjoys sports.	Not enough detail was provided about specific sports and level of participation.	Client enjoys hiking 1-2×/mo and skiing 10-12× during winter months.
5. Pt. cannot return to work 2° to architectural barriers.	Description of the architectural barriers is needed.	Pt. reports that 8 stairs in front entrance of office building limit her ability to enter the building with her wheelchair and thus are preventing her return to work.
6. Pt. was very active before her injury.	*Very active* does not provide enough detail. The type of activity the patient was involved in should be specified.	Pt. led a very active lifestyle before her injury—she bicycled 15 miles 3×/wk and played tennis 1 hr 2×/wk.
7. Pt. is in poor shape.	This statement has a negative connotation. There is not enough specific detail about the person's lifestyle or activity level that would be relevant to the rehabilitation program.	Pt. reports he has led a relatively inactive lifestyle and has not participated in a regular exercise routine for the past 5 yr.
8. Pt. lives in an apartment.	It is important to include whether there are stairs to enter, or stairs within the house, and with whom the patient lives.	Pt. lives alone on fourth floor of an apt. building, with elevator. No steps to enter building.
9. Pt. has a history of bad health habits.	Describing a patient's health habits as *bad* is making a judgment and does not provide useful information that is pertinent to physical therapy.	Pt. has hx of smoking 1 pack of cigarettes/day for the past 10 yr.
10. Pt. uses adaptive equipment.	The type of equipment used by the patient should be listed or described.	Pt. uses a raised toilet seat and a shower chair with handheld shower.

Exercise 8-5

Case Report A

Setting: Outpatient

Name: Terry O'Connor   **D.O.B.:** 3/23/57   **Date of Eval.:** 7/2/23

Reason for Referral

Current Condition. Right hip bursitis, onset around 5/10/23. Pt. is a 66 y.o. female who had a gradual onset of pain approximately 2 mo ago in her R thigh, which progressed to a continuous "throbbing pain." Pain radiates from the R hip to the R knee. Pt. does not attribute it to any particular incident.

Medications. Pt. has RA, diagnosed in 2001. Taking methotrexate 15 mg/wk; Humira weekly injection (unknown dosage). Pt. reports also taking 400 mg ibuprofen for pain every 6-8 hr for the past month.

PMH. L4-L5 discectomy Dec. 2010 secondary to herniated disk with radiating leg pain; right-hand surgery June 2022 -tendon transfer secondary to tendon rupture from RA.

Social History/Participation. Pt. lives with husband in a 2-storey house, 5 steps to enter, with bedroom on the second floor. Pt. is retired secretary. Volunteers 1 day/wk at the local hospital but has not volunteered since late May 2° to pain. Pt. reports that husband has recently been assisting with laundry and household cleaning. Sleep is frequently disturbed 1-2×/night, especially after rolling onto R side, and she has difficulty falling asleep due to the pain. Pt. enjoys cooking and golfing. Doctor advised her to discontinue playing golf until pain subsides. Pt. enjoys playing bridge with her friends once per week. She is still able to do this but has to modify her position (change from sitting to standing approximately every 10 min). Goes out to lunch or dinner 2-3×/wk with husband or friends; quality of this activity reduced due to constant position changes.

Prior Level of Function. Before the onset of hip bursitis, pt. was independent in all household activities and volunteered 1 day/wk at local hospital. Pt. also played golf and led an active social life.

Exercise 8-5
Case Report B
Setting: Inpatient Rehabilitation

Name:	D.O.B.:	Date of Eval.:	Admission date:
Tommy Jones	5/12/03	7/2/23	7/2/23

Reason for Referral
Current Condition. C7 incomplete SCI 2° to MVA on 6/15/23. Pt. was transferred this morning from County Acute Care Hospital, where he has been since his accident. Medical records reveal one episode of orthostatic hypotension upon coming to sitting and two episodes of autonomic dysreflexia. Pt. underwent surgery on 6/16/23 for anterior cervical fusion. Currently cleared for all rehabilitation activities per Dr. Johnston (per phone conversation this morning).

Medications. Unknown to patient; would be included in chart review

PMH. No significant PMH; no history of prior surgeries or hospitalizations

Social History/Participation. Before hospital admission, pt. lived at home with his parents while attending college full-time. His parents are very supportive, and his mother is able to stay home to assist with pt.'s care if needed.

Pt. was full-time engineering student on a large campus. He drove to school and walked long distances (10-15 min) between classes. Worked part-time at a local pub as a bartender 2 nights per week.

Prior Level of Function. Before injury, household responsibilities included doing laundry, cleaning room, and mowing lawn weekly. Pt. enjoyed running (completed several marathons), biking, and hiking. Very busy social life in college and with family. Enjoyed going out to dinner and to pubs and friends' homes. Described health as "good" before injury.

CHAPTER 9

Exercise 9-1

Statement	Rewrite Statement	Explanation
1. Able to walk 50 ft.	Pt. can walk a maximum of 50 ft I'ly, using str cane in hospital corridor; limited due to fatigue (HR ↑ from 78 to 115 mm Hg).	Context not specified; not enough detail. Describe where pt. can walk, such as surface conditions or specific environment. Also should indicate level of assistance and assistive devices, if applicable.
2. Able to eat with a spoon with occasional assistance.	Able to eat c̄ a spoon c̄ A required 25% of time to prevent spilling.	*Occasional assistance* is not measurable.
3. Pt. is confined to using a wheelchair for long-distance mobility.	Pt. reports propelling W/C I'ly for distances up to 1000 ft outside home.	*Confined* has a negative connotation; long-distance mobility is not measurable.
4. Able to climb a few stairs.	Pt. can ↑↓ 10 steps, step-over-step, c̄ 1 hand on R ↑ railing.	Not enough detail. Provide more details on capability. *A few* is not measurable. Indicates number of stairs, pattern of stair-climbing, or speed.
5. Can throw a ball but cannot catch one.	Can throw an 8-inch ball 5 ft 3/4 trials; unable to catch from 3 ft distance 0/4 trials.	Not enough detail; not measurable. Describe size of ball, distance thrown.
6. Can walk on uneven surfaces.	Pt. can walk outdoors on grass I'ly for distance up to 500 ft before fatigue reported (Borg RPE = 12).	The term *uneven surfaces* is not sufficiently detailed; not measurable.
7. Pt. is not motivated to walk.	Pt. would not attempt ambulation. Pt. reports he is not yet "ready to try to walk," despite advice by PT and MD that he is medically ready.	*Not motivated* has a negative connotation and is an interpretation by the therapist, not an objective statement.

(Continued)

Statement	Rewrite Statement	Explanation
8. Dresses upper body with difficulty.	Pt. needs min A to get arms through shirts and do most buttons.	*Difficulty* is not measurable; specify degree of difficulty—which components of dressing are problematic?
9. Walks slowly.	Pt.'s avg walking speed on indoor level surface is 60 m/min (avg. for an adult of her age is 90 m/min).	Not enough detail; not measurable; context not specified. Provide speed of ambulation to provide measurable data.
10. Pt. does not drive.	Pt. does not drive >20 min at a time 2° to pain in neck and R arm.	Not enough detail; specify why the patient does not drive.
11. C/o pain during standing.	Pt. is able to stand for max. 15 min. After this, pt. reports gradual increase in LBP (rated up to 4/10) and needs to sit after 20-25 min.	Focus should be on standing (an activity) not on pain (an Impairment). *Complains of* has a negative connotation and also is not measurable—specify time the patient can stand and where the pain is.
12. Transfers with assistance.	Transfers from bed → W/C c̄ max A using SPT.	*Assistance* is not measurable; not enough detail; specify how much assistance is required and the type of transfer.
13. Pt. can lift various-sized boxes.	Pt. can lift boxes up to 10 lb from floor to waist-height shelf.	Not measurable; provide more information about boxes (e.g., weight) and also to what height boxes can be lifted.
14. Pt. cannot get up from a low chair.	Sit → stand c̄ min A from 16-inch height chair.	Not measurable; quantify amount of assistance needed and height of chair.
15. Pt. is having trouble sitting for extended periods at work.	Pt. unable to sit at work desk for >20 min at a time 2° to back pain.	Not measurable; quantify how long patient can sit for and specify why he cannot sit longer.

Exercise 9-2

1. Ambulation
2. Self-care
3. Climbing stairs
4. NA—this information would be listed in Impairments section.
5. NA—this information would be listed in Reason for Referral, Past Medical History
6. Transfers
7. Standing ability
8. NA—this would be listed in the Impairments section
9. Traveling to work or traveling to school (or community mobility)
10. NA—this information would best be placed in Reason for Referral—Prior Level of Function
11. Dressing
12. Transfers
13. Food preparation

Exercise 9-3

Bus Driver
Sitting
Turning wheel
Operating doors
Shifting gears
Walking up and down stairs
Walking (approx. 50 ft)
Turning head to look behind both ways

Homemaker
Cooking—carrying pots and pans, standing to cook
Cleaning—mopping, vacuuming, washing dishes
Doing laundry
Managing finances
Shopping (walking, pushing cart, reaching to shelves, carrying groceries)

College Student
Sitting
Reading/turning pages
Traveling to and from classes
Traveling up and down stairs

Administrative Assistant
Typing
Filing
Using the computer
Sitting
Walking

Professional Basketball Player
Dribbling
Taking free throws
Running
Blocking
Jumping
Passing
Shooting
Walking backward and sideways

CHAPTER 10

Exercise 10-1

Impairment Category

1. Range of motion
2. Gait
3. Sensory integrity
4. Cognitive and mental functions
5. Range of motion
6. Cranial and peripheral nerve integrity
7. Anthropometric characteristics
8. Pain
9. Integumentary integrity
10. Balance

11. Mobility
12. Reflex integrity
13. Ventilation and respiration
14. Ventilation and respiration
15. Posture
16. Cognitive and mental functions
17. Aerobic capacity/endurance
18. Sensory integrity
19. Muscle performance
20. Cranial and peripheral nerve integrity

Exercise 10-2

Statement	Rewrite Statement	Explanation
1. Sensation is impaired.	Sensation impaired dorsal aspect R foot, 2/5 correct responses.	*Impaired* is not measurable. Not enough detail; describe where sensation is impaired; quantify extent of impairment.
2. ROM is moderately limited.	ROM R knee flexion 0°-85°.	*Moderately limited* is not measurable; ROM can be measured in degrees. Not enough detail; specify ROM of a specific joint and motion.
3. Pt. c/o excruciating pain.	Pt. reports pain in L shoulder at glenohumeral joint (stabbing), onset 3 days ago. Rates pain as 4/10 in AM, 8/10 in PM. Pain is relieved by lying down (2/10).	*Excruciating* is not measurable; describe location, quality, severity, timing, intensity, and what makes pain better/worse.
4. Pt. has L leg edema.	2+ pitting edema L ankle; circumference L ankle at malleoli 26 cm, R ankle 22 cm.	Not enough detail; specify where the edema is (ankle, calf, knee, etc.). Not measurable; quantify degree of edema.
5. Pt. demonstrates a significant ↑ in HR c̄ stair-climbing.	HR increases from 80-120 bpm p̄ pt. ↑ 24 steps.	*Significant* is not measurable; HR can be measured quantitatively.
6. Pt's. reflexes are hyperactive.	Patellar tendon reflex: L 2+; R 3+.	Not enough detail; specific reflex not identified. *Hyperactive* is not measurable; reflexes can be quantified.
7. Pt. does not know what is going on.	Pt. is alert and oriented ×1 (person).	Not appropriate; if patient's cognitive status is being documented, not enough detail is provided.
8. Pt. has abnormal gait pattern.	Pt. walks c̄ L Trendelenburg gait, indicative of gluteus medius weakness.	*Abnormal* is not measurable; should identify what is specifically not normal.
9. Pt. has poor endurance.	Pt. reports SOB (11/15 on Borg RPE) and has HR ↑ to 140 bpm p̄ amb 200 ft.	*Poor* is not measurable; not specific to an activity, which is important for endurance. Endurance can be measured on a perceived exertion scale.
10. Pt. walks c̄ L knee pain.	Pt. reports L knee pain began approx. 2 mo ago. Pain described as "sharp," located on the medial aspect of L knee. Pt. rates pain as 3/10 at rest (sitting or lying down), ↑ to 7/10 p̄ walking 5 min.	Not measurable; not enough detail. Focus is on walking and not on pain. For this statement to belong in the Impairment section, it should focus on the pain specifically. Describe location, quality, severity, timing, and what makes pain better/worse.

CHAPTER 11

Exercise 11-1
Case 1: Outpatient

Case Information	Assessment
59 y.o. man, s/p R THR 2° to osteoarthritis, 3 wk previous. Pt. past acute stage—no significant pain or swelling; incision well healed. **Participation:** Sales representative, travels by car, unable to work since surgery. **Activity Limitations:** Needs assist for transfers into car, walks slowly with walker, up to 100 ft at a time, and needs assist on steps. **Impairments:** Weakness in R hip flexors, abductors, and extensors; habitual gait deviations from preop antalgic gait. R hip √ and abduction ROM limited.	Pt. is a 59 y.o. male, 3 wk s/p R THR 2° to osteoarthritis. Incision is healing well, and pt. experiences no significant pain or swelling. Weakness in hip musculature, hip ROM limitations, and preop gait deviations have resulted in limited speed and distance for walking. Weakness also makes transfer in and out of the car impossible without assistance. Limitations in walking and car transfers are currently preventing pt. from returning to work as a sales rep. Pt. requires PT intervention to improve strength, ROM, and walking ability, facilitating pt.'s return to work.

Case 2: Outpatient

Case Information	Assessment
43 y.o. female with MS diagnosed 3 yr previous; recovering from recent exacerbation. **Participation:** Clerical worker in major downtown office building; rides train and bus to work; resists using cane. Pt. is fearful of falling during commute and needs extra time to commute. **Activity Limitations:** Requires assist to go up and down steps; walks slowly; walking difficulties exacerbated in crowded places. **Impairments:** Only mild weakness; standing balance easily disturbed, esp. when pt. is distracted. Pt. has particular difficulty with motor/cognitive simple and complex dual tasks.	Pt. is a 43 y.o. female diagnosed c̄ MS 3 yr ago. Pt. presents c̄ significantly impaired standing balance and cognitive/motor dual-tasking ability, resulting in slowed walking speed and difficulties walking in crowded places and negotiating stairs. These problems are limiting pt.'s ability to safely and efficiently commute to work. Pt. requires PT intervention to address balance and ambulation difficulties and improve the ability to commute to work.

Case 3: Inpatient

Case Information	Assessment
48 y.o. woman admitted to an acute care hospital with complaints of severe abdominal pain, diminished appetite with nausea and diarrhea for 4 days. PMH, end-stage liver disease; liver transplant 4 yr ago, end-stage renal disease with hemodialysis 2x/wk, hypertension, and a DVT with onset 4 mo ago; sacral onset x4 mo. **Activity Limitations:** Mobility limited to wheelchair. Mod. to maximal assistance for all bed mobility and transfers. **Impairments:** Muscle strength: 2+/5 gross lower extremity strength, 3−/5 gross upper extremity strength. Wound: 3.7 × 3.4 cm with 2-3 cm of undermining; 85% yellow rubbery eschar; 15% red granulation.	Pt. is a 48 y.o. female diagnosed c̄ end-stage liver disease. Pt. admitted to hospital for the current episode of care for abdominal pain, diminished appetite, nausea, and diarrhea. Pt. presents with upper and lower extremity weakness 2° to current medical conditions, which have led to significant mobility limitations, including dependence in all forms of mobility and transfers. This lack of independent mobility has led to further complications, including a sacral pressure sore. Pt. requires PT intervention to address strength deficits and deconditioning, treatment to facilitate healing of pressure sore, and functional training to minimize caregiver burden for mobility and transfers.

Case 4: Outpatient

Case Information	Assessment
39 y.o. female c̄ diagnosis of cervical strain. Onset of symptoms occurred 6 wk ago. **Participation:** CPA at local firm, currently unable to tolerate typical 8- to 10-hr workday 2° to symptoms. Majority of time typically spent on phone and computer. **Activity Limitations:** Occasionally requires pain medication to assist with sleeping at night. Unable to talk on phone 2° to pain with phone cradling position. Unable to tolerate computer work >2 hr 2° to increased pain. **Impairments:** Static sitting posture presents with a decrease in cervical lordosis and an increase in thoracic kyphosis. Limited AROM with R-side flexion and rotation at C-spine. Flexed, rotated, and side-bent left at C5 and C6. Weakness in bilateral lower trapezius: 3/5, bilateral middle trapezius/rhomboids: 4/5, and cervical extensors: 3+/5. Pain rated as 3/10 at rest and 6/10 after working 2 hr; described as throbbing and occasionally shooting.	Pt. is a 39 y.o. female with a recent diagnosis of cervical strain; onset of symptoms 6 wk ago. Pt. presents with poor cervical and thoracic postures, moderate ROM and strength deficits in the cervical and thoracic spine regions, cervical facet dysfunction, and increased pain that results in limited tolerance with computer and phone duties, as well as sleep disturbance. These issues are restricting the pt.'s work endurance and performance. Pt. requires PT to address postural dysfunction, ROM, and strength deficits, as well as facet dysfunction. Postural education, proper body mechanics, ergonomic assessment, and pain management would be addressed as well.

Case 5: Inpatient Rehabilitation—Burn Center

Case Information	Assessment
23 y.o. female college student sustained 11% TBSA full-thickness scald burn to right anterior thigh, anterior lower leg, and dorsal foot. s/p skin grafting surgery to excise burn eschar and skin graft the wound 5 days ago. **Participation:** Previously active in playing tennis weekly. Full-time graduate student; lives in apartment with 2 roommates; elevator to enter; all living on one floor. **Activity Limitations:** Able to amb. independently 20 ft in 19.5 sec; step to gait; Tinetti Gait assessment 7/12. Stands independently without support; independent and safe with transfers. **Impairments:** 11% TBSA, full-thickness burns to right anterior thigh, anterior lower leg, dorsal foot; potential for scarring after healing/surgery. Pain in right lower extremity: 4/10 at rest, 6/10 with movement. ROM: R knee ext/flex 0°-90°; right ankle dorsiflexion 5°, plantar flexion 20°. Edema noted right lower extremity.	Pt. is a 25 y.o. female s/p 11% full-thickness scald burn to right leg and foot and is 5 days s/p skin graft surgery. Pt. presents with wounds and grafts 2° to burn injury, which have resulted in significant pain and ROM limitations in R LE in addition to edema postsurgery. These impairments have led to limitations in ambulation speed and balance, which will limit pt.'s ability to function independently at home and return to previous active lifestyle and attend full-time graduate school. Pt. requires inpatient PT to address ROM limitations and edema, facilitate graft healing, and address ambulation and balance deficits, facilitating pt.'s return to independent and full participation in previous lifestyle.

CHAPTER 12

Exercise 12-1

1. **Independent in transfers in 2 wk.**
   Patient (A) will transfer (B) independently (D) bed → W/C (C) 100% of time (D) within 2 wk (E).
   Type: Activity — Problem: A, B, C
2. **Patient will be functional in ADLs within 3 wk.**
   Patient (A) will perform (B) all ADLs (C) independently (D) within 3 wk (E).
   Type: Participation — Problem: B, C, D
3. **Return to work in 3 mo.**
   Patient (A) will return (B) to work as kindergarten teacher (C) and be able to participate (B) in all required activities (C) within 3 months (E).
   Type: Participation — Problem: A, C, D
4. **4. Pt. will ↑↓1 flight of stairs in 1 min.**
   Pt. (A) will ↑↓ stairs (B) (1 flight, 7″ risers) (C) c̄ 1 rail (C) step-over-step pattern (D) in 1 min (D) I'ly (D) within 3 wk (E).
   Type: Activity — Problem: C, E
5. **Pt. will return to school.**
   Pt. (A) will return (B) to school (C), taking 2 classes (D) within 1 mo (E).
   Type: Participation — Problem: C, D, E
6. **Pt. will get from his room to therapy.**
   Pt. (A) will propel his W/C (B) from his room to therapy gym (approx. 250 ft) (C) in less than 3 min (D) within 2 wk (E).
   Type: Activity — Problem: B, D, E

EXERCISE 12-2

Statement	Rewrite Statement	Explanation
1. Pt. will experience less pain.	Pt. will walk >500 ft distance c̄ pain <4/10 4/5 days, within 2 wk.	Reports of pain are related to impairment goals. Focus should be on task or function. *Less pain* is not measurable. Where is the pain? During what activity?
2. Pt. will progress from a walker to a cane within 3 wk.	Pt. will walk 100 m at speed ≥0.80 m/sec in the clinic hallway using a cane in 3 wk.	Not enough detail regarding distance/speed or context. Reflects the process rather than the goal.
3. Educate pt. on hip precautions within 2 sessions.	Pt. will verbally demonstrate knowledge of total hip precautions when asked by therapist 100% of the time.	Educating the pt. is part of the intervention, not a goal. Reflects the process rather than the goal.
4. Pt. will walk with a normal gait pattern within 4 wk.	Pt. will amb 500 ft c̄ RW in hospital hallways c̄ CG, with adequate toe clearance to avoid tripping, in 3 wk.	Not measurable. *Normal* is a relative term and depends on status before recent injury.
5. ①ADLs in 2 wk.	Pt. will transfer W/C → toilet c̄ SB ① in <1 min in 2 wk.	Not enough detail; *all ADLs* is too vague.
6. Pt. will ascend and descend stairs within 3 days.	Pt. will ↑↓ 12 8″ height steps, using step-over-step pattern in 30 sec, within 5 days.	Not concrete; not enough detail. Height of stairs, time to complete, use of railing can all be used to clarify goal.

(Continued)

Statement	Rewrite Statement	Explanation
7. Pt. will not have pain when reaching.	Pt. will put away dishes from dishwasher to all shelves without report of pain (0/10), within 1 wk.	Emphasis is on pain, which relates to impairments; not enough detail describing functional skill of reaching; no time course.
8. Pt. will sit for 5 min.	Pt. will be able to sit on office chair for up to 30 min s̄ pain.	Sitting can occur in many different locations. Describe chair or surface and other conditions.
9. Pt. will improve standing balance.	Pt. will stand Ⓘ at kitchen counter for 5 min 2-hand support.	Need to be more specific about surface and task; time course not specified.
10. Pt. will transfer from sit → stand in 2 wk.	Pt. will transfer from sit → stand and min A 4/5 trials within 2 wk.	Describe conditions more specifically (e.g., level of assistance) and degree (e.g., success rate).

CHAPTER 13

Exercise 13-1

Statement	Rewrite Statement	Explanation
1. Practice walking.	Gait training within home from bedroom to bathroom, living room, and kitchen to address safety and teach compensatory strategies for visual field deficits and L spatial neglect.	Practice of a task does not mean the need for skilled services. Describe circumstances, type of walking, and type of training.
2. Apply hot packs.	Moist heat to cervical spine to promote relaxation and improve cervical spine flexibility.	Rationale not provided; not enough detail. Why is a hot pack needed? Specify to address pain, relax tissues, etc. Area of body needs to be stated. No indication of skilled services required.
3. Pt. will be able to walk 10 ft to the bathroom.	Gait training for short distances to bathroom using manual guidance as needed to improve foot clearance.	Not appropriate for this section. This is a goal, not an intervention. Need to state it in terms of what the pt. or therapist will do.
4. Pt. will be given strengthening exercises.	Pt. will be instructed in home program to include isometric strengthening for left quadriceps.	Not enough detail. Describe what type of strengthening exercises. Be specific to muscle group. *Instructed* is a better term than *given*.
5. Coordinate care with all nursing personnel.	Will review transfers and bed mobility strategies with nursing staff to facilitate pt.'s use of right side of body.	Not enough detail. What care will be coordinated? Clarify the PT-related activities you will coordinate with nurses on—transfers, bed mobility, etc.
6. Assess work environment.	Work environment to be assessed within 2 wk to make modification recommendations before returning to work.	Not enough detail. This could involve many different things; try to clarify which areas of the work environment will be addressed. What is the purpose of assessing the work environment?
7. Pt. will increase right hamstring strength.	Progressive resistive strengthening exercises for R hamstrings.	Not appropriate for this section. This is a goal, not an intervention. Need to state this as what the patient or therapist will do.
8. Balance training.	Training of sitting balance, including proactive (reaching, ball play activities) and reactive (response to perturbations in sitting, activities on therapeutic ball) to improve overall sitting ability.	Not enough detail. Need to identify what specifically will be addressed with this training.
9. Pt. will receive ultrasound at 1.0 W/cm², 1 MHz to R quadriceps (VMO), in a 10-cm area just proximal and slightly medial to R knee, moving ultrasound head slowly in circular fashion for 10 min, each session.	Pt. will receive ultrasound to R quadriceps (VMO) to improve mobility and promote tissue healing.	Too much detail is provided. It would be sufficient to eliminate some of the details; parameters could be specified in treatment notes. Rationale for the intervention is not stated.
10. Pt. will take pain relief medication as needed.	Pt.'s pain medication regimen will be coordinated with MD and nursing staff to be administered 1-2 hr before PT treatment for optimal exercise tolerance.	Prescribing or recommending medication is not within the scope of physical therapy practice. Therapists can discuss and coordinate with other health care personnel regarding a patient's medication management as it pertains to physical therapy.

Statement	Rewrite Statement	Explanation
11. Home evaluation.	Home evaluation will be conducted before D/C to evaluate pt.'s home environment and accessibility.	Not enough detail; rationale for doing a home evaluation not provided.
12. Reduce R ankle edema.	Ice to be applied to R ankle to ↓ swelling and pain.	Not appropriate for this section. This is a general goal, not an intervention. The method used to reduce the edema would be appropriate to document in the intervention section.
13. Teach family to care for pt.	Educate pt.'s family members on safe techniques for W/C transfers → car and bed.	Not enough detail; document specific skills being taught.
14. Practice pressure-relief techniques.	Educate pt. in effective pressure-relief techniques while sitting in W/C to prevent skin breakdown.	Not enough detail; not specific as to type of pressure relief.
15. E-stim to anterior tibialis.	E-stim to anterior tibialis for muscle reeducation.	Rationale not provided.

CHAPTER 14

Exercise 14-1

Statement	S or O	Rewrite Statement	Explanation
1. Pt. states he hates using his walker.	S	Pt. states that he "prefers to use a cane rather than a walker" because it is too difficult to carry things while using the walker.	Not enough detail. It would be helpful to know why he dislikes using his walker.
2. Pt. has an awkward gait.	O	Pt. walks on indoor level surfaces $\bar{s}$ assistive device decreased stance time on R 2° to pain in R foot on weight bearing.	Not enough detail; *awkward* is not measurable.
3. PROM at the knee is getting better.	O	PROM of R knee √ is 0°-95°.	Not enough detail; not measurable.
4. Pt. is very confused.	O	Pt. is alert & oriented ×1 (person). Mini-Mental State Examination score: 16/30.	Not enough detail. What is pt. confused about? If performing a mental status assessment, report findings in an objective manner.
5. Pt. reports that his son is concerned.	S	Pt. reports that his son is concerned about his ability to care for his father when he returns home. Son has a full-time job and 2 small children of his own.	Not enough detail. Need to document son's specific concerns.
6. Pt. c/o fatigue after walking for 5 min.	S	Pt. reports feeling fatigued (Borg RPE 14) $\bar{p}$ amb. 5 min outdoors.	*Complains of* has a negative connotation; fatigue could be quantified.
7. Pt. complains of pain in left shoulder.	S	Pt. continues to report pain in her L shoulder that radiates down to her elbow, 6/10. It aches all of the time, except when she is lying down.	*Complains of* has a negative connotation. Not enough detail about pain (location, quality, severity, timing, etc.).
8. Pt. performed 10 reps of knee exercises.	O	Pt. performed 10 reps of isometric quad sets.	Not enough detail; specific exercises should be documented.

Exercise 14-2

Statement	G, S, O, A, or P
1. Performed 10 reps SLR B.	O
2. Pt. reports she was able to walk with her daughter to get the mail yesterday and did not experience any dizziness.	S
3. Treatment next session will include progression to stationary bike ×10 min.	P
4. Pt. walked 15 ft from bed to bathroom without SOB in 30 sec.	O
5. Pt. states that she "felt sore" after the last treatment session.	S
6. Pt. is progressing well with increasing repetitions of LE strengthening exercises and has achieved goal 1.	A
7. Pitting edema noted in R ankle.	O

(Continued)

Statement	G, S, O, A, or P
8. Pt. was instructed to continue to maintain R leg in elevated position while sitting at the desk during the day.	O
9. Pt. will transfer from bed to wheelchair independently, 4/5 trials within 2 wk.	G
10. Pt. states she is anxious to return to work.	S
11. Pt. will continue with daily walking program at home during off-therapy days, progressing to 20 min each day by next week.	P
12. Pt. will stand s̄ A for up to 1 min within 1 wk.	G
13. Pt. reports pain in low back while walking as 5/10 and 8/10 while sitting at desk at work.	S
14. Pt.'s fear of falling is limiting his progress in improving his ability to ambulate in crowded environments and outdoors.	A
15. Pt. reports that she is going back to work on a trial basis next week.	S

CHAPTER 16

Exercise 16-1

Statement	Rewrite Statement	Explanation
1. The child was uncooperative.	Child refused to attempt several tasks on the evaluation, including hopping on one foot and skipping, preferring to play with the puzzles.	Describing a child as uncooperative has a negative connotation and is subjective. Instead, describe the child's behavior objectively.
2. John has poor strength.	John seems to have weakness of bilateral hip musculature: He could squat with only approx. 10° of knee flexion and demonstrated a + Gower sign upon coming from floor to stand.	Although *poor* is a muscle grade used in manual muscle testing, in this sentence it is used as a vague descriptor of strength. Rather, describe the child's ability to perform a task that is related to a particular muscle action.
3. Lucy has spasticity of B hamstrings and gastrocnemius.	Lucy demonstrates spasticity (increased muscle tone and reflexes leading to stiffness and involuntary muscle contraction) in both her hamstrings (muscle group in the back of the leg) and her gastrocsoleus (muscles of the calf).	*Spasticity* is a term that should be defined if the report is to be read by the parent (which in all likelihood it is). *Hamstrings* and *gastrocs* may also be unfamiliar terms to a layperson.
4. Kelly cannot walk and is currently wheelchair bound.	Kelly is able to stand for short periods (up to 30 sec) but has not yet demonstrated the ability to take steps. She uses a manual W/C as a primary means of mobility within the home, which she can independently maneuver. For community distance Kelly is pushed in her W/C by a family member.	This sentence has a very negative tone. It should include more information about Kelly's abilities, not just her disabilities.
5. Tommy can climb stairs but can only do so with one hand held by his mother.	Tommy is able to climb stairs with one hand held by his mother.	A child's abilities should not always be followed by a "*but...*" statement. This type of statement focuses the reader on what the child cannot do rather than on what he can do.
6. ROM R knee ✓ 100°.	Amelia demonstrates some limitation in range of motion (ability to move a joint) in her right knee (100°; typical range for a child of her age is 160°).	This statement uses abbreviations that will likely be unfamiliar to a parent or school personnel reading the report.
7. Samantha sits in W-sitting with excessive kyphotic posture.	Samantha prefers sitting in a W-sitting position (sitting on her bottom with her knees bent and feet out to either side of her hips) when playing on the floor. In this position, she tends to have an increase in normal thoracic kyphosis (outward curvature of the upper part of the spine), so that she appears very hunched over.	*W-sitting* and *kyphotic posture* are likely to be unfamiliar terms. They should be defined, and the tone of this sentence should be softened.
8. Timmy performed very poorly on the PEDI with a standard score of 20.	Timmy received a standard score of 20 on the Pediatric Evaluation of Disability Inventory (PEDI). This test has a mean of 50 and a standard deviation of 10, which means Timmy's score falls 3 standard deviations below the mean.	Report scores on standardized tests objectively without drawing judgment. Avoid abbreviations for tests or spell out the name.

Exercise 16-2
Examples of Possible Goals

1. Tim will walk in the school hallway with Lofstrand crutches and use a backpack to carry books from the classroom to lunchroom with avg. speed of 1.0 m/sec within 3 mo.

2. Tim will use the stairs (ascending) to get to art/music class 3×/wk.

3. Tim will amb. 200 ft from bus to school building with Pictorial Children's Effort Rating Table (PCERT) of <6/10.

Documentation Review Sample Checklist

The following checklist was developed by the American Physical Therapy Association (Alexandria, Virginia) as a guideline for key components to be included in medical records documentation.

Documentation Review Sample Checklist

⚕APTA
American Physical Therapy Association
The Science of Healing. The Art of Caring.

REVIEW FOR MEDICAL RECORDS DOCUMENTATION
Physical Therapy

Note: This is meant to be a sample documentation review checklist only. Please check payer, state law, and specific accreditation organization (i.e., Joint Commission, CARF, etc.) requirements for compliance.

Therapist reviewed: Privileged and Confidential

PT Initial Visit Elements for Documentation Date:	N/A	Yes	No
Examination:			
1. Date/time 2. Legibility			
3. Referral mechanism by which physical therapy services are initiated			
4. History – medical history, social history, current condition(s)/chief complaint(s), onset, previous functional status and activity level, medications, allergies			
5. Patient/client's rating of health status, current complaints			
6. Systems Review – Cardiovascular/pulmonary, Integumentary, Musculoskeletal, Neuromuscular, communication ability, affect, cognition, language, and learning style			
7. Tests and Measures – Identifies the specific tests and measures and documents associated findings or outcomes, includes standardized tests and measures, e.g., OPTIMAL, Oswestry, etc.			
Evaluation:			
1. Synthesis of the data and findings gathered from the examination: A problem list, a statement of assessment of key factors (e.g., cognitive factors, co-morbidities, social support, additional services) influencing the patient/client status.			
Diagnosis:			
1. Documentation of a diagnosis – include impairment and functional limitations which may be practice patterns according to the Guide to Physical Therapist Practice, ICD9-CM, or other descriptions.			
Prognosis:			
1. Documentation of the predicted functional outcome and duration to achieve the desired functional outcome			
Plan of Care:			
1. Goals stated in measurable terms that indicate the predicted level of improvement in function			
2. Statement of interventions to be used; whether a PTA will provide some interventions			
3. Proposed duration and frequency of service required to reach the goals (number of visits per week, number of weeks, etc.)			
4. Anticipated discharge plans			
Authentication:			
1. Signature, title, and license number (if required by state law)			

Develop a documentation review checklist. (Courtesy American Physical Therapy Association, Alexandria, Virginia.)

PT Daily Visit Note Elements for Documentation Date:	N/A	Yes	No
1. Date			
2. Cancellations and no-shows			
3. Patient/client self-report (as appropriate) and subjective response to previous treatment			
4. Identification of specific interventions provided, including frequency, intensity, and duration as appropriate			
5. Changes in patient/client impairment, activity, and participation status as they relate to the plan of care.			
6. Response to interventions, including adverse reactions, if any.			
7. Factors that modify frequency or intensity of intervention and progression toward anticipated goals, including patient/client adherence to patient/client-related instructions.			
8. Communication/consultation with providers/patient/client/family/significant other.			

9. Documentation to plan for ongoing provision of services for the next visit(s), which is suggested to include, but not be limited to:
     The interventions with objectives
     Progression parameters
     Precautions, if indicated			

10. Continuation of or modifications in plan of care			
11. Signature, title, and license number (if required by state law)			

PT Progress Report Elements for Documentation ** Date:	N/A	Yes	No
1. Labeled as a Progress Report/Note or Summary of Progress 2. Date			
3. Cancellations and no-shows			
4. Treatment information regarding the current status of the patient/client			
5. Update of the baseline information provided at the initial evaluation and any needed reevaluation(s)			
6. Documentation of the extent of progress (or lack thereof) between the patient/client's current functional/abilities and that of the previous progress report or at the initial evaluation			
7. Factors that modify frequency or intensity of intervention and progression toward anticipated goals, including patient/client adherence to patient/client-related instructions.			
8. Communication/consultation with providers/patient/client/family/significant other.			
9. Documentation of any modifications in the plan of care (i.e., goals, interventions, prognosis)			
10. Signature, title, and license number (if required by state law)			

** The physical therapist may be required by state law or by a payer, such as Medicare, to write a progress report. The daily note is not sufficient for this purpose unless it includes the elements listed above.

PT Re-examination Elements for Documentation Date:	N/A	Yes	No
1. Date			
2. Documentation of selected components of examination to update patients/client's impairment, function, and/or disability status.			
3. Interpretation of findings and, when indicated, revision of goals.			
4. Changes from previous objective findings			
5. Interpretation of results			
6. When indicated, modification of plan of care, as directly correlated with goals as documented.			
7. Signature, title, and license number (if required by state law)			

PT Discharge/Discontinuation/Final Visit Elements for Documentation Date: Note: discharge summary must be written by the PT and may be combined with the final visit note if seen by the PT on final visit	N/A	Yes	No
1. Date			
2. Criteria for termination of services			
3. Current physical/functional status.			
4. Degree of goals and outcomes achieved and reasons for goals and outcomes not being achieved.			
5. Discharge/discontinuation plan that includes written and verbal communication related to the patient/client's continuing care.			
6. Signature, title, and license number (if required by state law)			

PTA Visit Note Elements for Documentation Date:	N/A	Yes	No
1. Date			
2. Cancellations and no-shows			
3. Patient/client self-report (as appropriate) and subjective response to previous treatment			
4. Identification of specific interventions provided, including frequency, intensity, and duration as appropriate			
5. Changes in patient/client impairment, activity, and participation status as they relate to the interventions provided.			
6. Subjective response to interventions, including adverse reactions, if any			
7. Continuation of intervention(s) as established by the PT or change of intervention(s) as authorized by PT. Consultation with PT			
8. Signature, title, and license number (if required by state law)			

Sample Range of Motion and Strength Assessment Form

A sample form used for an examination of strength and range of motion. Norm values are from Randall et al. (1993).

Strength and Range of Motion

Extremities and Trunk			Strength		ROM	
			Left	Right	Left	Right
Neck	Flexion					
	Extension					
	Rotation					
Shoulder	Flexion	0°-180°				
	Extension	0°-45°				
	Abduction	0°-180°				
	Int rot	0°-70°				
	Ext rot	0°-90°				
Elbow	Flexion	0°-145°				
	Extension	0°				
Wrist	Flexion	0°-80°				
	Fingers					
Trunk	Flexion					
	Extension					
Hip	Flexion	0°-125°				
	Extension	0°-10°				
	Abduction	0°-45°				
	Adduction	0°-10°				
	Int rot	0°-45°				
	Ext rot	0°-45°				
Knee	Flexion	0°-140°				
	Extension	0°				
Ankle	Dorsiflex	0°-20°				
	Plantarflex	0°-45°				
	Inversion	0°-40°				
	Eversion	0°-20°				

ER, External rotation; *Int*, internal rotation; *ROM*, range of motion.

INDEX

Note: Page numbers followed by *f* indicate figures, *t* indicate tables, and *b* indicate boxes.

C